Praise for Anne Sarkisian's *Toxic Staple*

Toxic Staple is important reading for health professionals and the general public. Gluten intolerance heretofore was unrecognized as a possible factor in a spate of diverse health conditions. *Toxic Staple* presents reliable sources that show convincing evidence of connections. "Contains no gluten" or "gluten-free!" are phrases now found on numerous food product labels (although some of the products have never contained gluten). Nevertheless, this trend has developed a public awareness of gluten and the need for some individuals to avoid gluten-containing grains.

—Beatrice Trum Hunter, food editor, Consumers' Research Magazine
Pioneer writer on nutrition and healthy living

Toxic Staple is an exceptional and unique book integrating the vast amount of research on the gluten-related epidemic. The author balances the most complete synopsis of scientific knowledge published to date with eloquently written and compelling stories that make it accessible to anyone. Well-organized around a list of symptoms, the book provides remarkable evidence for the many health problems that may abate from following a gluten-free diet. It is a must-read, a gift for health care professionals, physicians, psychologists, or anyone looking to improve his or her own health or that of a loved one.

—Marie-Nathalie Beaudoin, PhD
Training Director, Bay Area Family Therapy & Training Associates
Author, The SKILL-ionaire in Every Child: Boosting children's socio-emotional skills using the latest in brain research *(www.skillionaire.org)*

Toxic Staple. The title of Anne Sarkisian's truly amazing book succinctly states the core issue: Mankind has mistakenly taken the safety of wheat for granted, even though gluten has now been shown to be toxic for many. Sarkisian guides us easily through a comprehensive catalog of gluten-related disorders enc[illegible]mpassing celiac disease, aty[illegible]pical symptoms, autoimmune problem[illegible] [illegible]itivity (also known as the gluten syndro[illegible] [illegible]es tell story after story of sickness, dismis[illegible] [illegible]gnosis, and finally healing when gluten w[illegible] [illegible]e source of

the problem. *Toxic Staple* is fully referenced, making it an invaluable resource for everyone who wants to get to grips with this emerging major health problem. All health professionals should read it cover-to-cover, because universal recognition of gluten-related harm will transform medical care. Like me, once you understand the implications which are so clearly documented in this book, you are unlikely to consume gluten ever again.

—Prof. Rodney Ford, MB, BS, MD, FRACP (paediatrician, gastroenterologist)
Christchurch, New Zealand (http://www.DrRodneyFord.com)
Author, The Gluten Syndrome

Not feeling quite right? Sick and tired of feeling sick and tired? Read on as you might just find a cure. Anne Sarkisian's highly researched book on celiac disease and gluten intolerance recounts her personal experience and that of many others who have discovered the benefits of eliminating the *Toxic Staple* from their diets. As a gastrointestinal surgical pathologist who routinely diagnoses celiac disease on tissue biopsies of the small intestine, and a mother of two children with celiac disease, I am awed by the detailed information presented in a user friendly format. Sarkisian raises valuable awareness not only about celiac disease, but about non-celiac gluten intolerance, putting this book on the cutting-edge of this topic, and a must read for physicians and patients alike. While a gluten-free diet may not help everyone, improvement in one's health and well-being without a prescription or operation is certainly worth the effort. Read on and learn how.

—Martha Bishop Pitman, MD
Associate Professor of Pathology, Harvard Medical School
Gastrointestinal Surgical Pathologist, Massachusetts General Hospital, Boston, MA

Toxic Staple is one of the most comprehensive and thoroughly researched books ever written about gluten sensitivity. As a practicing physician with tremendous success in diagnosing numerous patients with gluten issues, I highly recommend this book as a "must read" for all my colleagues, their patients, and families who want to expand their knowledge of gluten and its negative effects on one's mind, body, and spirit. Anne Sarkisian has done an excellent job of providing documented resources and presenting numerous case studies in a passionate, informative way. *Toxic Staple* provides a necessary and valuable awareness of the truth about gluten and empowers anyone reading it with knowledge that may help them achieve optimal health and well-being.

—Lawrence G. Miller III, MD
Henrico, VA (www.DrLarryMiller.com)

Toxic Staple is the big picture on why gluten can be so devastating to those who are intolerant of this common substance. Anne has done a wonderful job pulling practical information from the latest research and making it digestible for people to share with their health care professionals in the quest for a full and vibrant recovery. The stories are empowering and a great illustration of how medical miracles can happen.

—Christine Doherty, ND
Balance Point Natural Medicine, Milford, NH (www.pointnatural.com)

Anne Sarkisian's new book about the impact of gluten on human health has a visceral appeal that resonates with my own experience. Although justifiably frustrated with medical practitioners who are unschooled in the implications of gluten sensitivity, Anne's love is obviously the greater motive for this work. Her concern for her family and her sense of kinship with all those who struggle with the ravages of gluten reverberate from every page.

Each anecdote offers yet another insight into the many faces of this modern challenge to human health, while announcing the importance of gluten as a factor in the development of autoimmunity, neurological conditions, some cardiovascular diseases, many cancers, and a host of other ailments. Sarkisian cites and connects reports from the medical and scientific literature to numerous detailed case histories. She harnesses medical data in a way that top physicians do, but presents it in a plain-spoken style that is eminently readable. For your own good, read this book.

—Ron Hoggan, EdD
Co-author, Dangerous Grains: Why Gluten Cereal Grains May Be Hazardous to Your Health, *and* Cereal Killers: Celiac Disease and Gluten-Free A to Z
Author, The Iron Edge *(www.dangerousgrains.com)*

Anne Sarkisian, author of *Toxic Staple*, informs the reader about the myriad symptoms, health issues, and disease processes that may stem from gluten sensitivity. Along with summarizing superb research covering health issues related to celiac disease (CD) and gluten intolerance (GI), the author shares stories of individuals with CD or GI and their remarkable journey to diagnosis and improved health. The book is a must-read for anyone with chronic health problems, including autoimmune diseases, or for family members diagnosed with CD or GI. Health care providers also would benefit from reading about the multitude of health issues that may be due to undiagnosed CD or GI.

—Cheryl Gainer, MSN, RN, CNM
Clinical Instructor, UTA College of Nursing

An easy-to-understand, comprehensive book of patient and family journeys to restore and maintain health through a gluten-free lifestyle.

—Mary Schluckebier, Executive Director
Celiac Sprue Association (http://www.csaceliacs.info/)

Sarkisian has done an impressive job of organizing massive technical data into a readable and understandable format that neither speaks down to the medical community nor is beyond the capacity of interested laymen to find their way through medical jargon to an understanding of their own area of need or interest.

Obviously, the attitude of many medical professionals reading this book will be, "You have included every disease known to man." This is what I have often been told as I try to tell my peers about the data I have discovered on my own. They don't want to believe a staple as common as wheat has the potential to cause disease on so many fronts. Prior to my own experiences, I, too, was one of the naysayers, and even now I am often looked at with a cross-eyed stare when I relate my own family ordeal with gluten. In a culture accustomed to relieving symptoms with drugs, the concept that a simple dietary change can make such a difference seems, for many, too simplistic to believe. Nevertheless, I now have at my fingertips the ability to find not just the relief of symptoms, but potentially the root cause of my patients' concerns. Looking at gluten as a possible source of health-related issues can also point to the prevention of undiscovered medical problems for both patients and their family members.

—Gale Pearce, PA-C

Toxic Staple

Toxic Staple

How GLUTEN may be wrecking your health – *and* what you can do about it!

Best of Health
♡ Anne Sarkisian

Anne Sarkisian

Max Health Press, LLC
New London, New Hampshire

Max Health Press, LLC
New London, New Hampshire

anne@toxicstaple.com
www.toxicstaple.com

Edited by Susan Owens, Tales for Telling
Interior design and typesetting by Kitty Werner, RSBPress

Disclaimer: The author is a volunteer advocate, not a medical expert, and has made every effort to provide reliable, accurate, and up-to-date information to inspire the reader, in conjunction with his or her doctor, to solve some of their health issues that may be linked to gluten. The opinions expressed in this book are based on the author's personal experiences, copious research into conditions and testing related to celiac disease and non-celiac gluten intolerance (CD/GI), and the personal stories of patients. They are not necessarily the opinions of the storytellers or doctors/researchers quoted in this book. Although a gluten-free lifestyle has brought miracle results to many, the author, publisher, and storytellers do not guarantee any such results; each case is very different, and the gluten-free diet must be absolute. How the reader applies this information is NOT the liability of the author, publisher, or storytellers.

ALWAYS consult with your doctor or a medical professional to determine the appropriateness of this information in relation to your own medical issues. The information in this book is only an aid and should not be used as a substitute for competent medical expertise in the treatment and diagnosis of CD/GI. NEVER stop taking a prescribed medication without consulting a doctor. ALWAYS check with your doctor before taking supplements. Chapters 19 and 20 on the gluten-free diet are a great start, but are not all-inclusive. Knowledge in the area of gluten sensitivity is constantly changing, and some information in this book or on suggested websites may become obsolete.

The author is *not* financially associated with the labs mentioned in this book.

ISBN 978-0-9892392-0-2 (hardcover)
ISBN 978-0-9892392-1-9 (softcover)

Publisher's Cataloging-In-Publication Data
(Prepared by The Donohue Group, Inc.)

Sarkisian, Anne.
Toxic staple : how gluten may be wrecking your health-- and what you can do about it! / Anne Sarkisian.

p. ; cm.

Includes bibliographical references and index.
ISBN: 978-0-9892392-0-2 (hardcover)
ISBN: 978-0-9892392-1-9 (softcover)

1. Gluten-free diet. 2. Gluten--Health aspects--Popular works. 3. Celiac disease--Diagnosis--Popular works. 4. Diet therapy--Popular works. I. Title.

RM237.86 .S27 2013
613.26

To my beautiful and healthy daughters,
Tania, Daniele, and Jessica

My wonderful, loving, well-behaved, energetic,
And healthy grandchildren,
Nicholas, Brianna, Colby, and Alyxandria

My ever-supportive, spice-of-life, and loving husband,
Vahan

The storytellers in this book and people around the world
Who understand how gluten can slowly
Disintegrate
One's life and health

The forward-thinking, cutting-edge doctors and researchers
Around the world who "get it"

People who are "sick and tired of being sick and tired"
Who may find great resolve within these pages

Sickly children
Whose parents need to "get it"

May you always have the power within
To maintain a gluten-free lifestyle

Contents

Foreword

Anne Sarkisian's *Toxic Staple* began as a quest to gather information about celiac disease and gluten intolerance, which were affecting many members of her family. Nine years later, the author's extensive research has resulted in this incredibly-well-referenced book, an invaluable resource for anyone with a history of the myriad symptoms that may be related to gluten.

Most people incorrectly believe gluten-related disorders are always linked to gastrointestinal disease; in other words, if you don't have gastrointestinal issues you don't have a gluten problem. Because celiac disease/gluten intolerance is rarely considered by the vast majority of physicians, 97 percent of celiacs remain undiagnosed. The case histories in *Toxic Staple* add excellent examples of the chameleon-like nature of celiac disease and gluten intolerance. I applaud Mrs. Sarkisian for her dedication. Due to her efforts celiac, the most common autoimmune illness of humankind, and gluten intolerance will be increasingly diagnosed.

Cynthia Rudert, MD, FACP
Gastroenterologist: Specializing in Celiac Disease and Gluten Intolerance
Private Practice: Atlanta, Georgia
Medical Advisor: Celiac Disease Foundation
Medical Advisor: Gluten Intolerance Group

Acknowledgments

NINE YEARS AGO I discovered that gluten was shredding my health and the health of most of my family. Seven years ago I began to pour myself into the research, collection of stories, and writing of *Toxic Staple*. For the past five years this book has been a primary force in my life. As I pecked away on my Mac, sometimes past midnight, and took time away from lunch dates, reading, playing games, and helping with my grandkids as much as I would have liked to, my family was a constant source of support and encouragement.

To my three daughters, Tania, Daniele, and Jessica, and my four wonderful grandchildren, Nicholas, Brianna, Colby, and Aly, a huge thank-you for sharing your stories, for tolerating my mental absence even when I was physically present, and for putting up with my gluten talk as best you could. I realize my passion for this topic sometimes bordered on obsession; it was the only way I knew to bring this story to light.

To Vahan, my dear husband of 45 years, my deepest gratitude for believing in me and my determination to get the word out to the world. I thank you for allowing me the space I needed to complete this journey and for admonishing me to "stop doing the research and just get the book out there." I'm also thankful for your help on a more practical level. When the laundry piled up, the dishwasher needed emptying, or weeds in the garden threatened to multiply unchecked, you were always there to pitch in and lighten the load. For your indulgence and belief in this book and for your support for all my artistic endeavors over the years, I am deeply grateful.

I also owe a vote of thanks to my first editor, Deb McKew, who led me through the structuring of *Toxic Staple*. I had no idea what I was doing, but I was determined to do it. My second editor, Susan Owens at Tales for Telling, worked her magic polishing the text, giving the research a sense of flow, and getting rid of my anger and redundancy. I once wrote, "It would be insane to ever think of publishing a book without having an editor." After working with these two skilled professionals, I believe this statement more than ever. A huge thank-you to Kitty Werner at RSBPress for her continued support and hand-holding in getting *Toxic Staple* independently published and for the layout and design, and to Michael Manoogian, of Logo Design; you nailed the cover design with your creative genius. Thanks to Lisa Lirones, of LDesignerArtist for your computer expertise on the cover, and to Deb Vernon for editing the bibliography.

I am deeply grateful to my dear friend Kathleen Dunn, EdD and my daughter Jessica for proofreading *Toxic Staple*. Many thanks to friends Atty. Tom DeMille, Liz Meller, Sara Smith for your continued support, and to Noel and Cheryl Weinstein for helping with Mac issues.

I am most grateful for the vast amount of research available online and for forward-thinking doctors who comprehend the evolving epidemic of gluten sensitivity. A special thank-you to Dr. Kenneth Fine at EnteroLab. Without your cutting-edge testing, most of my family would have been on the medical treadmill for years. Instead, an accurate diagnosis gave us the opportunity to enjoy great health and renewed energy. I also owe a vote of thanks to Phyllis Zermeno at EnteroLab for her indulgence with my many questions and for previewing the chapters on testing.

A huge thank-you also goes to Dr. Ron Hoggan, coauthor of *Dangerous Grains* and *Cereal Killers*, for answering my many questions. Your efforts to spread the word that gluten sensitivity is so much more than celiac disease is making a difference in the lives of thousands of people around the world.

Last but by no means least, where would this book be without the stunning stories of renewed health brought about through a gluten-free lifestyle? Some storytellers have chosen to be identified in the text; others wish to remain anonymous. But each of you, by sharing your story, has become part of a larger story—the story of how a little-understood protein can cause untold misery and how eliminating it from one's diet may be a life-changing experience. The path so many of you walked was long, difficult, and sometimes frustrating beyond belief. If this book helps even one person avoid a similar fate, then all work we have done together will have been worth it.

Anne Sarkisian
2013

How to Get the Most from This Book

MAYBE YOU PICKED up this book because you're plagued by chronic health issues. Or maybe you're just "sick and tired of being sick and tired." In either case, I think you'll be both surprised and pleased at what you discover.

So how do you tackle this weighty tome? You could begin with the Introduction and read on through. Or you might want to turn directly to the chapter(s) that pertains to your particular issue(s). Here you will find a comprehensive list of symptoms, along with information about studies linking gluten to a variety of ailments, all conducted by well-respected institutions in the U.S. and abroad. When a study included concrete recommendations for action, I've noted these as well. For example: "People who have XYZ should be tested for CD"…or "XYZ cleared up on a gluten-free diet."

I've also included multiple stories—almost every chapter contains at least one—of folks just like you who suffered with undiagnosed or misdiagnosed issues, sometimes for decades, before discovering that gluten was at the root of their problems.

Detecting gluten sensitivity can be tricky, so it's important to read, and then re-read, Chapters 16 and 17 on blood and stool testing. Much current research supports the need for four blood tests, so it's vital you request all four, not just the one that's normally given. Still, even this combination is not foolproof. If your results come back negative but you're just not "feeling right," you may want to follow up with the more-sensitive stool testing.

You may wonder why you haven't heard more about the deleterious effects of gluten from your doctor, but the bottom line is that most health care professionals are woefully uninformed on this subject. Medical schools don't teach it; there are few continuing education courses that feature it, and there hasn't been a significant medical conference held for professionals in all facets of medicine since the CD Consensus Conference at the NIH in 2004, and even this event, which had a vast audience of patients, counted few doctors among the attendees. An international CD conference is held every two years in some part of the world, but this is not geared to educating our doctors here in the US on a wide scope. (There was to have been an international conference on gluten sensitivity—not just celiac disease, but the extended view of gluten intolerance—and associated inflammatory bowel diseases in Iran in spring of 2012, but it was cancelled due to political unrest in the region.) So do yourself, and your doctor, a favor by sharing with him/her what you learn from this book and from other sources you consult in your research.

Appendix C includes a list of acronyms and terms you will encounter as you read. I did not define every disease and disorder mentioned. After all, if you have one of them you know what it is! Appendix A provides many tips for doing more research on the subject of your choice. Appendix B provides a list of resources—books, websites, national support groups, and more—to help you on your journey to wellness. If anything you learn from this book is helpful along the way, I'd love to hear your story. Please send e-mail to anne@toxicstaple.com.

Introduction

WHEAT, ESPECIALLY WHOLE wheat, conjures up images of freshly baked bread, steaming pasta, crunchy cereal—wholesome foods that are plentiful, nutritious, and good for us. That these "amber waves of grain" flowing across much of North America's farmland and playing such a prominent role in the typical Western diet could be detrimental to our health is a very contradictory notion. Yet about 1 out of every 100 people in the United States suffers from celiac disease,[1] a malabsorption disorder resulting from intestinal damage caused by an autoimmune reaction to a protein called gluten found in wheat, rye, barley, and a variety of other grains. As surprising as this statistic may be, it pales in comparison with the findings of cutting-edge research. For example, Dr. Rodney Ford, a pediatric gastroenterologist from New Zealand, asserts that gluten affects 10 percent of the population.[2] The latest research by Dr. Alessio Fasano, a pediatric gastroenterologist and director of the Center for Celiac Research at Massachusetts General, in Boston, approximates that roughly 6 percent of the U.S. population is gluten sensitive (non-celiac gluten intolerant).[3] And Dr. Kenneth Fine, a gastroenterologist, medical researcher, and the director of EnteroLab, a clinical laboratory in Texas that specializes in the analysis of intestinal specimens for food sensitivities, has found that 30 to 40 percent of the U.S. population is affected by gluten sensitivity.[4]

It's difficult to believe such a seemingly benign protein could be so deleterious to one's health, yet extensive research substantiates that gluten can be toxic to those genetically predisposed to intolerance, and that the number of individuals who fall into this category is far larger than most people realize. Studies have shown gluten to be associated with—or a potential causative for—autoimmune diseases, many cancers, numerous neurological issues, organ problems (heart, pancreas, spleen, liver, lung, etc.), blood, bone, and skin maladies, and more.

As you might infer from its name, gluten is the "glue" that holds wheat and many other grains together. It's the sticky stuff that gives bread its wonderful chew and crunchy bite, but in those who cannot tolerate it, it can trigger an autoimmune response that damages the small intestine. This damage can lead to malabsorption of essential vitamins and minerals and, potentially, a hugely negative impact on the body.

Gluten is omnipresent in the American diet. It's found in cereals, bagels, toast, pancakes, sandwiches, subs, and hotdog rolls. It's part of breaded or marinated meats and fish. It's in pasta dishes and in the bread served with them. Cookies, cakes, pies, and most packaged snacks are laden with it. Wheat is ubiquitous in processed foods, too, an ingredient in nearly every canned or packaged item on grocery shelves and on the shelves in your kitchen cupboards.

Fortunately, gluten awareness is becoming mainstream. Gluten-free cookbooks are popping up everywhere and gluten-free products are multiplying exponentially. Having celiac disease or gluten intolerance 15 to 20 years ago was a hardship. Today, greater availability of packaged, gluten-free foods with improved taste and texture makes it much easier. There is still a long way to go, however, in getting health care providers to recognize the symptoms of gluten sensitivity and prescribe proper testing for diagnosis.

Until 2004 I'd barely heard of gluten intolerance. Then a grandson was diagnosed with celiac disease and I started to read. One day while scrubbing in the shower a light bulb went off. Consuming gluten, I realized, was a bit like ingesting tiny doses of arsenic, as in the old movie, *Arsenic and Old Lace*. You eat a little, then a little more, then a bit more. Before you know it you're quite sick (except with gluten it might take decades). Finally you die from toxic overload. In the years since that revelation I've seen so much gluten-related illness among family and friends and researched and read so much on the gluten issue that it's not a stretch for me to equate gluten with poison. Even researcher Dr. Fasano declared "gluten is poison to celiac patients."[5] In other words, gluten sensitivity is a serious health concern. As such, it needs to be addressed from a broader point of view than what you might learn from traditional media or expect your doctors to know.

I am an artist. I work with color and texture; I paint silk scarves and create jewelry from silk, fancy paper, beads and wire. I have been competing in interpretive floral design for 20 years. I had never thought of writing a book, let alone a book about medical research. Yet as I witnessed the role gluten played in the ill health of my own family and heard the stories of others negatively affected by this substance, I realized I had to understand more about this potentially life-threatening issue. Since 2004 I've made it my business to learn as much as possible about celiac disease (CD) and its companion disorder, non-celiac gluten intolerance (GI). In my research I've read extensively, reviewed more than 2,000 research abstracts and articles, and chatted with numerous people with CD/GI. I've attended the New England Celiac Conferences in Massachusetts in 2011 and 2009; The Gluten Truth Conference, in Dallas, Texas, in 2011; and The Higher Truth of Health Conference in Taos, New Mexico, in 2008. I've also attended the 12th International Celiac Disease Symposium in New York City in 2006 and the National Institutes of Health Consensus Development Conference on Celiac Disease in Bethesda, Maryland, in 2004. Some days I feel as if I've studied enough to earn a PhD in gluten. Now I want to share this information with others so they, too, can increase their chances for longer, stronger, and more productive lives.

Are you sensitive to gluten? How would you know? After all, you may have no symptoms or you may exhibit one or more of the 300-plus signs, symptoms, and maladies associated with gluten sensitivity.[6] (If you suspect gluten could be contributing to your health issues, the testing information included in Chapters 16 and 17 will help you track down potential gluten sensitivity, whether it's full-blown celiac disease or the often-more-elusive—but ultimately just as damaging—non-celiac gluten intolerance.)

Toxic Staple is a book of empowerment, intended to help readers learn about the devastating, far-reaching tentacles of CD and GI. Gluten sensitivity can affect any part of the human body, so if you, a family member, or a friend is suffering from chronic, eight-syllable ailments and/or degenerative health issues, or if you can't really put a name to what ails you but you're just "sick and tired of being sick and tired," the comprehensive, documented facts and real-life stories within these pages may inspire you to further investigation.

The stories in this book describe folks whose lives were negatively affected by a substance most people would categorize as beneficial—or at least benign. Yet when this substance was removed from their diet, almost all of them experienced positive results. I have witnessed this same transformation in my own life and in the lives of many members of my family. I know these stories are true, and I am passionately driven to share them for the benefit of others. If one of these tales leads you to seek better health for yourself or someone you love, I will have accomplished my goal.

Crazed 1

When the health of one's children and grandchildren is severely, negatively impacted and the doctors don't think anything is wrong, or can't find answers, or treat the symptoms with heavy pharmaceuticals that don't address the cause, then one can become a bit crazed. I don't mean crazed as in mentally unstable, I mean crazed as in *passionately driven* to learn as much as possible about the origin of the numerous and insidious maladies affecting not just members of my family but a huge number of people in families around the world. I also mean crazed as in determined to get the word out to the many folks who are finding no resolution to their ailments despite having had "every test there is"—except the right ones.

I am *saddened* to see the faces of thin, pale, sickly children and adults, especially older folks, whose bodies may be wasting away from the ravages of gluten consumption over the years. The health and future of our children depend on the wisdom, knowledge, and dedication of the adults in their lives—their parents, their teachers and, especially, their doctors. Yet who is educating the grownups?

I am *greatly saddened* to know that a large percentage of children with autism and Asperger's respond positively to a gluten-free/casein-free (GF/CF) diet, yet many of these children are being highly medicated with limited results. (Casein makes up about 80 percent of the proteins found in cow's milk, and studies have shown that eliminating dairy products also helps many who are gluten sensitive.)

I am *crazed* when I learn that many doctors know little or nothing about the ramifications of gluten on the human body. Celiac disease (CD) is the "end of the road" of gluten sensitivity, the consequence of an individual's health being negatively impacted by gluten for years, perhaps decades. People with CD have a damaged intestine; those with non-celiac gluten intolerance have not experienced intestinal damage. Accurate diagnosis of CD or GI has a very long way to go; few doctors understand how to adequately test for this condition, even with the tools now available. Moreover, there is very little talk in traditional medicine of the numerous maladies associated with gluten sensitivity that are affecting huge numbers of ailing folks.

I am *very crazed* to know how little is being done to educate our doctors in the face of the epidemic caused by gluten. In 2004 the National Institutes of Health held a conference on celiac disease. Although this conference was helpful for the many folks with CD/GI who turned out for it, the level of attendance by doctors and others in the medical field was disappointing. Although the National Foundation for Celiac Awareness has presented an on-line educational program for health care professionals since 2009, the program offers only 1.5 CME credits.[1] What could and should be happening is an expectation that all medical professionals take a two-day course that: (1) covers the deleterious ramifications of gluten sensitivity along with the adequate testing protocol of the four diagnostic blood tests currently available, and (2) provides an introduction to the wider view of non-celiac gluten intolerance.

I am *totally crazed* to learn that many autoimmune diseases, as well as orthopedic, hematological, tissue, skin, and organ maladies, are being highly associated with gluten. Yet few doctors consider, or suggest to their patients, that gluten could be contributing to their health issues.

I am *extremely crazed* to know that many neurological and cerebral maladies are now being linked to gluten by the rigorous research of Dr. Marios Hadjivassiliou, a neurologist from Sheffield, England, who is a pioneer in neurological research. Multiple sclerosis, schizophrenia, seizures, ataxia (lack of muscle coordination), neuropathy, attention deficit disorder (ADD), attention deficit hyperactivity disorder (ADHD), autism, dementia, migraines, headaches, and more are now being associated with gluten. If you or a loved one has any of these issues, has your neurologist ever suggested testing for celiac?

I am *absolutely crazed* to know that many types of cancer—stomach/intestinal, throat/esophageal, liver, blood, and others—are linked to gluten. This is little known and little talked about by doctors; they are too busy *treating* cancer. Ask anyone who has cancer if his or her doctor has ever mentioned testing for celiac disease or gluten intolerance.

I am *over-the-edge crazed* to know that pharmaceuticals are being prescribed so freely. Patients are often influenced by media ads to request drugs from their doctors without a true understanding of the effects of those drugs, yet many ailments could disappear or improve considerably with a gluten-free, and possibly a dairy-free, lifestyle. Has your doctor ever mentioned testing for gluten sensitivity or dairy intolerance, or are you plastered with meds and perhaps suffering from one or more drug-related side effects in addition to your original complaint?

Gluten sensitivity issues frequently affect more than one family member, and each person can exhibit multiple and totally different symptoms—or sometimes *no symptoms* at all. If you are gluten sensitive, ignoring a gluten-free lifestyle may lead to a warehouse of serious health issues over time. Yet few doctors are cognizant of adequate blood testing for CD/GI, and fewer still are familiar with the progressive stool testing that detects gluten *before it even gets into the blood.*[2] (Chapters 16 and 17 outline specific information about testing options.)

Now that I've hit age 70, why is it that I am in better health and have more energy and greater stamina than when I was 40? Without a doubt, it's my gluten-free lifestyle. These days you couldn't get me to consume a crumb of the stuff because for me, for most members of my family, and for many others, it's a toxic substance, and I know the damage it has done.

What you do with the information you read here is in your hands. Our bodies are meant to be healthy and, if given a chance, they are great at rejuvenation, but only you can alter the course of your health. If you choose to be tested for gluten sensitivity, and if this turns out to be your problem, do your body and your brain a favor: Begin a new lifestyle by getting rid of gluten. You just may see your life change, sometimes almost miraculously, before your very eyes.

2 Angry Gram: A Family Saga

THIS BOOK CONTAINS the tales of many individuals and families, but my initial impetus for writing it came from experiences in my own family. In February of 2004, my then five-year-old grandson, Nicholas, who'd been a sick little boy for quite some time, was diagnosed with celiac disease. Within months my husband and I; our three daughters, Tania, Daniele, and Jessica; and our other grandchildren, Brianna, Alexandria, and Colby, were also tested. Gluten sensitivity proved to be a problem affecting 100 percent of our immediate family. This chapter tells our stories.

Nick's Story

You bet I was angry! It was more like a stifled inner rage the first year or two after Nick's diagnosis. My husband and I had felt for a while that something was going on with our grandson; things just hadn't seemed right. "Honey, check with his doctor to make sure there's nothing serious developing," I would suggest to my second daughter, Daniele. "He's fine. Nothing is wrong," was the doctor's response.

At age two, Nick was a pudgy-cheeked, thriving child who was alert and content. As he became an active toddler he began to slim down as expected, but then the slimming continued. By age five he was pale, rib thin, and had little muscle tone. He became easily agitated and his muscles and bones ached. He couldn't eat much at the dinner table, but he was hungry all the time. His feet were ultra-sensitive to the stitching in the toes of his socks. He was always tired; when spending the night with my husband and me, he needed help getting into his pajamas and walking up the stairs. Eventually he began to have intestinal issues, and his lips were dry and cracked. On frequent visits to the doctor he was given a prescription for whatever ailed him—sore throat, cough, earache—the usual antibiotics for the usual childhood maladies.

Our extended family of aunts, uncles, and cousins gathers three times yearly to celebrate Thanksgiving, Christmas, and Greek Easter. Thank heavens for my cousin's wife, who has celiac disease. Listening to me describe Nick's symptoms at one of these family gatherings, she said they sounded a lot like indications of CD; she also told me about a simple blood test for diagnosis. As it turned out, at least 10 of Nick's symptoms suggested he might be gluten sensitive. Having just one or two of them should have been enough to indicate screening for the disorder, but Nick had never been tested. Had my cousin not shared her knowledge, Nick could easily have ended up in the hospital with heart fibrillation or any of a number of maladies caused by malabsorption.

Daniele immediately scheduled an appointment for her son to be tested. Although at the time the Celiac Disease Foundation recommended a panel of several different diagnostic blood tests, Nick was given only two, the tissue transglutaminase (tTG) and the antigliadin antibody (AGA: IgA and IgG). (Gliadin is part of the gluten protein.) His results were highly positive on the tTG, with a score of 49 (somewhere between 0 and 19 is considered normal), and mildly positive on the AGA: IgG. He was negative on the AGA: IgA. He was referred to a doctor at Children's Hospital for an endoscopic biopsy, the "gold standard" for diagnosing CD. For the endoscopy to be accurate, however, Nick's parents would have to continue feeding gluten to their highly gluten-sensitive child for four more weeks. You wouldn't do this to your dog!

Nick's parents chose not to do the endoscopy. The doctor respected their decision. He felt Nick's numbers were so high that if he responded to a gluten-free diet (GFD), this in and of itself would confirm the CD diagnosis.

Within two days of being put on a GFD, Nick's tummy felt better. Within two weeks his cheeks were rosy. After a couple of months he was developing muscles and swinging from the monkey bars. As his body began to heal, the intestinal issues subsided and the "real" boy began to emerge. His personality totally changed; instead of tired and irritable he was cooperative, bright, and energetic. We had our grandson back. Nick began eating a GFD in February 2004. Today he is an excellent student who loves to swim, kayak, play basketball and read. *And he is rarely sick.*

Brianna's Story

In 2001–2002, long before Nicholas' problems were diagnosed, Daniele's second child, Brianna, was having a terrible time sleeping. Daniele would prop Brianna in her car seat and drive around for a while to help the baby fall asleep. Still, many nights Brianna would awaken in the wee hours of the morning, terribly fussy and obviously uncomfortable. And during the day, due to her discomfort and irritability, she never napped, making the situation worse for parents and child alike.

Brianna's pediatrician diagnosed her with reflux and prescribed a heavy-duty drug, a diagnosis and treatment later confirmed by an ear, nose, and throat specialist. No matter how hard her beleaguered parents tried, however, Brianna simply would not take the drugs. Could they be that horrible? Daniele decided to taste them herself. The taste was awful. Almost immediately she changed her position on how she was going to treat her baby daughter. Although these days it seems almost the American way to address a medical complaint by simply ameliorating the symptoms with drugs, Daniele wanted to get to the root of the problem. She began to investigate food allergies and intolerances and to learn more about the impact of diet and proper nutrition on good health. Brianna was already consuming a wholesome diet, but Daniele learned that sometimes even foods considered "good for you" can be anything but.

Having read about how difficult it is for some people to digest wheat, she took Brianna off wheat products. The child's reflux issues disappeared within days. My granddaughter and her exhausted parents were finally able to enjoy a good night's sleep. After Daniele learned Nick had CD, she had Brianna tested as well. Although she tested negative for gluten sensitivity on the CD blood tests, she later tested positive on stool tests and has been on a GFD ever since (see Daniele's story following).

Brianna's problems however, did not end with gluten. Prior to beginning a GFD she had developed nut, soy, and dairy allergies that I highly suspect were caused by a leaky gut, a condition most likely resulting from gluten sensitivity and possibly exacerbated by the many chemical additives and/or colorants we all are exposed to in today's world.

Getting the toxins and allergens out of Brianna's diet has allowed her gut to heal. Gone are the dark eyes and the itchy and rough, pebbly skin that were so bothersome to her. Her behavioral issues have subsided as well. Today she is a bright, alert little girl, active in music, swimming, and gymnastics and thriving in a Spanish immersion class.

Aly's Story

Like her brother and sister, Daniele's third child, Aly (short for Alyxandria), appeared healthy at birth but, like her siblings, was born three weeks early. We later learned premature birth can be connected to CD (see Chapter 12). When Aly was an infant, it seemed as though Daniele never really had a full supply of breast milk (a circumstance also associated with CD), and Aly never nursed for long. In my eyes Aly didn't quite fill out to become a healthy, pudgy-looking baby, but, once again, when Daniele asked the doctor to double check that all was okay, the doctor assured her everything was fine. Most babies want to put weight on their legs by the age of six or seven months. Aly did not. She was a year old before she stood up and eighteen months before she learned to walk. She never babbled the way babies do, and it wasn't until the age of three that she began to say more than a few words. Even then, it was difficult to understand her. And, like her sister Brianna, she was plagued with itchy, rough, pebbly skin.

Aly was about a year old when Nick was diagnosed with CD. Six months later, Daniele also put the baby on a GFD. She didn't have Aly formally tested (she was too young for blood tests to return a reliable reading), but given the fact that both her siblings were sensitive to gluten, and that Aly herself was failing to meet various developmental milestones, switching her to a GFD seemed like a prudent choice. Later, tests revealed she also had allergies to nuts, soy and dairy.

I have no doubt that if Daniele had not taken Aly off gluten and dairy, she would be a developmentally delayed child, destined to spend her days in a special-education classroom and facing a dim future. Instead, as I write this she is a bright, alert youngster who plays very well by herself and interacts beautifully with others. She is vibrant and healthy, and her eyes sparkle. She has a learning disability in reading (see Chapter 9 for more on the link between gluten and some learning disabilities), but once she got the help she needed to be successful, she began to thrive. Soy and nuts still affect her, as they do her sister, but as the girls have gotten older both seem to be able to eat some dairy.

Daniele's children could not tolerate gluten in their diets. We had no idea why the same issue should affect all three of them, but we did know that some of the difficulties experienced by the children were also present in the adults. Could the problem be more widespread? We were about to find out.

Daniele's Story

After giving birth to Aly, Daniele never seemed to produce enough breast milk. She didn't fill out the way nursing mothers do and she had some awful bouts with mastitis. She had always been a sinuously lean young woman and had never put on excess weight during pregnancy, but after Aly was born she continued to lose weight. A few months later she looked almost anorexic, but she didn't have any symptoms other than a dull, gnawing pain in her right side and dark halos around her eyes.

Right after Nick was diagnosed with CD, Daniele's doctor tested her as well, but the blood tests were negative. In most cases doctors do not recommend an endoscopy if blood test results for CD are negative, but my daughter's doctor was concerned enough to advise her to see a gastroenterologist. She had the procedure (see Chapter 16 for more on endoscopic biopsy). It was negative as well.

Although she ate a very healthy diet, Daniele was becoming more and more emaciated, and none of the doctors could figure out why. It was about this time that my friend Sue (see Susan's story, *CD and the Family Tree*, in Chapter 16) told me about the more-sensitive stool testing pioneered by Dr. Kenneth Fine at EnteroLab. Because stool tests pick up the gliadin antibody before it gets into the blood, they can often provide an accurate diagnosis where other methods have failed.[1]

At this point it had been about seven months since Nick was diagnosed with CD. Given how much better he and his sisters (not to mention his grandmother—see Anne's story below) were doing on a GFD, and knowing there are genetic components to gluten sensitivity, I wanted to decipher who in my family had the genes. I also wanted to know who might even have CD and not realize it, since it's possible to have flattened villi—hair-like projections in the small intestine that absorb nutrients and that are considered the hallmark of celiac disease—and still exhibit *no symptoms*. Thus I offered to pay for a gluten-sensitivity panel of stool and genetic testing for our whole family.

Thank heavens they took me up on it! My husband and I, our three daughters, and two of our grandchildren had blood and stool tests. Nick and Aly did not, since Nick had already been diagnosed and Aly was too young. All of us (except Nick) also had a genetic test (from saliva gathered through a cheek swab) to determine if any of us carried a particular gene (or genes) that made us more susceptible to the disorder. My husband and I, as well as Daniele and her sisters, tested positive on the stool tests. Brianna and Colby tested positive as well, even though Brianna had been eating a (mostly) gluten-free diet. According to Dr. Fine, it's possible for someone to have a positive reading on the stool test for many months after he or she has adopted a GFD.[2] Although most of us tested *negative* on the blood tests, we tested positive on the stool tests. We also tested positive for a combination of genes indicating susceptibility.

Daniele's stool results were positive for the antigliadin antibody, and she was diagnosed as being gluten intolerant. She immediately began eating a gluten-free diet, and after a few months the dark halos and gnawing pain in her side disappeared. Even then, it took her nine months to put on four pounds. Today, she is svelte and has regained some lean muscle. With her beautiful shining hair, she is the picture of health, has great energy, and is rarely sick.

Tania's Story

When my oldest daughter, Tania, was in the first grade, she missed about four weeks of school due to a mysterious malady. Her doctor thought it was a lingering virus; she had a high SED (sedimentation) rate—a measure of inflammation—and her knees hurt. Finally I took her to a group of specialists. They talked about juvenile rheumatoid arthritis (JRA), but shortly afterward her symptoms disappeared. She had a similar joint issue in the sixth grade and once again missed three or four weeks of school. The scenario was the same: a trip to specialists, a mention of JRA, and symptoms that disappeared shortly thereafter. Rheumatoid arthritis (see Chapter 10) is an autoimmune disease, and autoimmune diseases are now being associated with celiac disease. In fact, many people suffering from diseases of this type improve on a GFD.

As a child Tania often had sore throats, many diagnosed as strep, and she often felt sick enough that she didn't want to go to school. After having her tonsils out, sore throats and strep were less frequent, but in college she went through a bout of mononucleosis.

Always actively involved with swimming, skiing, and tennis, Tania has dealt with aches and pains in her knees off and on throughout her life. At the age of 36 she suffered from a debilitating neurological condition that caused extreme fatigue and left her legs so weak she could barely walk. After about four weeks her symptoms slowly subsided and she regained her normal stride, though the fatigue remained.

At the time of this incident, Tania had already tested positive for gluten sensitivity on Dr. Fine's stool test and had been eating a GFD for over two years. Prior to the two months it took to get an appointment at one of New Hampshire's finest hospitals, I called the offices of two of the gurus of gluten to see if they knew of any neurologists in New England that were up on gluten and its devastating neurological consequences. The answer was no. I then contacted Danna Korn, author of *Wheat Free, Worry Free.*[3] She was very sympathetic, but she really didn't know anyone, either. Since few doctors have been trained on how damaging gluten can be, I was not surprised. I then started researching the issue on the Internet myself, compiling information relative to neurological issues caused by gluten that I took to Tania's doctor. A few weeks prior to the visit I also called and politely requested the doctor do a bit of research on gluten and neurology in case he was not familiar with this connection.

When Tania finally got to her appointment, everything checked out fine neurologically. An earlier MRI showed no brain lesions, fortunately ruling out multiple sclerosis. The doctor, knowing Tania was following a gluten-free diet, suggested she continue to do so. He seemed to be aware of the damaging affects of gluten, but to what extent I don't know, since by the time we arrived for the appointment Tania was pretty much back to normal.

When Tania became debilitated, I asked her if she had been following the GFD faithfully. "Yes," she answered, but when I asked if she always checked salad dressings and marinades for gluten she said no, which meant she wasn't being *absolute* with the diet. Unfortunately, for those of us who cannot tolerate this substance, the littlest bit of gluten—I'm talking crumbs—can keep the small intestine damaged and sustain the antibody reactivity that can cause harm to any part of the body, even the neurons and cerebrum.

Some months later, as I was relaying Tania's story to a friend, she mentioned a similar incident of severe muscle fatigue that had turned out to be associated with adrenal fatigue. Interestingly, Tania felt that a frightening "fight and flight" reaction she'd had when swimming in deep water with her son and nephew might have triggered her problem. Later I found an article connecting adrenal exhaustion to gluten.[4] It's also known that an accident, illness, divorce, or other stress can kick-start CD that's been lying low in the body—"the straw that broke the camel's back," so to speak.

It's been several years since Tania's debilitating episode, and although we may never know its cause, I continue to hope she follows her GFD diligently.

Colby's Story

When the "family" tests for gluten sensitivity were done in 2004, Tania's son, Colby, was three years old. At the time he tested positive on the antigliadin stool tests; he also tested positive for dairy intolerance. His main symptoms were blotchy cheeks and behavioral issues in the form of meltdowns. Dairy would bother his stomach, bring on diarrhea, and keep him stuffed up. Bright red chin and cheeks would blossom. After the tests he was off dairy for three to four years; it was then reintroduced and he now seems to be able to handle some. He continues to eat a GFD.

Jessica's Story

Jessica, our youngest daughter, appears to have been the least affected by gluten. However, in 2004 she, too, tested positive on Dr. Fine's stool test. Looking back, Jessica claims she had "ants in her pants" in school, not being able to sit still; and she reminds me she used to get earaches and strep throat often.

Today she's a commercial pilot who treasures her eyesight and mental acuity. Knowing the ramifications of consuming gluten, she takes the GF lifestyle seriously and enjoys a very healthy diet. And since she's been gluten free, the colds she used to get every two to three months, along with annoying problems of excess mucus and postnasal drip, have disappeared.

Anne's Story

When we first learned that our grandson, Nick, had celiac disease, it was crushing news, but at least we had a name for what was draining his emaciated body. Shortly thereafter (a few months before I was tested), I, too, began to follow the GF diet. As far as I knew, I had no medical reason for doing so—I just felt compelled to offer support to Nicholas as he adapted to his new lifestyle.

I'd always thought I was relatively healthy; other than my ob-gyn I'd never even had a regular doctor. Yet, thinking back, I realize I'd had several chronic complaints. In my thirties and forties I'd been plagued off and on with bronchial and urinary infections. In my forties I was tormented with extremely heavy periods and eventually had a total hysterectomy, which included removing a fibroid the size of a grapefruit. About age 50 I was diagnosed with hypothyroidism, but I'd been "always tired" for years—not excessively fatigued but tired enough to be a drag, yawning in people's faces and needing an afternoon nap. My hay fever got worse as I aged, and I became allergic to whatever was flying in the air, from pollen to cat and dog dander to dust and mold. Fall was particularly irritating, but I never liked taking drugs unless I was quite miserable. Then, in my mid-50s, sinus infections landed in my chest and led to reactive airway, an asthma-like condition. I would rest, flood myself with liquids, and sometimes manage to avoid the nasty puffers that let me breathe when the wheezing got too bad. It's incredible what people will tolerate and still think they are healthy!

Amazingly, within three to four weeks of starting on a GFD in 2004 I began to feel like dynamite. As I learned later, my body was beginning to absorb all those vitamins and minerals that had been slipping out the back door through malabsorption. I dropped 10 to 15 pounds without even trying. My hay fever became practically nonexistent (though it reappears if I eat dairy during allergy season) and, after being on the diet for about a year, my cat/dog and mold/dust allergies disappeared. These days I rarely pick up a cold or bug and if I feel one coming on, I know it's directly related to the energy I've expended. In other words, sometimes I push myself too far because life is so wonderfully full and because, with so much energy, I can!

As part of my education process after Nick was diagnosed, I also read Danna Korn's *Wheat Free, Worry Free*, which helped me realize how toxic a substance gluten is for huge numbers of people, as well as how many symptoms and maladies can be tied to it, many of which are often misdiagnosed.

By this time I knew a little about testing, so I requested the three blood tests I had read about:

- The tissue transglutaminase – tTG: IgA and IgG
- The endomysial antibody – EMA: IgA
- The antigliadin antibody – AGA: IgA and IgG

(Four blood tests are now available. For more information about them, see Chapter 16.) My doctor agreed to my request and ordered the tests. The tTG and the EMA tests were negative, which meant I didn't have CD. The AGA: IgA and IgG, tests that measure the level of the gliadin antibody, were positive. (Gliadin, as mentioned earlier, is the nasty little protein found in gluten.) A separate allergy test for gluten and wheat was also positive. My doctor wanted to treat my problem as an allergy. I could have a little gluten every four days, on a rotational diet, the doctor said. I don't think so! Gluten intolerance is not an allergy; it's a system-wide intolerance and it lasts a lifetime. Yes, one can be allergic to gluten, but the main focus here is on celiac disease and non-celiac gluten intolerance, not on a gluten allergy (for more on the interaction between gluten and allergies see Allergies and Asthma in Chapter 8). And besides, by this time I had read enough to know that consuming gluten for a person who is gluten sensitive is not a healthy idea.

Through further reading, I realized the results of my tTG and EMA blood tests might have been negative because I hadn't eaten any gluten since shortly after Nick had been diagnosed with CD. In order for the blood tests to produce valid results, the patient must be consuming gluten at the time the tests are given. No one had mentioned this important fact prior to testing, so I decided to try it again. This time I lined up an appointment with "the best in Boston" for a couple months later. To prepare for the tests, I began to eat wheat.

This process of deliberately eating wheat after having removed it from the diet for several weeks or more is called a gluten challenge. This approach is sometimes recommended by alternative practitioners to see how a patient responds, but you should never do so without first consulting your doctor, especially if you know you are gluten sensitive. In my case, a challenge is exactly what it turned out to be. No sooner had I returned to a "normal" diet than my energy level began to fall. I put on weight, and my elbows and knees became so sensitive it hurt to kneel, even on my bed. This aggravation was something new to me, and it greatly interfered with gardening, because I like to garden on my knees. These symptoms told me my body was rebelling against gluten, but I was bound and determined to stick it out long enough to repeat the blood tests. I wanted to see the proof for myself in black and white.

I had the blood tests again. The results were unchanged. The tTG and EMA were negative, and the AGA: IgA quite positive, with a score of 76 (the normal range is 0–19). My doctor left a message saying my test results were "consistent with celiac disease." There was no message about nutritional counseling or an endoscopy to examine the villi in my intestine for damage, the "gold standard" for CD diagnosis. I would have declined an endoscopy anyway. I already knew I was extremely gluten intolerant and that I needed to live a GF lifestyle if I wanted to get healthy and be able to function optimally at my ripening age. I went back on my gluten-free diet immediately after the testing. The proof, as they say, is in the pudding!

It was shortly thereafter that I discovered Dr. Fine's more sensitive stool testing at EnteroLab (see Chapter 17). My stool test came back positive on both the tTG: IgA (the tTG stool test is more sensitive than the tTG blood test) and the AGA: IgA. I also had a malabsorption test, which measures the amount of fat in the stool; an elevated fat content may indicate a high level of malabsorption.[5] The results showed I was malabsorbing quite a bit. No wonder I'd been tired most of my life. In my eyes, this information—yet another indicator of CD—was enough to indicate my villi probably were damaged.

The news that everyone in my immediate family, including my husband, was sensitive to gluten was shocking, but it made me determined to learn all I could about this condition. As I studied I discovered the blood test on which I'd tested positive, the AGA: IgA and IgG, was not specifically recommended by the National Institutes of Health (NIH) and thus not on the radar screen of many doctors. Yet it was this test that had confirmed why a GFD, which I'd adopted originally strictly out of sympathy for my grandson, Nick, made me feel so much healthier and more energetic.

Nearly everything I could find on the topic of gluten sensitivity was geared toward CD. If someone didn't have flattened villi (villous atrophy) as confirmed by an endoscopic biopsy, he or she wouldn't be classified as having the disorder. For example, since none of my family had an endoscopy, except for Daniele, who was negative anyway, none of us can be considered as part of any CD statistical calculations, nor can we offer to join a study, since participants must be confirmed as having flattened villi through a positive endoscopy.

Still, many people were testing positive on the AGA: IgA and IgG test and negative on the biopsy. As I continued to do research I learned there was a lot more to celiac disease than intestinal damage, yet intestinal damage is what the tTG and EMA antibody blood tests are designed to detect. I began to question the credibility of the endoscopy and blood-test regimens.

For the most part, celiac was the hot topic of conversation, but I soon discovered another whole dimension of gluten sensitivity, a dimension without gut damage called non-celiac gluten intolerance (GI). Few people in the medical profession were talking about GI in 2004, a situation that remains basically unchanged as I write this in 2012. Yet millions of people who were not exhibiting damaged villi in the small intestine and who might never test positive on the tTG or EMA blood tests (because their gut wasn't damaged—or wasn't damaged enough) were suffering from gluten intolerance. Many of these folks were sick as dogs, with symptoms affecting multiple organs and other parts of the body, but rarely was gluten considered in diagnosing their ailments. Then, as now, many of these individuals are being plastered with prescriptions that often come with a list of nasty side effects—just turn on your TV to listen to the disclaimers—and no one in their medical hierarchy is recognizing that gluten could be the real culprit.

Once I became aware of the reliable, serious research available online, I bought my first computer so I could study in the comfort of my own home (see Appendix A for tips on how to do research and Appendix B for a list of resources you may wish to explore). The more I read, the more annoyed I became that so much valuable information, especially data about the devastating effects of gluten sensitivity and how to test for it, was not being made readily available to our pediatricians, hematologists, neurologists, obstetricians, gynecologists, infertility specialists, osteologists, oncologists, psychologists, cardiologists, you name it. Since any part of the body can be affected by gluten, doctors in every medical specialty need to be educated on its potentially negative effects. Primary care physicians, especially, need to be made aware of this disorder and how to test for it.

If I had my wish, I would make it mandatory for every doctor in this country to complete at least a two-day course on (1) how to adequately test for CD/GI, and (2) the consequences of gluten consumption for those who are sensitive to it. Since this is not about to happen, I'm hoping this collection of stories, complemented by some well-documented research to substantiate the various and highly different scenarios of individuals whose lives have been negatively affected by gluten, may lead you to explore your own physical, mental, and emotional health and well-being.

The short-term results of a gluten-free diet for each member of my family were dramatic. Our allergy symptoms, along with numerous other ailments, gradually disappeared, and each of us experienced an improvement in energy level and general well-being. These same positive results continue to this day, which, of course, only fuels my passion for getting the word to others through this book.

In this great country, especially given the ever-escalating costs of health insurance, it is unfortunate that we need to become our own health advocates. Still, no matter when we begin, each of us has within our hands the power to start turning our health around.

3 A Whirlwind of Illnesses

Recently I heard someone refer to gluten and celiac disease (CD) as the "latest buzzwords." Maybe they are. Perhaps these words are surfacing, after decades of lying dormant, because gluten sensitivity is finally beginning to be recognized as a major contributor to ill health around the world.

In the mid-1940s, an astute Dutch pediatrician named Willem-Karel Dicke noticed that some children who were very ill got better during periods of strict flour rationing and relapsed when bread was again readily available. This connection helped to establish gluten as the cause for what we now know as classic celiac disease, a condition first described centuries ago by the ancient Greek physician, Aretaeus of Cappadocia. After Dicke's observations, scientists began to study the effects of gluten on the body, but it wasn't until the 1990s that significant research started to be done in this area. Twenty years later, most doctors still don't understand the serious ramifications of gluten on the human body and mind, nor do they understand the need for adequate testing. Why not?

Part of the answer lies with the fact that celiac disease was once thought to be very rare—1 in every 4,600 people, according to a 1991 study lead by Dr. Peter H. R. Green,[1] director of the Celiac Disease Center at Columbia University and co-author of *Celiac Disease: A Hidden Epidemic*. Later studies have proven these numbers to be grossly understated, but many medical professionals, unaware of current research, still think CD is an uncommon medical condition. Many doctors also believe that CD can be classified solely as a wasting disease with a short set of classic symptoms. As a result, screening for CD is not likely to be on their radar screens.

Celiac disease, as it turns out, is far from rare. Rather, it is one of the most common genetically influenced disorders, and the symptoms and maladies associated with it extend far beyond the classic symptoms of diarrhea, weight loss, and failure to thrive. James Braly, MD and Ron Hoggan, EdD in their eye-opening book, *Dangerous Grains: Why Gluten Cereal Grains May Be Hazardous To Your Health*, list over 200 symptoms and maladies associated with gluten.[2] *Recognizing Celiac Disease*, by Cleo Libonati, RN, BSN, lists more than 300.[3] This is a "happening" dilemma for the health care industry, but it's one that is far from being adequately or appropriately addressed.

Current scientific thought suggests that approximately 1 of every 100 people has CD. Given a U.S. population of 311 million as reported in the 2010 census, this translates, statistically, to 3.1 million U.S. residents. Even more startling is the fact, according to Dr. Green, that "97 percent of these folks are undiagnosed."[4] These numbers, as significant as they are, address only individuals who have been (or would be if they were tested) diagnosed by endoscopic biopsy as having celiac disease. They do not reflect the multitude of those with non-celiac gluten intolerance (GI), folks with no intestinal damage who nonetheless may be very sensitive to gluten.

Research lead by Dr. Fasano detects non-celiac gluten intolerance in about six percent of the U.S. population.[5] This translates to 18.6 million people. And gastroenterologist Dr. Kenneth Fine claims that nearly one-third or more of the U.S. population may have gluten sensitivity.[6] Much more research is needed, but regardless of what the final numbers turn out to be, by any calculation there is an astronomical number of ailing folks with CD/GI literally *dying* to be diagnosed.

In the United States, the average time from the first signs of a problem indicating celiac disease to a diagnosis is 11 years.[7] Imagine being sick for one or two decades before detecting celiac disease or non-celiac gluten intolerance.

A study by Dr. Fasano and colleagues found that for those with CD, the chance of their first-degree relatives (parents, siblings or children) developing the disorder is 1 in 22; among second-degree relatives (cousins, aunts and uncles) it's 1 in 39. For those in the general population exhibiting CD-like symptoms, chances that they have the disease are about 1 in 56. Compare these numbers with statistics that indicate approximately 1 in 133 people in the U.S. population at large (approximately 1 percent) have celiac, a prevalence similar to populations in Europe.[8] A recent overview from Finland found the occurrence of CD increases as people age: "1.5% in children, 2% in adults and 2.7% in the elderly."[9] "Up to 2% of some European populations" may develop CD, notes another study.[10] And still another study claims the incidence of CD to be nearly 10 percent among first-degree relatives.[11]

Even more disturbing, a recent Mayo Clinic study led by Dr. Joseph Murray found CD is more than four times more prevalent now than it was 50 years ago, and that in the group studied, those with CD were almost four times more likely to have died in the past 45 years than those without the disease. The study also concluded that for every person diagnosed with CD, there may be 30 more who are undiagnosed.[12] *And this number doesn't even include those with GI!*

We have barely scratched the surface when it comes to understanding the harmful effects of gluten and how drastically it can affect our health and productivity at home, in school, and on the job, not to mention our happiness, mental stability, and emotional well-being. And since gluten has the capacity to affect "any organ or body system,"[13] we've a long way to go before its role is recognized by *all* doctors in *all* disciplines of medicine.

Even many doctors familiar with celiac rely on only one blood test for diagnosis, most commonly the tissue transglutaminase (tTG: IgA). There is no standardization among the national support groups and university research center websites; however, there are now *four* separate tests and it is important to have all of them. Offering a panel of tests provides more opportunity to detect gluten issues. The need for this comprehensive testing is reiterated in a 2003 article titled "Coeliac Disease" in *The Lancet*, one of the world's foremost medical journals.[14]

The good news is that these four blood tests are readily available if you know to ask for them. The bad news is that even if your doctor agrees to order them, you may test negative on all four and *still* be gluten intolerant. Luckily, more progressive testing is offered by Dr. Kenneth Fine. Both the stool tests available at Dr. Fine's EnteroLab, and the antigliadin antibody (AGA: IgG and IgA) blood tests so helpful in detecting non-celiac gluten intolerance (available through your doctor), may identify gluten sensitivity where other tests have failed. (For specific details, see Chapters 16 and 17.)

It isn't long ago that CD was thought to be associated only with its most commonly recognized symptoms of diarrhea, weight loss, and failure to thrive. Today researchers are finding this form of the disease, now termed classic CD, to be in the minority. The three more common forms of the disease—atypical, silent, and latent—may produce a wide variety of symptoms or, in some cases, no symptoms at all. And even when doctors are aware of this fact (and many are not), it's easy to see how such a diversity of reactions to gluten sensitivity can present a diagnostic challenge. "The rate at which celiac disease is diagnosed depends on the level of suspicion for the disease," says Dr. Joseph Murray.[15] If doctors are relying on classic symptoms to raise that suspicion, they're unlikely to check for CD in a patient who is not exhibiting them. It simply doesn't occur to them.

These days the problem of celiac disease (though not gluten intolerance, which is still in its infancy) is finally getting some press. On rare occasions there's even something on TV. True, much of the media coverage relates to gluten-free (GF) recipes, GF products and new GF restaurants and bakeries, but at least articles are hitting magazines and newspapers. Most people I talk with have heard or read something about celiac disease or gluten; they may even know of a relative, friend, or neighbor who was recently diagnosed.

What isn't being reported is information on how to properly diagnose gluten sensitivity or facts about the numerous distressing and serious consequences of gluten ingestion for people who cannot tolerate it. After all, aren't our doctors supposed to know that stuff? One would think so, but in reality the level of awareness in the medical profession is minimal in relation to the devastation being wrought.

On December 9, 2005, the front page of the *Wall Street Journal* reported that in the U.S. (unlike in Europe where CD has long been recognized) "the perceived rarity [of CD]...depressed interest among researchers." Since a GF lifestyle is the only treatment necessary, CD "attracted little attention from drug companies"–not too many money-making opportunities exist for "surgical or drug treatments" related to CD[16] (except for the huge number of ailments being cause by gluten).

Dr. Peter Green at Columbia University found that "the long duration of symptoms was mostly due to a physician delay in reaching the diagnosis rather than a patient delay in seeking medical attention."[17] So whose job *is* it to educate doctors about gluten, and what will those studying medicine now and in the future be taught about it? Hopefully, someone is working on these questions, because the lack of education on this topic among our health care professionals is keeping people sick.

If you think a sensitivity to gluten might be your problem, it's easy to rule it in—remember, simply "feeling good" doesn't rule it out—by seeking the traditional and progressive tests outlined in Chapters 16 and 17. If it turns out you are sensitive to gluten, living a gluten-free lifestyle will not only improve your health, it may also increase your energy and vitality, lift your spirits, and possibly extend the years you have left to spend on planet Earth with those you love.

4 Gluten 101: A Primer on Intolerance

Gluten Sensitivity

Although the term *gluten sensitivity* is sometimes used interchangeably with gluten intolerance, I (and many others) define it to include the manifestations of both celiac disease (gut damage) and non-celiac gluten intolerance (no gut damage). Gluten sensitivity can manifest itself in a vastly complex continuum of symptoms from very mild or almost non-existent to severe and even life-threatening. These symptoms can affect almost any part of the body (and consequently, the mind) on multiple levels over a long period of time. Gluten sensitivity may also be revealed by an allergic response to gluten.

In trying to clarify the "broader field of gluten sensitivity," author and educator Ron Hoggan, EdD, notes, "Celiac disease is just one sub-set of a rather large and growing continuum of illness that require a life-long gluten free diet."[1] It was less than two decades ago that Dr. Marios Hadjivassiliou and his research team found that "gluten sensitivity was shown to manifest solely with neurological dysfunction....The concept of extraintestinal [outside the intestine] presentations without enteropathy [intestinal damage] has only recently become accepted."[2]

Celiac Disease

Celiac disease (CD) is the end of the road of gluten sensitivity. Also known as celiac sprue, gluten-sensitive enteropathy or nontropical sprue, CD is an autoimmune response to gliadin, a protein entity of gluten found in wheat, rye, and barley, as well as in contaminated oats and a few lesser-known grains such as spelt, kamut, triticale, etc. CD damages the villi, tiny, finger-like projections in the small intestine that aid the body in absorbing vitamins and minerals. When villi are functioning normally, nutrients can be absorbed easily. Spread your fingers apart and imagine they're villi. Notice how much open space there is up and down each finger. Now make a fist. When villi are inflamed or diseased, they become flattened—like the fingers in your closed fist. Flattened villi can no longer absorb enough nutrients to keep the body operating optimally.

By the time an individual is diagnosed with CD, damage to the villi has usually occurred over a period of time—often years, sometimes decades. For some people, the resulting symptoms and maladies are significant and affect multiple systems within the body. Others experience no symptoms at all.

CD is *not* an allergy but, rather, an *intolerance*, an autoimmune disease where the body's immune system attacks the intestinal villi, leading to symptoms on the inside that may not become apparent on the outside until the results lead to some other malady or condition. As an autoimmune disease, CD lasts a lifetime.[3] It's not something you can outgrow, but it *is* something you can manage because—at least so far—it is the single autoimmune disease with a known cause: gluten. The only effective treatment is an *absolutely* gluten-free lifestyle. Fortunately, following a gluten-free diet (GFD) to the max has the potential to improve one's health in multiple ways.

It's also possible to be *allergic* to wheat and gluten (see Chapter 8 for more information on allergies). In fact, like some folks who are allergic to peanuts, there are people so allergic to gluten that ingesting it can cause an anaphylactic response (a reaction so severe it can cause death). However, allergies and intolerance are two different things. One can be *allergic* to wheat/gluten, experiencing symptoms such as hives, runny nose, itchy eyes, etc., without having gluten intolerance. One also can be gluten intolerant without being allergic to the substance.

The *gold standard* for diagnosing CD is an endoscopic biopsy to see if the villi are damaged. By inserting a tube down a patient's throat into his or her small intestine, a doctor can take snippets of the mucosal (intestinal) wall for observation under a microscope. Doctors normally recommend an endoscopy if a patient tests positive for CD on blood tests.

Although there are *genetic* components that predispose some people to CD (see Chapter 18), having the genes does not mean they will develop the disease. A trigger such as an accident, illness, divorce, pregnancy, financial issues, or other major stressors may also bring on CD. And since we are a society that overindulges in wheat from infancy, I expect there are times when the excess just catches up with us.

In addition to *genes, gluten,* and a *trigger* being contributors to the development of CD, it also appears a condition known as permeable gut may be involved. Celiac researcher Dr. Alessio Fasano and his colleagues at the University of Maryland discovered a protein known as zonulin that "works like the traffic conductor or gatekeeper of our body's tissues." Folks with CD have "an increased level of zonulin, which opens the junctions between the cells," giving gluten and other allergens access to parts of the body where they don't belong, "like the blood brain barrier." These invading antigens then provoke an autoimmune attack by antibodies, not only on the intestinal villi, causing CD, but on other tissues and organs as well. Conditions such as diabetes, multiple sclerosis, and rheumatoid arthritis (and possibly other autoimmune diseases) also may be linked to this permeable-gut process.[4]

When a patient is diagnosed with CD, doctors in the know will recommend that his or her parents, siblings, and children also be tested. If second-degree relatives have any symptoms, it behooves them to be screened too.

Four Classes of Celiac Disease: Classic, Atypical, Silent, and Latent

Classic—Failure to thrive (not growing), weight loss, diarrhea and/or constipation, foul-smelling, clay colored, or floating stools (steatorrhea), gas, bloating, distended tummy, vomiting, and/or abdominal pain are recognized symptoms of this form of CD. However, this "classic mode of presentation has become less common, with diarrhea or a malabsorption syndrome as the mode of presentation in fewer than 50% of individuals."[5] In one study, the "classic mode of presentation" was 67 percent in children under the age of three, but atypical gastrointestinal issues and the silent form of CD were more common in older children.[6]

CD also could be rearing its ugly head if your child (or you) exhibits any of the following:

- Grumpy, clingy, or irritable behavior
- Pale face; dry or cracked lips
- Depression, lethargy, or unexplained fatigue
- Achy muscles and bones; low muscle tone
- Allergies, developmental issues
- Disinterest in eating (anorexia) but hungry all the time

My grandson had 10 or more of these symptoms, but his doctor didn't recommend testing until we asked.

Ignoring these symptoms in children may lead to growth/stature issues, delayed puberty, and a miserable, unhappy, and unhealthy childhood. If CD is allowed to reign undiagnosed, the potential exists for infertility and pregnancy problems; numerous neurological, endocrinological, and skin issues; autoimmune diseases; and cancers to rob you or your child of good health.

Atypical—In atypical CD, blood test and endoscopic biopsy results are positive but gastrointestinal symptoms are often not apparent. As a result, the disease may be suspected (and therefore, tests performed) only at "an advanced stage and advanced age."[7] In a Finnish study done by Dr. Anitta Vilppula and colleagues, "the prevalence of celiac disease was high in elderly people, but the symptoms were subtle."[8] Over the time it takes to finally reach a diagnosis (sometimes many years), patients may complain of one or more of the following *atypical* symptoms and maladies:

- Dermatitis herpetiformis or Duhring's disease (an itchy, blistery rash on both sides of the body: elbows, knees, feet, buttocks, or back), eczema, psoriasis, and many other skin issues.
- Delayed puberty, infertility (males and females), endometriosis, miscarriages, early birth, low birth weight, other pregnancy issues, birth defects, and learning disabilities.
- Dental enamel and discoloration problems, striations and malformed, skewed teeth, gum issues, mouth sores (aphthous stomatitis), and/or swollen tongue.
- Neurological and cerebral issues: depression, migraines, headaches, ADD and ADHD, ataxia (balance), neuropathy, schizophrenia, seizures, brain fog, irritability, and/or muscular issues.
- Osteopenia, osteoporosis, bone pain, connective tissue disorders, various types of anemia, and other blood diseases.
- Thyroid, adrenal, pituitary, heart, liver, eye, and other organ and endocrine issues.
- Allergies, asthma, chronic cough, and other lung ailments; fatigue, sinus issues, and feeling chronically sick.
- Weight gain, vitamin and mineral deficiencies, short stature, and on and on.

Believe me, this is the short list! Over 200 symptoms and maladies associated with gluten sensitivity appear in the appendix of Braly and Hoggan's book, *Dangerous Grains: Why Gluten Cereal Grains May Be Hazardous To Your Health.*[9] *Recognizing Celiac Disease* by Cleo Libonati lists more than 300.[10] Many sufferers may find many of their health problems improve or even disappear on a gluten-free diet.

Throughout this book you will find a diverse array of atypical CD manifestations, along with research to support either a causal link or strong association with gluten.

Silent—Silent or subclinical CD (CD not detected by the usual lab tests) was found to be the most prevalent form of the disease, though why this is the case is not known.[11] One study found CD to be "24–48 times more frequent in the siblings of celiac patients than in the general population,"[12] Such numbers further support the recommendation that at least first-degree relatives of CD patients also be screened. Individuals with the silent form of the disease have positive blood-test and endoscopy results (thus, flattened villi) but exhibit either no symptoms or symptoms that are barely noticeable. In other words, you can have full-blown celiac disease with *no apparent symptoms.* Or, as Dr. Peter Green reported, silent CD without diarrhea may appear as anemia, irritable bowel syndrome, malignancy, neurologic disorders, and/or osteoporosis.[13]

Latent/Potential—In latent celiac disease, patients with positive blood test results, even those with a normal gut (no villous atrophy) are at "increased risk of future CD." Such patients may also have "CD-like symptoms and a family history of CD."[14] Given the continued consumption of gluten, histologic (tissue) changes may occur and symptoms begin to develop over time. In other words, the *potential* to develop CD exists. Those at risk for latent or potential CD are family members of CD patients as well as individuals with other autoimmune diseases and those with Down's syndrome. To avoid long-term complications, it is vital to identify the atypical symptoms and signs of CD.[15] In this case, a GF lifestyle could be *preventive* medicine.

A study done in 2001 found "abdominal symptoms in the absence of mucosal abnormalities [damaged villi] are features of both irritable bowel syndrome (IBS) and latent/potential celiac disease (CD)."[16] Counting the intraepithelial lymphocytes in the tips of villi (white blood cells that go on the defensive in the presence of an antigen) helps identify individuals with latent or potential CD.[17] When test results are borderline, "villous tip analysis" is a good tool to recognize early CD.[18]

The title of a recent study conducted in Finland poses a thought-provoking query: *Latent coeliac disease or coeliac disease beyond villous atrophy?* The researchers conclude: "Gluten-induced mucosal deterioration [villous atrophy] may take years or even decades [to occur] in some individual cases."[19] In other words, gluten sensitivity is on a continuum. Latent or potential CD, seemingly non-existent, may be developing for years before it morphs into the full-blown version of the disease.

Non-Celiac Gluten Intolerance

Since CD was first recognized by modern medicine in the mid-1940s, doctors have focused on the "gold standard" of diagnosis, the endoscopic biopsy, to confirm the presence of the disease. The purpose of an endoscopy is to identify intestinal damage in the form of villous atrophy. However, a huge number of folks adversely affected by gluten have *no* intestinal damage. Not surprisingly, such individuals often show negative results on the transglutaminase (tTG) (the test most commonly given) and/or endomysial (EMA) antibody blood test, because these tests are designed to find evidence of intestinal damage.

When these patients learn from their doctors that they do not have celiac disease, little or no mention is made of non-celiac gluten intolerance (GI) and its potentially devastating health consequences. And, of course, without dietary changes their symptoms continue. Some are handed a prescription to treat the symptoms (but not the cause). Others are told to see a shrink to deal with their "bellyaching."

Many disorders that respond to a gluten-free diet do not qualify as celiac disease. For example, abdominal pain with symptoms much like irritable bowel syndrome, fatigue, "foggy mind," headaches, or tingling extremities are some of the more prevalent ailments associated with GI.[20] A recent study reported that differences between CD and GI "remain poorly defined,"[21] but some health care professionals are beginning to recognize that gluten sensitivity goes far beyond the classic definition of CD as villous atrophy (intestinal damage). As a wider view of gluten sensitivity is embraced by forward-thinking doctors, the need for a positive endoscopic biopsy to confirm the presence of CD may become obsolete. Eventually this *gold* standard may become the *old* standard, replaced by a broader, widely accepted group of diagnostic tools that can identify the full spectrum of gluten sensitivity. In the meantime, the antigliadin antibody (AGA: IgG and IgA) blood tests, as well as specialized stool tests, can be helpful in detecting GI in those for whom traditional diagnostic tools have failed.

Some broad-minded doctors already recognize the value of AGA testing and—if results are negative—may even suggest the cutting-edge stool test (see Chapter 17). Some alternative health care professionals simply recommend trying a gluten-free diet (GFD), though I would encourage you to get tested if at all possible. If it turns out you're not gluten-sensitive, you won't have to worry about it. If the results are positive, seeing them in black and white can be a strong incentive to adopt and stick to a GFD.

Results of recent research by Dr. Alessio Fasano and his team "have proven that gluten sensitivity [non-celiac gluten intolerance] is different from celiac disease at the molecular level and in the response it elicits from the immune system,"[22] but GI research is still in its infancy. Dr. Peter Green claims that "research into gluten sensitivity [non-celiac gluten intolerance] today is roughly where celiac disease [research] was 30 years ago."[23]

The first-ever non-celiac gluten intolerance conference was scheduled for 2012 in Iran. Unfortunately, it was cancelled due to unrest in the region, but it was a beginning nonetheless. As research findings reach many more doctors, the doors to diagnosis will open wider, but it's a slow process. It's hard to teach old dogs new tricks, especially when the old dogs aren't tossed any new bones.

Gluten sensitivity is a complicated subject; one that patients, researchers, and health care professionals will continue to learn about for years to come. Someday we may know how to diagnose this disorder with 100 percent accuracy and/or how to prevent it altogether. In the meantime, if you believe you or a loved one may be suffering from CD/GI, I strongly encourage you to educate yourself on the many facets of this complex condition.

Misdiagnosed from Coast to Coast 5

CELIAC DISEASE (CD)/NON-CELIAC gluten intolerance (GI), with its extensive list of symptoms and related maladies, has been misdiagnosed and underdiagnosed for far too long. Worse yet, folks in this misdiagnosed or underdiagnosed category are often "overdosed" as well, as they try to ameliorate their symptoms with one of the many prescription or over-the-counter pharmaceuticals advertised on TV. While some of these drugs provide temporary relief, few claim to get to the bottom of what ails us, and many have side effects that can be quite harmful. If this scenario rings true for you or someone you care about, read on.

I met Les in 2006 at the International Celiac Disease Symposium in New York City. His "classic" story—a testament to the pervasive lack of knowledge about gluten sensitivity—highlights the importance of early intervention. If a seemingly healthy child is not achieving normal developmental milestones like walking and talking, or if he or she is losing ground in these areas, it may be cause for concern. And if these issues are accompanied by intestinal problems (they aren't always), don't wait to talk with your doctor about the possibility of gluten sensitivity. (Also see *Aly's Story* in Chapter 2.)

There is so much gluten-related illness that one would think doctors should test for gluten sensitivity as part of a first response. To do so, of course, they need to know the numerous signs and symptoms of this disorder, along with which tests best track down the stealthy gliadin protein. After reading this book you'll be in a better position to discuss these issues with your health care professionals, especially if they're not up-to-date on the subject. Think of the billions of testing dollars expended in vain, the unnecessary prescriptions, and the time wasted in doctors' and hospital waiting rooms, precious hours lost from work and play. How many misdiagnoses does one have to have before a proper diagnosis is reached?

Misdiagnosed Time and Again, by Les Doti

In 1945 I developed a sickness that was diagnosed as celiac disease. Apparently I'd been a normal kid until the age of 18 months or so, at which time I developed a bad case of diarrhea. Everything I ate ran right through me. My mother said my abdomen was so distended I looked like one of those starving babies from regions of the world that suffer from famine. I was so weak I stopped walking. I stopped talking. I stopped growing. She took me to several doctors; none had a clue what was wrong. Finally one doctor diagnosed me with celiac sprue. "If he survives," he told my mom, "he will grow out of it." For a time after that, all I ate was bananas, nuts, and ketchup. I survived. Then, sometime between the ages of four and six, I distinctly remember my mother feeding me farina. I didn't like it, but it was shoveled down my throat. Although I had no choice, I also had no ill effects from it. Perhaps I'd "outgrown" my celiac disease as the doctor predicted.

Having nothing to compare it with, I thought I had a relatively normal youth, adolescence, and early adulthood. I know now my bowel habits were far from normal. I vacillated between relieving myself anywhere from several times a day to once or twice a week. By my late twenties or early thirties, I had begun to adjust my lifestyle to accommodate bouncing between constipation and diarrhea. In addition, I became very gassy; the odor was most unpleasant. I spoke to my doctor about these habits, but I had no recollection of what my mother had once told me about having celiac disease.

Over the course of the next 15 years I was diagnosed with nearly every large bowel disease in the book: irritable bowel syndrome (IBS), colitis, Crohn's disease, colon polyps, and infections. I had upper GIs, lower GIs, and rigid sigmoidoscopies (flexible endoscopes to check for damaged villi were not available at the time). After a given treatment things would settle down, but within a few weeks the symptoms always returned.

When I was about 45, I lost a great deal of weight in a single week. I also became quickly fatigued. My associates thought I'd developed cancer. When I saw a gastroenterologist, he scheduled a colonoscopy and an endoscopy the very next day. The evening before the procedures I had dinner with my mother. More accurately, she had dinner; I was not eating. When I told her about my scheduled tests she asked if the doctor knew I'd had celiac. "No," I replied. After all, it ***had*** been about 30 years since Mom had mentioned it. I'd completely forgotten.

She insisted I call the doctor and tell him—right then. Since in my family one always obeys one's mother, I excused myself and made the call. The nurse checked the doctor's records. His notes showed he suspected celiac!

It took about six months to get a grip on a strict GF lifestyle. Once I did, the results were miraculous within a week's time. I felt so good I dreaded having to eat out due to cross-contamination issues. After ingesting just a pinch of gluten, it would take me five to seven days to feel better.

Is the foundation of most of these debilitating intestinal maladies being laid by the nefarious gluten? CD is often difficult to distinguish from disorders with similar symptoms: chronic fatigue syndrome, Crohn's, depression, diverticulosis, intestinal infections, IBS, and ulcerative colitis.[1] Could some of these diseases also be influenced (or even caused) by gluten? No one knows for sure—at least not yet—but it's indisputable that many people, including some whose stories are detailed on these pages, experience significant improvement on a gluten-free diet.

"Most cases [of CD] remain currently undiagnosed in North America, mostly due to poor awareness of CD by primary care physicians."[2] In one study where the favored diagnosis was IBS, the majority of doctors never thought to reevaluate the case or consider CD. Given this approach, it's not difficult to understand why the average time to diagnose CD was *13 years.*[3]

Taking years—sometimes decades—to be diagnosed with gluten sensitivity "can result in significant immune and nutritional consequences, many of which are irreversible even after treatment with a gluten-free diet. Some of these disorders include loss of hormone secretion by glands (hypothyroidism, diabetes, pancreatic insufficiency, etc.), osteoporosis, short stature, cognitive impairment, and other inflammatory bowel, liver and skin diseases... Only with early diagnosis can these problems be prevented or reversed," according to Dr. Kenneth Fine.[4]

Remember, one does not outgrow CD/GI. If you are sensitive to gluten, it's for life!

6 Systemically Intrusive, Ever Elusive

A DISEASE IS defined as "systemic" when it affects anything from several organs or tissues to the entire body. Examples of diseases in this category include chronic fatigue syndrome, diabetes, Grave's, lupus, rheumatoid arthritis, and, of course, celiac disease (CD). One study found that "celiac disease is a common systemic disorder that can have multiple hematologic [blood-related] manifestations."[1] Cleo Libonati, in her well-documented, outlined reference, *Recognizing Celiac Disease*, lists numerous systems that may be affected by CD and associated conditions, including blood, body composition, cardiovascular, digestive, glandular, immune, integumentary, lymphatic, muscular, nervous, pulmonary, reproductive, sensory, skeletal, and urinary. A fetus also can be affected by a number of these conditions, sometimes as early as the zygote stage, and the disease can have an impact on the organs of both children and adults. Often more than one organ or part of the body is involved.[2]

It's not rocket science to understand that if someone is deficient in vitamins and minerals due to malabsorption caused by celiac disease, the body can be adversely affected in numerous ways on many different levels. A quick glance at one of the A-to-Z encyclopedias on chronic illnesses, with its accompanying lists of vitamins and minerals needed to keep the body healthy, makes it easy to realize how serious a depletion of these nutrients can be.

In addition to the malabsorption resulting from CD, immunological reactions to invading antigens (gluten, dairy, viruses, etc.) result in the production of antigliadin antibodies and other autoantibodies that may lead to major damage in the body. "The cytokines (and chemokines) produced by the T cells in the IgA [immune] reaction can travel to any part of the body to cause problems, and they usually attach themselves to an area that is already displaying some type of problem or weakness (tissue damage, infection, inflammation, mutated cells, etc.)."[3] Cutting-edge research by neurobiologist Dr. Aristo Vojdani asserts antibody tests can show organ damage "up to 10 years before the onset of disease"—in other words, before a major assault takes place and the disease manifests itself.[4] As a result, testing to see if an individual is exhibiting certain antibodies could literally provide a glimpse into the future, uncovering an illness that might have been brewing for years and possibly triggering a change in lifestyle and/or medical treatment that could significantly affect a patient's long-term well-being.

I watched impatiently for 10 minutes after seeing the waiter bring a gluten-free menu to a diner at a nearby table. Finally I drummed up the nerve to go over and introduce myself and my endeavor. Bridget, the woman who had requested the special menu, was thrilled to be able to share her long and arduous journey to health. She had suffered for more than 15 years with a multitude of ailments affecting many different bodily systems. After adopting a gluten-free/dairy-free diet, all of her symptoms miraculously cleared up. She now has her life back. Bridget's incredible story is an example of a trigger, a major traumatic event that may have brought on celiac disease—in other words, "the straw that broke the camel's back." Her plethora of symptoms and maladies speaks to the widespread lack of knowledge among far too many doctors about the travesties of gluten and dairy consumption and how these proteins can have a negative impact on the human body.

A Healing Journey, by Bridget Skjordahl

The Trigger—It is a perfect summer day in 1992, and suddenly I am wondering why my car is moving. The last thing I remember was being stopped at a traffic signal waiting for the light to change, and now my car is heading into oncoming traffic. I struggle to reach the brake and steer the car away from a collision, or, as it turns out, another collision. As I'll discover later, the reason I can't control the car is because the bolts holding the driver's seat to the floor have sheared off and I'm situated nearly in the backseat of my Mercedes sedan, out of reach of the steering wheel and pedals. The car finally comes to rest just as a woman runs up, shouting at me to get out if I can, that fuel has spilled all over and there's immediate danger of a fire. Conveniently, all this has happened directly in front of a fire station.

Eventually it becomes clear to me that while I was waiting for the light to change, an SUV traveling at high speed had rammed into the rear end of my car, pushing me into oncoming traffic. The SUV had finally come to a halt against a fence several hundred yards down the road; the driver never even applied the brakes. He must have been asleep at the wheel—literally, and perhaps figuratively as well.

After the accident, in addition to the expected neck and back injuries (and symptoms consistent with mild traumatic brain injury), I began to experience a number of puzzling symptoms, and ever since I've been on a roller coaster of diminishing and occasionally improving health. I've felt the frustration of being shamed and dismissed by a series of traditional medical professionals. I've been admonished to "just learn to live with it" and even told I was "crazy." The worst, of course, was being told the doctors could find nothing wrong, when I knew something was very, very wrong.

Perhaps even more troublesome were the diagnoses—often misdiagnoses—along with subsequent treatments for disorders and syndromes that were really symptoms, not underlying causes. I have been treated for fibromyalgia, chronic headaches and migraine, post-traumatic stress disorder, clinical depression, ADHD, Hashimoto's hypothyroidism, chronic bladder infections, severe PMS, adult acne, candida overgrowth, head injury, and irritable bowl syndrome. Many times I feared I was bipolar, schizophrenic, had an anxiety disorder, and/or was obsessive-compulsive.

For years I couldn't put a name to what was wrong with me, but I knew without question that whatever "it" was began on that sunny day in 1992 when my car was rammed by the SUV. Many others with whom I have spoken also believe their disease process was somehow triggered by a physically and/or emotionally traumatic event. Perhaps such an event serves as the "last straw," creating an imbalance severe enough to trigger a cascade of malfunctions that manifest themselves as disparate but intricately related symptoms. So often, it seems, the same "group" of diseases or diagnoses will turn up in some combination, i.e., fibromyalgia, chronic fatigue syndrome, hypothyroidism, adrenal burnout, candida, food and environmental sensitivities and allergies, sleep disorders, autoimmune diseases, emotional and behavioral disorders, malnutrition, autism, hormonal imbalances, signs of accelerated aging, etc.

My Cup Runneth Over—In 2005 I moved across country, then moved again in my new location. At the same time I changed careers and started a new business. Within the first six months of all these changes, it became increasingly difficult to summon the energy I needed to execute my business plans. I found myself breaking down in tears, unable to sleep at night, and thoroughly fatigued during the day. I had chronic bowel problems that were becoming more and more severe and had started to disrupt my business schedule and personal life. I felt a profoundly heightened level of anxiety and started to experience panic attacks.

Some days I felt absolutely catatonic, unable to think or do anything that wasn't absolutely urgent, at which point I would fall into habitual learned behavior just to get through the next interaction until I could be alone and just sit and stare, browse the Internet, or do other mindless busywork. Completing a load of laundry or bringing in the mail each day started to feel like a major accomplishment.

Life had again brought me to my knees. Out of sheer desperation I followed up on a suggestion I'd heard from three or four sources: I ordered the gluten sensitivity stool panel and milk protein sensitivity and genetic tests from EnteroLab. The results were positive for both gluten and dairy sensitivity. Immediately I started to rid my diet of all gluten and of all dairy products except butter. I would discover later that it was not milk sugar but the protein called casein that caused my reaction. About this time, I was also divinely guided to a physician who has the gift of looking at the whole picture and the wisdom to look for root causes rather than treat symptoms. Under the guidance of this physician, patients are encouraged to help heal themselves.

My Prayers Are Answered—After listening to my story, my new doctor was able to explain a disease process that had been in the works since my car collision over a decade earlier and which had resulted in a cascade of endocrine system failures: adrenal, thyroid, pituitary, and hormonal deficiencies (DHEA), damaged immunity, candida overgrowth, and concomitant nutritional deficiencies (severe B12 and iron deficiencies), all of which were either caused or made worse by food intolerances and possible environmental sensitivities. It all became a vicious cycle.

The analogy that resonates as truth for me is that our body/mind/spirit system can take only so much stress in any given period. In order to recover and be available to survive the next stressful event, our system requires periodic nourishment and rest. Suppose the stress on your body/mind/spirit could fit in a cup. How full is your cup? Some stressors are chronic, things like unaddressed food allergies, low-grade infections such as candida or gum disease, diseases like diabetes. Then there are prescription medications, junk foods, and pollution. What else fills our cups? Perhaps it's a workaholic, rush-aholic, over-schedule-yourself-within-an-inch-of-your-life-aholic lifestyle, and the subsequent sleep deprivation common to most Americans, not to mention the emotional gremlins we all travel with from time to time—unfulfilling relationships and jobs, guilt, and unreleased grief. Do you tend to be a perfectionist? Throw that in the cup, too.

If your cup is just under half full, everything might seem to be working well enough not to attract much attention on a day-to-day basis. However, if your cup is nearly half full and you're hit with a major life event or witness something traumatic, it can overflow in an instant and your health—either quickly or over time—can suffer significant negative consequences. Of course, not everyone's cup has the same capacity. For example, the pituitary damage I sustained in my car accident is likely the reason my cup now looks more like a demitasse than a coffee grande.

My doctor thought I had a severe case of adrenal burnout, or hypoadrenia. She referred me to an endocrinologist, who concurred and put me on a radical program involving strict nutritional guidelines and supplementation and drastic lifestyle changes. In other words, I started working to empty my "cup" of the toxins and stressors that were making me sick. Two of those toxins were gluten and casein.

After initiating a gluten-free, dairy-free diet I began to feel better, dramatically better, almost immediately, and it's been a process of trial and error and continual refinement ever since. As new information comes in, more and more less-obvious gluten is eliminated, and with each such elimination my health improves incrementally. For instance, I recently discovered the brand of rice milk I've been using for ages contains gluten. Once I switched to a different brand I started to see a dramatic improvement.

The list of symptoms that quickly diminished or disappeared altogether with a gluten-free/casein-free lifestyle includes anxiety, panic attacks, acne, itchy skin, bloating, gas, abdominal cramping and pain, bowel irregularity, exhausting and painful diarrhea, depression, diminished libido, lack of initiative, profound fatigue, iron and B-vitamin deficiencies not explained by food intake, hypothyroidism, hypoadrenia, hypoglycemia and the accompanying feelings of starvation and impending doom, inability to make decisions and analysis paralysis, irritability, fear-based thinking, bitterness, anger, hair loss, heartburn and acid reflux, premature/accelerated aging, brain fog, susceptibility to upper respiratory infections, frequent and severe nosebleeds, eczema flare-ups, ringing, itching and fluid discharge in my ears, sleep disturbances, overly emotional reactions to situations or events, sugar cravings, inability to respond to stress, self-loathing, social avoidance . . . the list goes on and on.

Despite the physical and emotional pain of my ailments and the search for their cause, the last few years have been an incredible journey of discovery, a journey that has awakened me physically, mentally, emotionally, and spiritually.

It has given me a strong determination to never slip into that dull, numb sleep of unawareness ever again. I have been blessed to find myself surrounded by caring, supportive, loving people and to have my healing facilitated by some of the finest, most divinely and genuinely gifted healers, coaches, and miracle workers in the state of Colorado, if not the world. It is due to these gifts and blessings that I again experience joy and see endless possibilities for myself and for the future. I know I will persevere, and my wish for you is a healing journey of your own toward your own vastly improved health.

B. B. J. is another courageous woman whose story illustrates the systemic damage undiagnosed gluten sensitivity can inflict on the human body. Before being diagnosed in 1981 she had endured celiac disease on many levels for decades: digestive, hematologic (blood), osteological (bone), cerebral/neurological, cardiac, endocrinological, autoimmune, and cancerous affecting many different organs and bodily systems. In the intervening years, she and her ever-smiling and supportive husband have continued to learn about celiac disease and the gluten-free lifestyle and to enthusiastically share their knowledge with others. When I met B. B. J. at a CD support meeting, she readily agreed to share her story. Her husband served as the e-mail go-between for capturing her tale.

From Night to Day, by B. B. J.

My symptoms ranged from fatigue, weight gain after pregnancy, iron deficiency anemia, and hypothyroidism (prescription meds had no effect), to aphthous ulcers (mouth sores), joint pain, weight loss, and depression, accompanied by odd mental behavior (I was flaky and vague about many things). My periods were irregular and at times included excessive bleeding, my hair was thinning, and my fingernails were tender and tore easily. Diarrhea was common for me, and I had clay-colored stools with a foul odor.

With my first child, I had preeclampsia [a serious complication of pregnancy]. I also experienced a number of issues with other pregnancies and births.

In 1974, I had a heart attack. A bone marrow test showed pernicious anemia, but the B12 shots prescribed for my condition were not working.

Over the years I was told my problems were the result of colitis or nerves. My doctor suggested I had a malabsorption problem, but he had no idea why. He just didn't know what was wrong. He gave me several series of Prednisone shots, which did relieve some of the symptoms; however, the basic problems remained. Clearly I was getting worse. At one point I became very ill and, because my doctor was out of town, I went to an endocrinologist. This specialist immediately admitted me to the hospital, where I continued to worsen. Finally, the doctor ordered an endoscopic biopsy to check my small intestine. "I don't think you have celiac disease," the gastroenterologist said, "but I'll do it anyway."

Voila! It *was* celiac. I finally had an answer and was discharged with a gluten-free diet. By this time, however, I looked and felt like a frail, little old lady. I was 49 years old.

At that time there was virtually no help available when choosing gluten-free food. Doctors knew nothing; nutritionists had no clue; and package labels weren't nearly as comprehensive as they are today. My husband and I were calling companies for lists of ingredients. Finally, Ener-G Foods started making gluten-free products. I thought I was doing well, but after I found a support group in Wayland, Maryland, I learned I was eating many things that were not gluten free. With more research and support groups, things finally got better.

I believe I've had celiac disease since I was a child, when I had pneumonia and jaundice of unknown origin. I also believe my pregnancies triggered the serious onslaught of CD complications. As an adult I've had heart problems, hypothyroidism, colon cancer, photosensitivity, Sjögren's syndrome, osteopenia, Asperger's, cholecystectomy (removal of the gallbladder), and a hysterectomy.

By the time I was finally diagnosed with CD, I weighed only 112 pounds and could barely function. My husband and I were both convinced I'd be dead within a short time. Today I'm in my mid-seventies and lead an active and healthy life. Adopting a gluten-free lifestyle has changed my life from night to day!

Both Bridget and B. B. J. were bombarded in just about every bodily system with multiple, degenerative, and life-threatening health issues, yet each has experienced extraordinary resilience and improvements in her health by following a gluten-free lifestyle. The devastating effects of CD are multiple and far-reaching and "can manifest as a disturbance of function of virtually any body system. A priori, there must be many other associations yet to be discovered."[5]

7 More than a "Gut Feeling"

THE GASTROINTESTINAL TRACK, which runs from the mouth to the anus, can play host to a variety of symptoms and disorders of which irritable bowel syndrome (IBS), colitis, Crohn's disease, intussusception, lactose intolerance, gastritis, constipation, and, of course, celiac disease (CD) are only a few. It is surprising how many of these conditions can be linked to gluten.

For three decades, Lisa, a holistic health nurse practitioner, suffered horrendously from many of the typical symptoms of celiac disease. After being diagnosed and adopting a gluten-free lifestyle, her health has improved dramatically, as has the health of her sister and other family members who also banned gluten from their diets. Lisa finally has her health back and, as a result of her experiences, is better able to recognize symptoms of gluten sensitivity in her patients, leading them to better health as well.

Finally, at Almost 40, by Lisa Vasile, Holistic Health NP

At the age of 38 I was diagnosed with celiac sprue. The one thing I've been asked, again and again, is, "Why did it take so long?"

For as long as I can remember I've struggled with bowel problems. For months I would have constipation, followed by days of diarrhea. In the constipation phase bowel movements became a difficult, dreaded task. During the diarrhea phase I'd become so sore from using the bathroom non-stop I'd often end up sitting on pillows.

One day when I was 16 and complaining to my mother, yet again, about a stomachache, she said, "You always have a stomachache! When is the last time you went to the bathroom?" I couldn't remember. As it turned out, it had been almost two weeks. I don't blame Mom for not noticing sooner. She was busy taking care of the whole family, and at 16 I wasn't exactly forthcoming about my bowel habits. That day, however, I certainly got her attention. A trip to the pediatrician yielded a referral to a gastroenterologist, who put me through a barium enema and an upper gastrointestinal tract exam. The results came back "normal." Basically, I was just weird, I was told; I'd just have to struggle with ways to make my bowels work (raisin bran, Metamucil, prunes, and other such remedies became my friends).

As I grew older, I got used to having IBS, though I'd get discouraged each time I watched my husband walk into the bathroom at the same time every day. I would be out somewhere (in a restaurant, at the beach, on a long drive) and have horrendous heartburn or gas pains; I lived my life on over-the-counter remedies, antacids, and on foods like high-fiber cereals and crackers. These "therapies" worked sporadically at best. Plus I was always tired, not just a "didn't-get-enough-sleep-last-night" kind of tired but a heavy, constant, overwhelming exhaustion that left me dragging and cloudy.

In the summer of 2006 my sister began to experience bloating that was so severe it affected her quality of life. Some days it was so bad she had trouble taking care of her five children. She sought evaluation from her primary care physician (PCP) and her gynecologist but got little support. She had her IUD removed, thinking it might be the cause, but noticed no improvement. She was told she had a one-centimeter ovarian cyst, yet as a nurse practitioner (NP) I knew a cyst this size would not affect her waistline. She complained about new, unexplained skin disorders and about exhaustion her medical providers blamed on having five children. She spoke about a racing heart doctors blamed on stress; they'd suggested counseling. Traditional medicine was offering no answers and even homeopathic remedies, which she'd used for some time as she sought a more holistic approach to health, provided no relief.

On a trip to Niagara Falls with her in September of 2006, I had the chance to witness the full extent of the problem. When I saw her abdomen swell to the point she looked six months pregnant, I really became concerned. Given my medical training, I was thinking the worst.

When we got back from our trip my sister returned to her PCP, but still she got nowhere. She decided to take her health (and, as it turned out, mine) into her own hands, researching every article and every website mentioning bloating until she came across a description of celiac disease. When she reviewed a list of some of the subtle, atypical symptoms, she realized she had 85 to 90 percent of them. She returned to the PCP's office and asked them to "appease" her by ordering celiac lab tests. She even cited research and told them the best blood test to run.

A week later she had an explanation for her bloating, rashes, headaches, and exhaustion: She had celiac sprue. Two weeks later one of her daughters was diagnosed. A month after that she found out—at the age of 35—she had osteopenia. Other than bloating, she fortunately had no gut/intestinal issues, but she had so many other complications of CD, including "soft" teeth, brittle nails, horrendous environmental allergies, and a long list of food allergies.

After just *two days* on a gluten-free diet (GFD), her bloating was significantly reduced. In less than *two weeks*, it was gone entirely and her heart had stopped racing. If left untreated long enough, one of the quirky things about celiac disease is that it causes the body to be in a hyperallergic state. So as my sister started to feel better than she had in years, she sought allergy testing to find out what else her body might be fighting. It turned out to be a fairly sizeable list of food allergies. While some people find this type of information to be frustrating, others discover that knowledge is power. My sister is happy to be armed with this "power" and to make the best food choices she can for her body. Does she feel deprived? No! If you know something will make you feel bad within minutes or hours of ingesting it, it's pretty easy to say "no thanks."

My sister's son had had horrible bowel explosions, starting at four months of age. At the age of two-and-a-half he was tested for celiac, but the tests were inconclusive. [Many times younger children will not have had enough time to develop the relevant antibodies and thus will not test properly.] Until he could be tested again when he was a little older, my sister was instructed to "just let him eat whatever he wants." However, from her own experience she knew what celiac symptoms could feel like. She also knew the damage the disorder could cause, so she put her son on a gluten-free diet (GFD) right away. The difference was so phenomenal she decided to have all her children tested for the celiac gene through EnteroLab. Four out of five were confirmed as positive; all are now thriving on a GFD.

As I helped my sister with research in learning to adjust her shopping, eating, skin care choices, etc., I began to realize I, too, had many symptoms of CD, including IBS, unexplained infertility, GERD (gastroesophageal reflux disease), headaches, exhaustion, rectal bleeding from hemorrhoids, and lifelong anemia.

As a nurse practitioner, perhaps I should have recognized the connection. But although CD was mentioned in our training, we were never taught just how common it really is. Medical providers are taught to listen to all areas of concern when a patient comes in with a problem, e.g., the onset of the issue, the location, how long it lasts, what makes it better or worse, how it's affecting their lives, and what treatments they have tried. After listening to the patient, we do a thorough examination to help guide us toward the top five things or "differential diagnoses" his or her problem might be. Believe me, CD never made it to the top five.

Once I began to understand how common CD actually was and how often it was misdiagnosed or underdiagnosed, I told my PCP I, too, wanted the lab test. One week later I had the results: celiac sprue.

Like my sister, I immediately changed my diet to be absolutely gluten free. Within a week I felt less tired and, wonder of wonders, I started to go to the bathroom every day! Some time later I realized my fatigue had also disappeared, along with the daily aches and pains I'd come to regard as almost normal. And I hadn't had a headache or heartburn in two months. My tTG went from 75 to 4 (normal is 0 to 19), and for the first time in my life I wasn't anemic. I even gained 10 pounds in three months. Since I wasn't trying to gain weight, this part concerned me a bit, but the doctor just shrugged. "It's because your gut damage is repairing, and you are now absorbing nutrients from food," she explained. And she was right; the weight gain stopped once my body adjusted to actually using the food I was eating.

Once my sister and I began to feel better, we started thinking about my mom's health. Mom had worn dentures since the age of 36, when she'd lost all her teeth. She'd also had lifelong IBS, and she occasionally battled with exhaustion and depression. Within the past five years she'd shrunk three inches. Initially she was confused as to why we wanted her to be tested for CD, but when we explained it was a genetic disorder, she agreed. She, too, tested positive and has felt much better since adopting a GFD; her IBS resolved itself and her tTG numbers are now within normal range.

Other family members who passed away before we knew the toll CD can take were not so lucky. Looking back, we're sure my grandmother had undiagnosed celiac which most probably contributed to her diabetes, osteopenia, depression, and heart disease. And my mother's brother was never seen without Tums in his hand. We'll never know for sure the cause of his obvious ongoing intestinal issues, or how much damage resulted from them. What we do know is that he died of duodenal cancer before he turned 59.

One of my daughters has both genes for celiac—one from me, one from my husband—and by the age of four she was beginning to exhibit some of the telltale symptoms: stature issues and tummy aches. However, she tested negative on the tTG blood test. Like my nephew's doctor, my daughter's physicians told me to "wait until her antibodies are positive before changing her diet so drastically" and that there was "no research to show if being on a GFD before a positive antibody [test result] really improves long-term health." My reaction was that of my sister. Why wait for a positive lab result when I could help my daughter feel better *now* and avoid continued damage? None of us chose to have an endoscopy; for us the proof was in the reversal of nasty symptoms and a lower tTG score.

My husband and I had our three children tested through EnteroLab; all were positive for antigliadin antibodies in the stool and, since January of 2008, all have been gluten free. These days, if my younger daughter has the tiniest amount of gluten she has a stomachache and often vomits (sometimes violently). Since being on a GFD she is growing, has finally gained weight, and has no more daily stomachaches or abnormal stools. My son used to have trouble "getting the poop out" but now has no problems. He has ADD, but we are hoping never to use meds. My older daughter also has ADD, but by combining a GFD with acupuncture we've been able to take her off Ritalin, and we've seen dramatic improvements in her ability to pay attention. She loves not having to take medication that made her feel "flat." She also grew four inches in a single year and has a great appetite.

There may be many in our extended family yet to be diagnosed, but there are also people who live their whole lives with ailments and never get a diagnosis, or never *want* a diagnosis due to the "restrictions" of a gluten-free diet.

One good thing that has come from my diagnosis is that my colleagues and I now recognize many of the symptoms of gluten sensitivity. In fact, since learning about the extent of this disorder, we have identified seven patients who tested positive for celiac disease. I also teach at a nurse practitioner master's program, and because of my diagnosis many more up-and-coming NPs (and faculty) have CD much more focused on their radar. With each subject we discuss, I incorporate celiac as a differential diagnosis and discuss how easy it would be to add a celiac panel to routine lab work.

Numerous gut issues associated with (or indirectly caused by) gluten resolve themselves when someone is on a GFD. Lisa and her sister were smart not to wait for their children to test positive on a blood test before initiating a GFD. Why wait until gluten sensitivity has progressed to the point the patient tests positive on a test that only recognizes full-blown CD?

Irritable Bowel Syndrome

Irritable Bowel Syndrome (IBS) is a chronic ailment that can cause bloating, constipation and/or diarrhea, fatigue, and pain, symptoms that can interfere greatly with quality of life in work and play. One study found the prevalence of IBS to be approximately 10 to 15 percent in the Western world, but more than 75 percent of sufferers may be undiagnosed.[1]

Another study showed an extraordinary improvement of intestinal symptoms in most patients diagnosed with CD once they began following a GFD. (Among those who don't respond to the diet, poor compliance is often the reason.) This same study suggested IBS was not the cause of the symptoms that responded so dramatically to the removal of gluten.[2] What was the cause? Under the circumstances, it certainly seems reasonable to assume it may have been gluten itself.

According to Dr. Joseph A. Murray and colleagues at the Mayo Clinic, patients later diagnosed with CD reported the symptoms listed below at some time before diagnosis.[3]

Common Gastrointestinal Symptoms of Celiac Disease

Symptom	Percentage of Patients Experiencing Symptom
Recurrent abdominal pain	79
Diarrhea at least monthly	75
Abdominal bloating	73
Urgency	64
Flatulence	61
Postprandial diarrhea (following a meal)	More than 50
Underweight (adults); failure to thrive (children)	50
Daily diarrhea—more than 50% had buoyant and malodorous stools (suggesting steatorrhea)	47
Nausea	42
Lactose intolerance	39
Constipation	38.6
Fecal incontinence	38
Tenesmus (straining; feeling need to pass stools)	31
Vomiting	20
Bloody diarrhea	12

Of course, someone may have no symptoms and still have CD, but if you or a loved one has one or more of the symptoms listed in the table above, it would behoove you to get screened.

A recent Italian study found IBS to be more than five times as common in those with CD than in the controls.[4] Another study found IBS was often diagnosed when CD was the real problem; this research suggested CD should be "considered in the differential diagnosis of IBS," especially when IBS is resistant to treatment,[5] and also considered when a patient experiences "persistent IBS-like symptoms after an episode of infectious gastroenteritis."[6] Still another study suggested that "gluten can induce symptoms similar to FBD [functional bowel disorder—pertaining to IBS]," even when villous atrophy is not fully established.[7]

Could IBS be a catch-all phrase for a group of symptoms with no known cause? Some websites and informational material on IBS suggest there is no cure for this condition. However, there is much supportive research to suggest gluten may be a causative factor in IBS patients. For more information, see the research on small intestinal bacterial overgrowth in Chapter 13.

Bev is a good friend of my sister. When we met recently at a party, I hadn't seen her for decades, but it turned out we had a lot in common—gluten sensitivity—and a lot to chat about. Since adopting a GFD, Bev's IBS is a thing of the past, and she related a story about a man who suffered from diverticulitis and was slated for surgery. A week before he was to have been admitted to the hospital, he discovered he was gluten sensitive, adopted a gluten-free diet, and experienced a miraculous recovery. The surgery was never needed.

Miraculous Results, by Bev Olean

Over 40 years ago I began to have gastrointestinal problems—diarrhea, abdominal pain, and heartburn. I was only 20 years old and thought my medical issues would go away. They never did.

Twenty years ago my mother was diagnosed with colon cancer. Her doctor suggested I start having colonoscopies to catch any abnormalities at the earliest possible stage, so I saw a gastroenterologist. When I told this specialist about my digestive problems, he diagnosed me with IBS (also known as spastic colon) and suggested I take Metamucil every day. No nutritional information was ever mentioned.

As the years passed, I went to two other gastroenterologists; both said to continue with the Metamucil. I had colonoscopies every third or fourth year and twice had polyps removed, but nothing else was ever found.

Then one day my son and I compared notes. He'd been doing a lot of research on intestinal disorders, and some of the articles he'd read linked the symptoms I was experiencing to gluten. "Why don't you try a gluten-free diet to see if it helps your IBS?" he suggested.

Having nothing to lose, I decided to give it a try. The results were miraculous. Within a short time I had no symptoms at all. I felt like a new person. As I write this it's been four and a half years, and I continue to be symptom free. No doctors were involved in my diagnosis thanks to my son's research.

I continue to see a gastroenterologist, but he only wants to prescribe medication. When I told him I had become gluten free he asked how that was working for me. "Good!" he answered when I explained the astounding results. "See you next year."

Inflammatory Bowel Diseases

Inflammatory bowel diseases (IBDs) affect the colon and small intestine and include ulcerative colitis and Crohn's disease. They are autoimmune in nature and can take a huge toll on one's health and quality of life. Interestingly, one study found IBD was 10 times more prevalent among patients in the study with CD than among those in the control group.[8]

Ulcerative Colitis—A 25-year-old study revealed a greatly increased risk of developing celiac disease and ulcerative colitis among siblings of those with CD; other family members also had a higher chance of developing these two disorders.[9] A recent study by Dr. Peter H. Green and colleagues found that CD patients had "a 70-fold increased risk" of developing microscopic colitis.[10] A recent German study found ulcerative colitis is similar genetically to other autoimmune diseases such as celiac, Graves', psoriatic arthritis, rheumatoid arthritis, and type 1 diabetes.[11] There is scant research going back to the mid-1980s suggesting a gluten connection to colitis but, still, don't you wonder why you or your doctors haven't heard more about this?

Due to a high prevalence of CD in patients with lymphocytic and collagenous colitis, it's important to screen these patients early for CD.[12] Another study proposed that "collagenous enterocolitis represented a diffuse manifestation of gluten sensitivity."[13] As early as two decades ago, a study suggested gluten may be an antigen causing colonic lymphocytosis.[14]

Crohn's Disease—A recent study from Great Britain found that participants with celiac and Crohn's disease had a similar genetic background, which made them susceptible to other, related ailments.[15] In another study, celiac disease was found to be quite common in patients with Crohn's disease, nearly 26 percent.[16]

As one report stated, "The diarrhea stopped only after maintaining a gluten-free diet." Crohn's usually develops after celiac disease has been diagnosed, but in this case latent CD was identified years after Crohn's was diagnosed.[17] If the patient had been given the antigliadin antibody test years earlier, one can't help but wonder if CD would have been diagnosed that much sooner.

Another study revealed there is "a significant correlation between anti-tissue transglutaminase and Crohn's disease…" and that tissue transglutaminase (tTG) levels reflect the degree of disease.[18] How interesting that the tTG is also one of the antibody tests used to detect celiac disease.

As a case in point, a young woman named Maggie was diagnosed with Crohn's disease at age 16. Her doctor wanted her to lead as much of a "normal" life as she could, so he prescribed meds and told her she could eat what she wanted. Two years later she had a bowel resection. Following the surgery she was still on meds and had no food restrictions. She also was still having symptoms of Crohn's, with diarrhea nearly every day. Needless to say, she didn't feel well.

One day her mom was chatting with a pharmacist who had a naturopathic background and happened to ask if he had any ideas that might help her daughter. He suggested Maggie adopt a gluten-free, dairy-free diet. Maggie opted not to go dairy free, but within a few days of getting the gluten out she felt much better and her diarrhea had disappeared.

Lactose Intolerance

My mother lived quite well to age 80; she died at age 82 before I had ever heard of gluten. Looking back, I expect she was gluten sensitive; she had a perennial weight problem, had had her thyroid removed, suffered from high blood pressure and heart issues, and had an enormous amount of gas. This abundant flatulence, often associated with lactose intolerance, cleared up for me and for one of my grandchildren within a few days after we began a GFD.

A 2008 study found lactose intolerance was "due to genetic expression or mucosal injury," resulting in a low level of lactase that leads to lactose or dairy intolerance, and that 10 to 15 percent of northern Europeans endure it.[19] Symptoms can include abdominal pain, bloating, diarrhea, and/or mega flatulence. Another recent study reported about "70% of the world population" has a low level of the lactase enzyme.[20] It's interesting to ponder to what degree this condition may be the result of damaged villi. A deficiency in lactase can be the sole sign of CD. Due to the high number of CD patients who test positive on an H2-lactose breath test, testing for CD is now recommended for "all patients with a positive H2-breath test" prior to starting a dairy-free diet.[21] Likewise, a "lactose breath test should always be included in the diagnostic work-up" for IBS.[22] The evidence that IBS and gluten are often connected is overwhelming, yet many lactose-intolerant patients are being diagnosed with IBS without first testing to see if, in fact, they may be gluten sensitive. Is this a multi-ring circus—gluten causes damaged villi, which leads to low levels of lactase, which leads to poor absorption of dairy, which leads to intestinal symptoms, which results in a diagnosis of IBS?

Since lactase, the enzyme needed to break down the lactose in milk, is produced in the tips of the villi, it stands to reason that someone with lactose intolerance might very well have flattened villi and thus, celiac disease. Yet a recent TV program that addressed lactose intolerance made not a single mention of gluten or of the fact that if an individual has CD, he or she may not be able to produce the lactase enzyme.

Gastritis

Gastritis, an inflammation of the stomach lining, can cause pain or discomfort in the upper abdomen, as well as nausea and/or vomiting. Symptoms can be chronic or acute.

A number of studies have identified gluten as one cause of gastritis. In a study of children with CD, about half had lymphocytic gastritis that disappeared after being on a GFD.[23] In another study, a patient with collagenous gastritis became symptom-free on a GFD and showed some improvement in pathology findings after only three months.[24] "There is a high prevalence of lymphocytic gastritis in untreated celiac disease associated with elevated gastric permeability."[25]

Since so much research is being done on CD and the numerous ailments it is causing in children and adults, you may wonder why testing for gluten sensitivity isn't at the top of the heap of diagnostic options. I believe one reason is that many doctors still consider CD a rare disorder with classic intestinal symptoms that affects mainly children. There is a lot happening among grassroots support groups and through websites and books to dispel that image among potential sufferers, but who is educating our doctors? Even in the field of gastroenterology, let alone across multiple disciplines of medicine, there hasn't exactly been a groundswell of conferences for physicians and other healthcare professionals on this topic.

Malabsorption caused by CD can have disastrous consequences if not recognized and treated, so if your child is exhibiting any of the symptoms

reported in the next two stories, please pay attention to them. Fortunately, Bryanne's health turned around with the help of dedicated parents and a gluten-free lifestyle.

Saving Bryanne, by Bonnie Zonghi

My life was almost perfect. That's how it seemed after the birth of my second child. The actual delivery was a nightmare, but Bryanne was well worth the misery. The nurses all told us she was the prettiest baby they'd had in the ward in a long time. I was married to a loving and devoted family man who also happened to be my best friend. We'd been together for 11 years, married for the previous five. Our two-year-old son was sweet and wonderful, with no signs as yet of the inevitable, terrible twos, and he welcomed his new sister into the family with open arms.

Unfortunately, our idyllic existence soon began to deteriorate. For one thing, Bryanne didn't sleep through the night. Even after months she'd be up for hours at a time, sometimes two or three times in a single night. We were changing diapers up to seven times a night and were completely sleep deprived. At first we were told we'd been spoiled by our first child—that not all babies sleep through the night. Then, when visiting the doctor for one of Bryanne's regular checkups, I was told my eight-month-old was "stubborn," that she had a different disposition than her even-tempered brother. The wiggling from side to side while she rubbed at her belly was "behavioral," a sign of her discontent. She wasn't in pain, the doctor told me; she just didn't want to sit in her high chair or be buckled into her car seat.

One Mother's Day morning, my husband brought the kids to his parents' house for a visit. The baby became so distressed in her car seat that he raced her to the emergency room, sure she was struggling to breathe. The ER doctor examined her and took X-rays, but found nothing.

As time passed, I was beginning to really worry about my daughter's behavior. *Was* something wrong? My fear was growing, yet I often found myself defending the physician's point of view. I wanted to believe Bryanne was all right, that nothing was physically wrong with her.

One afternoon I took her to the doctor for a sick visit for some usual childhood malady. Her primary physician wasn't in that day, so another doctor examined her. As part of the exam, the doctor put a stethoscope on Bryanne's stomach. She never told me what she was listening for and she sent us home without a word, but I could tell by the look on her face she was concerned. I had a sinking feeling in my gut.

At some point during the next few months, Bryanne stopped growing, even though she ate like a horse. She learned to stand and walk, but everything seemed to take more effort than she wanted to expend. Often she would stand for 15 minutes before sitting down again without taking a step. I loved taking videotapes of the children playing, but when I played them back what I saw was my four-year-old son running circles, literally, around his baby sister. He'd be talking non-stop and she would smile and watch him go.

It wasn't until Bryanne's 15-month checkup that her pediatrician became alarmed. By this point, my beautiful child had skin the color of milk and a belly distended like that of a starving baby. It had been three months since her last routine visit, and the difference in her appearance was dramatic. The doctor examined the baby's abdomen and told me she was concerned about a possible tumor. She set up an emergency ultrasound for later that day. My husband met us at the hospital, where the sonographer found an intermittent intussusception in Bryanne's small intestine. In other words, one part of her intestine was slipping in and out of another part, and the problem couldn't be corrected unless the two parts got "stuck." When and if this happened, doctors would have 24 hours to operate or Bryanne would die. We were told to take our child home and watch for symptoms indicating she needed emergency surgery. I've experienced a number of frightening moments in my life, but this was the worst.

Within a few days, we were sent to Children's Hospital to try to find the reason for the intussusception. Bryanne was given a barium swallow and multiple X-rays, but the doctors could find nothing out of the ordinary, not even the intussusception. Apparently, the protruding part had slipped out again. In a moment of irony, we were grateful to have the first ultrasound report as proof the condition existed at all. The radiologist said he was at a loss for what could be causing the weakness in Bryanne's bowel. The only thing he could think of was a rare condition he'd recently seen a segment about on TV called celiac disease. It was the first time we'd ever heard these words.

We were referred to a specialist who took one look at our daughter and told us she had all the classic symptoms of CD: milk-white skin, distended belly, wasted buttocks and, believe it or not, very long eyelashes. An endoscopic biopsy confirmed the CD diagnosis. We must have looked devastated, but he assured us that if our child had to have a disease, this is the one we would want her to have.

Finally we had a name for what was wrong with her and, more important, a treatment: A gluten-free diet would make her better. Bryanne would have to follow this diet to save her life, and for the rest of her life. We took our daughter home to begin this new chapter in our lives.

In the years since that time we've had plenty of ups and downs, but being absolute with the gluten-free diet has always been worth it. Within three days of removing gluten from Bryanne's diet, we saw an overall improvement in her health and disposition. The pain went away and she began running after her brother. She started laughing all the time and her vocabulary tripled in two weeks. The transformation was so gratifying it made the work involved in becoming familiar with the GFD almost inconsequential. And the intussusception never came back.

As I write this Bryanne is 10 years old, an enthusiastic figure skater and basketball player with a first-degree brown belt in karate. She's a bright and beautiful little girl and, most importantly, she's healthy.

Intussusception

Intussusception is a condition of the intestine where one part of the bowel slips into another, similar to the manner in which the extending components of a telescope slip into one another. A number of studies point to an association between this condition and CD. The combination of failure to thrive (a common symptom of classic CD in children) with cramping stomach pain should be a red flag to investigate for CD and intussusception.[26] When celiac disease was discovered in a three-year-old child who was failing to thrive and the child was placed on a GFD, her intussusception issue completely healed.[27]

One study concluded that "the finding of transient small bowel intussusception . . . should prompt investigation of celiac disease." The three children with intussusception in this study also healed after being placed on a GFD.[28] In adults this all-too-common disorder is often linked to both CD and Crohn's disease.[29]

Is your child unhappy, tired, or cranky—colicky comes to mind for babies? Does he have constipation, diarrhea, anal fissures, or vomiting? Is her appetite waning? Or perhaps she's hungry all the time or doesn't feel like eating much at the dinner table? Are his nails brittle or is his hair drab and flat? Madi's mom noticed her daughter's teeth were *gray*! These are a few more of the many manifestations of CD.

Madi's Turnaround, by Heather Carneiro

My daughter, Madison, was diagnosed with celiac disease in November 2004 at the age of two and half, but she'd started showing signs of the disorder when she was only 12 months old. Up until her first birthday she'd been a fantastic eater, eating everything I gave her and often wanting more. But about the time she turned one her good eating habits started to fade, making every meal a frustrating battle that left us all exhausted. She started to get thinner, losing all her baby fat except for her belly. She became so constipated she developed anal fishers. "Put more fiber in her diet," advised her pediatrician, "and use natural laxatives." When I did what he suggested, Madi's system went from one extreme to another; she had diarrhea for two solid weeks. She also started throwing up at least once a week. Her toenails were so brittle they would break off, and her teeth were gray.

"She must have a virus," the doctor said when I took her back. "It just needs to run its course." Weight loss, brittle toenails, vomiting, diarrhea, loss of appetite, and gray teeth all due to a virus? This seemed too much. I told the doctor I wasn't going to wait any longer and asked for a referral to a gastroenterologist. The doctor looked at me strangely but went along with my request.

The gastroenterologist came highly recommended, and Madison and I waited patiently for over an hour, only to get a 10-minute consultation. After taking a quick look at Madi the doctor immediately diagnosed her with CD. The look on my face must have said it all; I had no idea what he was talking about. He quickly explained the basics of the disease and scheduled Madi for an endoscopy. The results confirmed the doctor's suspicions: Madison's small intestine had been damaged. We needed to eliminate all dairy products and put her on a GFD right away.

I signed up for every support group I could find and was eventually introduced to a wonderful woman who'd been gluten free for years and who had extensive knowledge of what to do and where to shop to make life easier. She stopped by my workplace to drop off two bags filled with gluten-free flours, cake mixes, and snacks for children. For the first time since Madi's diagnosis, I felt I wasn't alone.

Madi's intestinal problems cleared up within a year, and she became a happier child. Her teeth were no longer gray, her fatigue disappeared, and she experienced a huge growth spurt. Since that time our family has banded together to protect Madi from unsafe food. She's going to be all right!

From the time of Madi's diagnosis she followed a strict GFD. Then, at the age of eight, she developed type 1 diabetes. CD and type 1 diabetes are intimately related, as are many other autoimmune diseases, and the mechanisms for their pathology are not fully understood. For more information on type 1 diabetes, CD, and autoimmune disease, see Chapter 10.

Constipation

Constipation should not be a part of anyone's daily routine; yet, if you or your child is constipated it could be caused by gluten sensitivity. You can even have normal stools and have CD.

A 2011 study of 41 different populations found the "pooled prevalence of CIC [chronic idiopathic constipation] was 14 percent" and revealed a significant link between CIC and IBS.[30] Another recent study from the Netherlands found a strong association between the early introduction of gluten and cow's milk allergy and constipation in young children.[31] Since gluten sensitivity and an intolerance of casein, the protein in dairy, often go hand in hand, be sure to read Chapter 21 for more information on dairy intolerance.

Most doctors have much to learn about the particulars of celiac disease and non-celiac gluten intolerance (CD/GI), including how to recognize the symptoms and how to test for these disorders. I have many friends and acquaintances with medical conditions potentially resulting from gluten sensitivity, yet their doctors either haven't offered to test for CD/GI or haven't offered *enough* testing—not because they're insensitive or unwilling but because they simply don't know how. As an example, I recently ran into a woman who has had IBS for 65 years, ever since she was seven years old. Due to her condition, her activities have been curtailed throughout her life, and she's had *every test* there is. She recently saw a gastroenterologist from a prestigious hospital who definitely should have known more about the IBS/CD link and the newly expanded view of CD, but he didn't. I expect this woman is one of millions with similar complaints.

If you or a loved one has any of the symptoms mentioned in this book and your doctor has never suggested testing for gluten sensitivity, requesting the appropriate tests is a good first step for both you *and* your doctor. The more medical professionals learn about this disorder—from their patients if need be—the more quickly they'll be able to recognize its diverse symptoms. Chapters 16 and 17 provide information on the latest testing options, including stool testing for those whose blood test results are negative but who are still plagued by various unresolved ailments. Insurance may cover most of these tests but even if you have to pay for some of them out-of-pocket, it may be the best money you've ever spent. It certainly was for me and my family.

8 Typically "Atypical" Symptoms

A 2008 STUDY reveals that "up to 85% of patients with histologically proven coeliac disease have no gastrointestinal symptoms."[1] Thus, the picture of celiac disease (CD) is changing rapidly from a smaller percentage of classic gastrointestinal symptoms to a barn filled with *atypical* (not intestinally related) ailments including, it seems, just about everything else. I've had friends say, "Anne, you think everything is caused by gluten." If I even suggest some symptom or disorder they are suffering from is associated with gluten—even when my suggestions are supported by major research—they quickly chop me off at the knees. Of course, not all ailments are caused by gluten, but a huge number disappear or get much better when gluten is removed from the diet. By the time you finish this book, you just might agree with that statement. Below are some of the more typical atypical symptoms of gluten sensitivity.

Anemia

The most common atypical symptom found in adult CD patients is iron deficiency anemia (IDA). **One study found that 66 percent of CD patients had anemia and that, for some patients, anemia was their only symptom.** The conclusions of the study stressed the importance of CD screening for patients who have gastrointestinal symptoms or IDA for no apparent reason.[2] Anemia may result from the malabsorption of vital nutrients—"iron, folic acid, and/or vitamin B12."[3] In fact, another study found anemia to be linked to "folic acid deficiency rather than iron deficiency,"[4] and that after adopting a gluten-free (GF) lifestyle, it can take between six and twelve months for the intestine to heal enough to return to normal absorption.[5]

Fatigue and weakness are the most common signs of anemia. If you've been diagnosed with IDA, you may want to do additional research on the Internet or at your public library to explore this condition.

Seth is married to a longtime high school buddy of mine. When I learned of his health issues I immediately sent some testing information to him. After testing negative on the tissue transglutaminase (tTG)—the one blood test he was offered—he decided to try progressive stool testing. His positive results and the gluten-free diet (GFD) he adopted thereafter brought tremendous relief to this retired hospital executive who'd been ill for decades. His story screams of the lack of knowledge about gluten sensitivity, the numerous ailments connected to it, the inadequate testing protocols, and the enormous waste of time and money spent on mega testing that often resolves nothing.

A Celiac Disease Case History, by Seth Ames

At the suggestion of my hematologist and primary care physician, I presented myself in the office of a Portsmouth, New Hampshire gastroenterologist. At the time I was 69 years old and outlined the following symptoms and lab findings:

1. Periodic micro and macro anemia
2. Past IgG spikes [IgG spikes indicate antibody immune response]
3. Periodic IgG-mediated anemia indications
4. Chronic gas and abdominal bloating
5. Dull pain on the right side of my abdomen
6. Ringing in my ears
7. Chronic steatorrhea (floating stools, oily slick on surface of water, foul odor, pale tan in color, and with an appearance of undigested food in stools)
8. Neuropathy in my feet and legs and loss of feeling and temperature sense in my hands and feet (also: extreme burning-foot syndrome)
9. Frequent muscle cramps
10. Chronic, unexplained joint pain in my knees and back
11. Flushing of skin around my head, face, and shoulders
12. Dry skin (with peeling on my hands predictably every six to eight weeks)
13. Chronic body temperature regulation malfunction (worse in hot weather or with exercise)
14. A feeling of internal chilling (with shivering) at night
15. A catarrh (buildup of mucus), with constant gulping and clearing of my throat

16. Elevated blood platelets (thrombocytosis) that was 100 percent responsive to Prednisone, and moderate splenomegaly (abnormal enlargement of the spleen)
17. Significant memory problems (investigated by psychologists in Boston—no known cause)
18. The need to sleep 12 hours a night
19. Low total cholesterol (130 to 140 range)
20. Chronic fatigue and weakness (in the form of a "very deep fog")

The physician was sympathetic, but he didn't feel justified in ordering an intestinal endoscopic biopsy since my tTG blood test came back negative.

I then enlisted the services of a computerized symptom-review organization. The report indicated malabsorption problems with thyroid involvement and also mentioned I might have essential thrombocythemia (a high number of blood platelets, another name for thrombocytosis) in addition to other potential disorders. Five prominent medical centers stamped their approval on the essential thrombocythemia diagnosis, and one treated me with oral chemo for six years.

A friend then referred me to EnteroLab in Texas, run by Dr. Kenneth Fine, a research-oriented, board-certified gastroenterologist. Dr. Fine's lab specializes in assisting with the diagnosis of malabsorption conditions, and many professionals hail his methods as being more effective than the more traditional blood-test-and-biopsy approach in diagnosing celiac disease.

I submitted both gene swab and stool samples for analysis. The results showed I have two DQ3 genes. While DQ2 and DQ8 genes are markers for CD, DQ3 genes are "copy marker genes" for gluten intolerance. The stool analysis indicated major malabsorption issues, with the IgA for gliadin being positive, yet both the tTG blood and the tTG stool test were *negative*.

I immediately started a gluten- and lactose-free diet. The results were swift and dramatic. My steatorrhea and gas problems cleared up within three days. The chronic fatigue and fog improved by 75 percent. The peeling skin on my hands was healing.

Over the past 30 years I've been seen and tested by 37 physicians, including 9 specialists, and I've expended $175,000 to determine the cause of my ailments, $150,000 from insurance companies and an estimated $25,000 out-of-pocket. In addition:

- The failure to diagnose my gluten intolerance resulted in early retirement, costing me thousands of dollars in lost income.
- I was refused long-term care insurance.

- I spent countless hours in clinics, waiting rooms, and labs in four different states.
- I went through three painful bone marrow exams, numerous X-rays, and hundreds of blood tests.

It has been a long and costly diagnostic journey.

Think about it. Are some of these symptoms plaguing you as well? If you are suffering from gluten sensitivity, early detection is key to preventing serious health issues and the related financial, professional, and social hardships that may accompany them.

I often hear people say, "Anemia runs in my family." Precisely! So does celiac disease, and many forms of anemia are connected to chronic diseases, including CD. (For a lengthy list of anemia types you won't believe, search http://www.wrongdiagnosis.com.)

Of course, for those with both conditions, the perennial question remains, "Which came first, the chronic disease or the gluten sensitivity that caused anemia and other nutrient deficiencies and led to the chronic disease?" What is the instigator? Please don't tell me it is old age! I am much healthier now than before going gluten free, and I'm *certainly* much healthier than I was 30 years ago.

Here are some significant examples of research indicating a link between various types of anemia and gluten:

- **Aplastic anemia (AA)**—This study, one of the first to link aplastic anemia to CD—warns doctors to be on the lookout for fatigue and malaise, signs of CD often observed in AA patients.[6]
- **β-thalassemia major**—This study suggests CD might be a potential issue among those with this disorder. Screening is recommended.[7]
- **Chronic heart failure**—A new study has discovered that "anemia is associated with an increased risk of mortality and rate of hospitalization for heart failure."[8] More information on potential connections between heart issues and gluten can be found in Chapter 14. This is an area of much-needed research.
- **Idiopathic pulmonary hemosiderosis (IPH)**—There is a strong association between IPH, a serious lung condition, and CD. Screening for CD in IPH patients is highly encouraged.[9] For more on this topic, see *Lung Problems* in Chapter 14.
- **Hemolytic anemia**—A study of an 11-year-old girl with a severe

case of hemolytic anemia demonstrated a causal link to gluten when her anemic condition disappeared after she adopted a GF lifestyle. Thus, patients with "Combs negative 'immune' hemolytic anemia" may also want to be screened for CD.[10]

- **H. pylori**—In patients with CD, one study found an important association between H. pylori and iron deficiency anemia.[11]
- **Hypochromic anemia (paler red blood cells)**—An important finding of this study was that hypochromic anemia may be the only symptom of CD.[12]
- **Microcytic hypochromic anemia and dimorphic anemia**—In a study of children with CD, these two types of anemia were found in 80 percent and 20 percent of participants, respectively. After following a GFD, only "19% had microcytic anemia and in 81% the hematological picture" returned to normal size and color.[13]
- **Neurodevelopment**—Iron deficiency causing "central nervous system alterations and deficits in behavioral functioning," in spite of iron supplementation, may negatively affect infants.[14]
- **Refractory IDA**—IDA, which is difficult to treat, may result from CD and H. pylori gastritis, a chronic inflammation of the stomach lining. For patients suffering from refractory IDA, supplementing an iron-rich GF diet with iron and folic acid, along with treating the H. pylori infection, will "optimize their mental and psychological functions."[15]
- **Type 1 diabetes**—It is vital to screen for CD in patients who do not respond to treatment for IDA, especially those with type 1 diabetes.[16]

Even after following a GFD and supplementing it with iron, the iron-deficient condition may continue for a time, so early screening for CD and following a GFD is important.[17] In one study, a link was found between "abnormal intestinal changes and low ferritin levels" in CD patients; both conditions showed improvement when patients adopted a GFD. This study, dating from 1982, went so far as to suggest intestinal biopsies to diagnose CD could be eliminated by assessing ferritin levels and white blood cell migration.[18]

If you have anemia or borderline anemia, your health is already compromised. Has your doctor shown any interest in what could be *causing* your condition, or is he or she prescribing giant iron pills that may not be absorbed if you are gluten sensitive? (By the way, do not take iron pills on your own without checking with your doctor; too much iron can be toxic.) If you do have anemia, you just might be able to do something about it. By getting screened for CD, you could be doing your body, your mind, and your future health a big favor.

Thrombocytosis

In one study 60 percent of the participants who'd been diagnosed with CD also had thrombocytosis, a high platelet level. Following a GFD led to a speedy recovery of the thrombocytosis in nearly all patients (the numbers shrank to less than 3 percent) "as well as [improvement in] most of the nutritional and hematological parameters."[19] "Extreme thrombocytosis and severe anaemia—considered in an elderly patient to be typical of myeloproliferative disorders [bone marrow disorders such as leukemia][20] or neoplastic conditions [conditions related to abnormal new growth of tissue][21] can be due to celiac disease."[22] Thrombocytosis reflects an advanced stage of CD and "may indicate a major risk of associated autoimmune disease."[23] With results like these, doesn't it make sense that patients diagnosed with thrombocytosis should be screened for CD?

As far back as 1976 a study revealed that **over half of the CD patients had "peripheral blood thrombocytosis"** and suggested that CD and inflammatory bowel disease should be taken into account in the "differential diagnosis of thrombocytosis" and that blood platelet levels may be helpful in identifying CD patients.[24] Other blood disorders that may occur in connection with CD include hyposplenism, IgA deficiency, leukcopenia, thrombocytopenia (low blood platelets—see Chapter 10), and venous thromboembolism.[25] Is there a common theme here? Could gluten be the *root cause* of these blood disorders? So far, the experts don't know, but it is obvious much more research is warranted.

Osteoporosis

Osteoporosis can be assaulting your body for years without you knowing it. You can't feel it happening and then, all of a sudden, you have it. Your bones have become frail and sponge-like, ripe for fractures. The boss of a friend of mine was having terrible pain in her feet. It turned out she was suffering from stress fractures caused by using a treadmill. She wound up testing positive for CD, is now on a GFD, and her pain has disappeared.

If you've been diagnosed with osteoporosis, osteopenia, osteomalacia, bone pain, or too many broken bones, has your doctor suggested testing for

CD? Most people think of osteoporosis or related disorders as old people's diseases, but if someone is malabsorbing due to CD, bone disease can develop at any age, even in the very young. The story below is a great example of osteoporosis *not* due to aging.

Broken Bones, by Jim Moriarty

Over the years I'd broken dozens of bones, the result, I thought, of my enthusiastic participation in action sports (skateboarding, snowboarding, etc.) Then, I was informed I had osteoporosis and the bones of a 70-year-old man. I had always been active, gotten plenty of exercise, and eaten a reasonable diet. Thus, the question quickly became "why?"

When I met with the doctor who was going to perform the tests for celiac he said, "I can tell you right now you have celiac disease."

"You know that before I even take a seat?" I replied. "Aren't you going to let me sit down, take some blood, do some tests, and send me a bill?"

"I can do all that, but I'm telling you up front; you have celiac disease. You are obviously active, in your 40s, blue-eyed, prematurely greying, probably originally from a Celtic nation, and *very slim.*"

Can you relate to any part of Jim's story? Are you also very slim? Are you getting hunched over, breaking a few bones, or can't put on weight no matter how hard you try? If so, your body's sending you a wakeup call to get tested for both CD and osteoporosis!

Osteomalacia, osteopenia, and osteoporosis are atypical disorders associated with CD. In fact, the link between CD and bone disorders was identified nearly five decades ago—that's half a century![26] Newly diagnosed CD patients often have reduced Bone Mineral Density (BMD) that may be caused by malabsorption of calcium and vitamin D and "proinflammatory cytokines." In adults who adopt a GF lifestyle, BMD may improve, but it hardly ever returns to normal. If diminished BMD is diagnosed in children before they reach puberty, those on a GFD may fully recover from the loss of bone mass.[27] One study stressed the importance of the pediatrician's role in recognizing CD and suggested less focus on monitoring bone damage and more focus on following an *absolute* GFD, since it may take as little as 6 to 12 months for children's bones to normalize.[28] Another study found that at the time of diagnosis "children and adolescents with celiac disease have remarkably reduced lumbar spine and whole-body bone density."[29] Osteomalacia may present as the only symptom of CD. In one case study, a

59-nine-year-old woman who was wheelchair-bound due to weakness and severe pain in her lower limbs saw her condition improve drastically within 3 months on a GFD. She was able to walk free of pain with a cane.[30]

A 2009 study reports that the increased production of cytokines also enhances the breakdown of bone, "which is further accelerated by hyperparathyroidism connected with malabsorption of calcium and vitamin D." The bottom line: Patients with "unexplained hyperparathyroidism...or...various autoimmune disease" should be screened for CD, along with "premenopausal women and men, who did not reach the appropriate peak bone mass."[31]

In a 2006 study, **"fifty-nine percent [of CD] patients had either osteoporosis or osteopenia.**"[32] This is huge! I wonder what percent of osteoporosis cases are related to CD. Setting up a study to find out should be fairly easy to do. **Osteoporosis may also be the only presenting sign of CD**. Early menopause and amenorrhea in women and hypogonadism in men, along with a growth hormone deficiency, are also associated with osteoporosis.[33] (See Chapter 12 for information on infertility.)

One study concluded that all patients with osteoporosis should be screened for CD. It found that "the antitissue transglutaminase levels correlated with the severity of osteoporosis...demonstrating that the more severe the celiac disease the more severe the resulting osteoporosis..."[34] Some osteoporosis drugs come with a warning that they could cause seizures if taken by a patient with a malabsorption problem. So if you've been diagnosed with osteoporosis or a related disorder, it's doubly important to know if you also have celiac disease in order to avoid potential side effects from a drug intended to treat your condition.

Esophagitis and Reflux

Symptoms that Magically Disappear, by Maria E. Willinski

As far as I can remember, I have always had anemia. I've also been underweight for the most part of my life and have frequently had diarrhea.

When I was 16 I had an endoscopy because of acid reflux, and my doctor in Spain, where I grew up, found I had esophagitis (inflammation of the esophagus). He said my esophagus was being scratched due to the reflux, causing small bleeding irritations that led to the anemia. He also believed I wasn't eating right or consuming enough meat and that my periods were "heavy," although I told him at every visit this wasn't true.

By the time I was an adult I came to believe my condition was "just the way it was." I pictured myself being forever tired, taking iron supplements for the rest of my life, and periodically getting sick. I was always the one in my family catching the airborne viruses, sore throats, flu, and colds, not to mention stomachaches, headaches, and yeast infections.

I'd been in the United States less than a year when, in May 2006, my new doctor suggested I might have celiac disease. It was only my second consultation with her! A blood test showed extremely high levels of antigliadin antibodies and a subsequent endoscopic biopsy revealed the second and third parts of my duodenum were affected with celiac sprue. The endoscopy also revealed I have a hiatal hernia, and a bone density test revealed I have osteoporosis in my back. (Unfortunately, some of the consequences of having undiagnosed CD for decades are going to be with me for the rest of my life.)

After starting on a GFD, most of my symptoms magically disappeared. And after following the diet for about six months, although I still needed to take supplemental iron, I recovered from my anemia and was able to exercise five times a week.

A couple years after being diagnosed with CD I was diagnosed with a degenerative hip condition that had most likely been developing for years. I was 39 years old.

Are you having hip or knee pain due to a degenerative condition and your doctor is talking replacement? This condition, and the resulting physician-patient conversation, is becoming altogether too common. Yet there is little talk of gluten sensitivity being associated with degenerative hips and knees—it's so new many doctors don't even realize CD could be causing osteoporosis or anemia—but I have read a couple stories where a replacement was put off because the person, having been diagnosed with CD and now on a GFD, was beginning to heal, and the pain was subsiding. Let's use a bit of common sense here. If your body could develop osteoporosis due to malabsorption of vital nutrients needed to keep your bones healthy, what do you suppose could be happening to the joints, cartilage, and ligaments holding your hips and knees together? Perhaps these parts of the body are not suffering exclusively from wear and tear due to age (especially if you didn't spend your youth battering them by running track or getting pummeled on the gridiron). Perhaps, for some people, celiac disease is playing a part as well.

In a 2007 Swedish study, Ludvgisson, et al., report: "Individuals with celiac disease, including children with celiac disease, may be at increased risk of hip fracture and fracture of any type."[35]

Hopefully, with diet, exercise, and supplements, Maria will heal sufficiently to avoid becoming one of the "hip replacements" and reduce her risk of hip fracture. However, to heal the body from damage caused by gluten, one must become vigilant in pursuit of a gluten-free lifestyle. Even the littlest bit of the substance can hurt. *There is no room for error!*

New studies are examining a potential connection between CD and esophageal/reflux issues. Some conclusions indicate a gluten-free lifestyle may help prevent reflux, Barrett's disease, and other esophageal disorders, as well as some throat-related cancers. However, gluten may not be the only irritant. If you have any of these troublesome ailments, you may want to consider allergy and intolerance testing for a wide swatch of other allergens, especially dairy.

A 2010 study suggested eosinophilic esophagitis may exist along with CD and that a biopsy of the esophagus should be taken along with an endoscopic biopsy, even if the esophagus otherwise appears normal.[36] Another recent study concluded that "all adult patients with cervical esophageal web and iron deficiency need screening for celiac disease even in the absence of chronic diarrhea."[37]

Another 2010 study found that gastroesophageal reflux disease (GERD) is prevalent with classic CD and is more severe than with atypical or silent CD; **nearly a third of classic CD patients had "moderate to severe GERD."** Patients following a gluten-free lifestyle for three months experienced rapid improvement in reflux symptoms.[38]

In a first study involving non-erosive reflux disease, researchers found that following a GFD decreased GERD symptoms and helped prevent them from recurring.[39] For example, I have a friend who developed a very raspy voice; at times it sounded as if he had marbles in his throat. When he went to the doctor's he was diagnosed with a type of reflux that doesn't cause the usual discomfort of GERD but, naturally, he was given a prescription for meds. After explaining that reflux, throat and esophageal cancers, Barrette's disease, esophagitis, and more can be associated with gluten sensitivity, I suggested he get tested. He agreed and tested positive, but he didn't believe the results. A year later he was tested a second time; the results were still positive. This time he started on a GFD, and after a few weeks his voice improved. He also no longer deals with bloating after eating a meal of GF pasta; his flatulence has subsided; and his waistline has trimmed way down.

Patients with CD have been noted as having an "increased prevalence of esophageal metaplasia" that may be linked to sensitivity to gliadin.[40] One study concluded that "cervical esophageal web and iron deficiency" are indicators for CD screening. Patients in the study were free of symptoms of dysphagia, difficulty swallowing, after being on a GFD from 3 to 16 months.[41]

A deficiency of vitamin A may be at the root of esophageal cancer, says one study, and "carcinoma of the pharynx and oesophagus..." occur more commonly in CD patients.[42] "Barrett's esophagus (i.e., columnar epithelial metaplasia in the distal esophagus) is an acquired condition that in most patients results from chronic gastroesophageal reflux...[and] is associated with a 30- to 125-fold increased risk for adenocarcinoma of the esophagus."[43] One might surmise that gluten is an irritant leading to reflux, thus causing metaplasia (a change of one kind of tissue into another...it may be pre-cancerous...)"[44] in the esophagus and eventually leading to esophageal cancer. (See Chapter 13 for more on cancer.)

Fatigue, Insomnia, Anemia, and Depression

Extreme lethargy is a significant symptom of celiac disease and can miserably affect one's quality of life.[45] In one survey **fatigue was reported to affect 82 percent of adults with CD.**[46] Another study suggested physicians need to be open to screening for CD in the differential diagnosis of patients who present with "non-specific complaints of arthralgia, myalgias, and fatigue."[47] The title of one study, *Fatigue in primary care. Test for celiac disease first?* says it all, and not just for fatigue. If patients were tested for CD/GI first, my hunch is that billions of dollars worth of other tests might be avoided.

Along with fatigue, insomnia is another sign of celiac disease that plagues millions of people. Yet both fatigue and insomnia seem to miraculously clear up with a gluten-free lifestyle, once the body has a chance to heal. Before eliminating gluten from my diet, I'd been tired for most of my adult life—not extreme fatigue, but definitely in need of an afternoon nap. Now I have great energy, no need for a nap, and generally burn the midnight oil. And I sleep very soundly. (Many others on a GFD have told me they sleep soundly as well.)

Since starting a website reviewing gluten-free products, Tiffany Shaw-Diaz has written *Pinching Pennies: You Can Cut Your Gluten-Free Grocery Bill* for the nationally distributed magazine, *Gluten-Free Living.* Her own story is typical of an overlapping array of classic and atypical symptoms of CD.

A Food Critic's Story, by Tiffany Shaw-Diaz

When I was growing up, I vividly remember snack time at Grandma's. Grandma had celiac disease, and as a decades-old veteran of a gluten-free diet, she kept her fridge and pantry stocked with rice cakes, hard-as-brick bread, and utterly bland cereal. Even as an eight year-old, I often opted for a raw carrot over anything else in her kitchen.

When I wasn't at Grandma's I was an addict of all things wheat: macaroni and cheese, sandwiches, cookies, and foods containing soy sauce. *I'll never be forced to eat gluten free,* I told myself. There's no chance. Unlike my maternal grandma, I have always been a healthy weight and, besides, the medical community considered celiac disease a "rare" condition.

At the same time, I unknowingly had many classic and atypical CD symptoms: iron-deficiency anemia, abdominal pain, depression, insomnia, and constipation. But since I wasn't skinny (meaning I wasn't malnourished), no doctor—despite my family history—ever mentioned the possibility of CD to me. I spent my high school years so anemic I was nearly hospitalized. When I was sixteen, I remember taking three iron pills a day yet still managing to fall asleep in every class. And then there were the stomach pains, gut-wrenching, hours-long discomfort that occurred—not so surprisingly—whenever I'd eat pasta or other gluten-containing foods. I never knew why I was anemic, or why my stomach hurt so much. I just figured I ate an unhealthy diet and was under too much stress—that in some way I had a control over my chronic ailments. My assumptions turned out to be far from the truth.

My obsession with food, and my love affair with gluten, continued into my twenties. Then, while working as a freelance writer, I was offered a chance to review food after the previous critic stepped down. I jumped at the opportunity and served as a bi-weekly food critic for nearly eight months. Then I received an unexpected phone call from my mother, who'd been struggling with IBS for several years. "Tiffany," she said, "I've been diagnosed with celiac disease, and since you have many of the same symptoms, my specialist suggests you get the blood test immediately."

I was so shocked I practically dropped the phone. There's no way I wanted to believe I had this disease; the memory of Grandma's cupboards still loomed large! At the same time, I knew I couldn't ignore the possibility. Two weeks later I had a CD blood panel. The phone call that followed would change my life.

At first I was devastated by my positive results. *How could a rising food critic lose her job to a crippling food intolerance?* I thought. The whole scenario was too ironic, like one of those plot twists found only in sitcoms and movies.

I was saddened by the loss of my part-time job, but soon after adopting a GFD I felt better than I'd ever felt before. Instead of needing three plates of food to satisfy my hunger, I only needed one. Instead of falling asleep everywhere I went, I now had energy. For the first time, I wholeheartedly embraced life.

There are times when I look back and think, "What if I'd never gotten that blood test?" On the one hand, I would still be a food critic in the traditional sense; on the other, I'd be so exhausted my quality of life, not to mention my well-being, would surely be suffering. Although there is no question my GFD is a lifestyle change, I am elated to reclaim my health, and most importantly, my zest for life. (Read *Thriving at Ninety-two,* the story of Tiffany's grandmother, Barbara Wasson, in Chapter 24.)

Do you wake up tired, need an afternoon nap, or feel exhausted all the time? Could you have a chronic disease but think your symptoms are just part of getting older? I wish I'd kept a log of all the people I've spoken with over the years who suffer from fatigue, reflux, anemia, and/or osteo and thyroid issues—to name just a few of CD's more insidious symptoms—and still think they're healthy. They couldn't possibly be sensitive to gluten, they tell me. And of course, they might not be, but only adequate testing (and a positive response to the GFD) can tell for sure, and burying one's head in the sand has never been an effective diagnostic tool.

Allergies and Asthma

I'd been prone to bronchitis and plagued with allergies—hay fever, dust, mold, and animals—for years. In the 10 years prior to ditching gluten it seemed as if every sinus cold landed in my chest and turned into reactive airway, an asthma-like condition. After living a gluten-free lifestyle for just over a year, I realized my allergies were greatly lessening. Today they are nearly non-existent. I can rake leaves without sneezing my guts out and enjoy spring and fall without scratching my eyes out. And my bouts with reactive airway and bronchitis are a thing of the past.

Dairy creates mucus for me, along with the need to constantly clear my throat and sniffle. It also makes my body very stiff after sitting for a while, so I have basically given it up. One day during hay-fever season I got into some cheese (I really miss cheese), and within 20 minutes my eyes were itching unbearably. As I've mentioned before, gluten isn't the only irritating protein in town.

My immune system is in tip-top shape now that my villi have healed and, since I no longer have a permeable gut, I'm absorbing all those vitamins and minerals that once went out the back door. On the rare day I feel as if I'm catching a cold, it's because I've been burning the candle at both ends. The "cure" is simple: I kick back, take a vitamin booster and get in a few more fruits and veggies.

Allergies and asthma are plaguing an enormous segment of our population. Just ask any school nurse or teacher. Something is *causing* these health issues; they don't just happen, and when the cause (the irritant/s) is removed, the problem gets better.

Wendy Cohan has created two websites, www.glutenfreechoice.com and www.wellbladder.com, to help others navigate the practical considerations of diet-related health problems. She's also written the *Gluten-Free Portland [Oregon] Resource Guide*. Before detecting gluten sensitivity, she suffered for years with allergies and interstitial cystitis (see Chapter 14 for her interstitial cystitis story, *They Said, "No Cure!"*). Since adopting a GFD Wendy feels much better, although she still has numerous food sensitivities. For some people, gluten is just one of many irritants that cause them trouble.

Choices, by Wendy Cohan, RN

I eliminated gluten from my diet more than a decade ago and have been following a GFD ever since. Although I know I am highly gluten sensitive I am not officially diagnosed with CD. (Testing options a decade ago were not as sophisticated as they are today.) However, as my overall health has improved my body has become even more sensitive to various substances. These days, I can tell by the response I get when I eat a particular food whether my system will tolerate it or not, as well as how much of it I can tolerate. For me, the response is highly individualized. Oats make me itchy on the insides of my eyebrows. Dairy hits me right between the eyes with a headache, along with the usual runny nose and gastrointestinal symptoms. Oranges, chocolate, red wine, and dark-skinned plums contain vasoactive amines that can trigger migraines, and I react to all of them within minutes. So while I dislike the fact I'm so sensitive and would like to be able to eat anything I want, I've come to accept I may always be highly sensitive to a variety of foods. Rather than reaching for my migraine medication, I've learned not to reach for the chocolate or the red wine. But I can eat a coconut macaroon and enjoy a glass of white wine, or I can have a peach instead of a plum. In other words, in spite of limitations I still have choices, and that's important to me.

Consuming the littlest bit of gluten can keep the degenerative process going, so contamination is a big issue (see Chapters 19 and 20). Mimi's story below is a good example of what can happen to those with gluten sensitivity if a gluten-free lifestyle is not followed 100 percent. I met Mimi at a bakery where the baker goes out of her way to create delicious gluten-free products. Fortunately, more and more such establishments are springing up around the country.

Tidbits of Gluten, by Mimi Tracy

We have a family history of an allergy to penicillin, and I am allergic to gluten and dairy. I stopped eating gluten about 25 years ago and just this year eliminated dairy. I do my best to exclude these substances from my diet, but I'm not always totally successful. Sometimes I get symptoms that bother my breathing: wheezing, stuffiness, runny nose, and itchy eyes, ears, and nose. Often I develop a migraine. If I eat enough gluten or dairy I develop allergic bronchitis. I'm often surprised at how little it takes to provoke some sort of a reaction.

Many people think they may have a food allergy, but, in fact, "fewer than 1% have true allergies." *Intolerance* to corn, dairy, and wheat/gluten generate most of what appears to be an allergic response.[49] Many people who are tested for allergies are not tested far enough to determine if they have an intolerance. For example, when I had allergy tests, one doctor told me I was *allergic* to gluten and could have a little on a rotational diet. Further testing revealed I was also *intolerant*, which meant I should never consume gluten again. If you test positive for being allergic (IgE antibodies) to some food, you may want to undergo intolerance (IgA and IgG antibodies) testing for that food as well.

One 2004 study found that "baker's asthma" (an allergic response to inhaled wheat flour)[50] and "classical allergy to wheat proteins" are types of a gluten allergy, but these are different from CD (an intolerance). Reactions to these allergies may be anaphylactic, dermatological, intestinal, and respiratory.[51] "Over 90% of food allergies in childhood are caused by eight foods: cow's milk, hen's egg[s], soy, peanuts, tree nuts, wheat, fish and shellfish.... The main principle of food allergy management is avoidance of the offending antigen."[52] In other words, *remove the irritant!*

"**Food-dependent, exercise-induced anaphylaxis is a severe form of allergy**" that has been recognized for over a decade. It is difficult to diagnose since "neither the ingested food nor the exercise alone induces the symptoms."[53]

Jess, a graphic designer and editor, is creative, passionate about education, and well traveled. She loves life, has a positive attitude, and enjoys good wine and delicious food. For years her doctors thought she was a hypochondriac; now that she has found an answer to her asthma and other health problems she can finally breathe easy.

Profound Results, by Jess M.

I have had health problems since the day I was born. As a small child I had issues with chronic insomnia and other sleep problems such as somnambulism (sleep walking) and nightmares, as well as frequent illnesses such as tonsillitis, sinusitis, and a case of pneumonia that landed me in the hospital nearly every December. As I headed into my twenties, I developed endometriosis, a painful condition research has shown may be an autoimmune disorder and which required me to have annual surgeries to reduce scarring. I was also getting sick frequently and was suffering from asthma, forgetfulness, mood swings, water retention, and dry, swollen hands and feet. All this illness was affecting my performance at work.

I visited several physicians, but they could find nothing wrong with me. My frustration mounted as doctor after doctor told me I was perfectly fine and several suggested therapy, saying they believed my symptoms were a result of high levels of anxiety due to an overwhelming schedule. I began seeing a therapist, who said my feet were firmly planted on the ground and believed there was no reason to medicate me. She asked if I'd tried Eastern medicine or homeopathic remedies.

One day I was visiting a close friend who had recently completed acupuncture training and was in the midst of extended studies in traditional Chinese medicine. She took one look at me and told me my problem was food—specifically, wheat and other grains with gluten. She placed me on an elimination diet that involved consuming only water, unprocessed meat, vegetables, and fruits. All processed sugars and high-carbohydrate foods such as rice, potatoes, and corn were cut as well.

After several weeks on the diet I was sleeping through the night. I'd lost 12 pounds—ostensibly all water weight, since the swelling in my body disappeared. I also was calmer, had much greater clarity of thought, and had ceased to experience any gastrointestinal discomfort when I ate.

At the time I write this I've been gluten free for seven years, and my *endometriosis and the asthma are gone*. However, any time I ingest even the tiniest bit of the substance by accident (I've even learned to take my own soy sauce to sushi bars), I immediately become bloated, short of breath, and uncomfortable for several days. Removing gluten from my diet was a difficult life change for me. It took me almost three years to completely eliminate it, but the reward has been profound. Not only am I now living a much healthier, higher quality life, but I'm eating homemade, whole foods that are much tastier and nutritionally superior to what I was eating before. I have a more fulfilling, deeper connection with food and am more conscious now of all substances, edible and otherwise, with which my body comes into contact. Becoming gluten free has enriched my life beyond measure.

"Flour is still one of the most common causes of occupational asthma worldwide," gliadin being the *inhalable irritant causing the asthma.*[54]

One researcher reported, "Those [children] who go on to develop chronic asthma most likely have a genetic predisposition and exposure to various environmental factors resulting in chronic inflammation of the lower respiratory tract."[55] A decade-old study found that asthma can coexist with CD, rheumatoid arthritis, and type 1 diabetes, suggesting a "common environmental denominator" may be involved in the disease mechanisms.[56] A 2011 study revealed that "celiac disease confers a 1.6 fold increased risk of asthma," which may be a ramification of low levels of vitamin D (found in 60–70%) due to malabsorption.[57]

Don't mess around with asthma. I can remember once spending two weeks on the couch drinking tea and juice and resting while waiting for my reactive airway to lift, just because I didn't want to take the puffers. It finally did, but looking back, I was a fool. It could have killed me. Fortunately, with my gluten-free lifestyle I no longer have the problem.

I am disgusted by the asthma medication ads on TV that make it seem almost cool to have asthma, like it's no big deal. Don't be fooled! Asthma is a serious disease, and as such it should be taken seriously. If you or your child has asthma or bad allergies, you may want to consider testing for gluten and dairy allergies or intolerance. The longer such allergies and/or intolerances are ignored, the worse life can get.

In a 2007 news release, the National Institutes of Health (NIH) reported that "more than 22 million people in the United States have asthma, including 6.5 million children under age 18,..."[58] Although these are informative statistics, the remainder of the report focused almost exclusively on treatment, controlling with drugs, and monitoring, as opposed to presenting information about prevention, cause, or the effects of gluten.

Weight Loss/Gain

Weight loss is a typical sign of classic CD. Surprisingly, weight gain may be an atypical sign. By the time I joined my grandson, Nick, in a gluten-free lifestyle, I had gained 50 pounds since giving birth to my first child. Over the years I'd tried various diets, but none of them worked, and I continually found myself drawn to the cookie jar.

Three weeks after beginning the GFD, I not only had much greater energy, I'd lost more than 10 pounds without thinking about it. Many overweight people have spoken of how excess weight has peeled right off after they eliminated gluten. Some folks I've talked to have lost as much as 30 to 40 pounds living a gluten-free lifestyle, without really trying to diet. Of course, part of the secret to losing weight is to avoid replacing traditional junk food with gluten-free junk food. A healthier diet based on lean protein, fruits, and vegetables will help your body get the nutrients it needs.

If you've been a beanpole (due to undiagnosed CD), eating voraciously to fill your body with nutrients but unable to put on weight no matter how hard you try, things may change once you adopt a GFD. As your body heals and nutrients are being absorbed, you may put on a few pounds. If you are putting on too much weight then you may need to check your calorie intake against your exercise output.

Marcy and I had chatted about gluten a number of times before she finally took me seriously. A friend of hers says she can tell immediately if Marcy is hit with gluten. Her face puffs up and she clears her throat a lot.

Over the Course of Time, by Marcy Vierzen

I had been experiencing a slow weight gain over the years, nothing very dramatic, but a few pounds a year, and my face was frequently puffy. I assumed it was my sinuses reacting to seasonal allergies. I also had some skin problems (breakouts), postnasal drip, dull headaches, and allergies from April through October. And I was forever lethargic.

I decided to do a fall cleanse program with a local nutritionist, just to get me back on a healthier footing. During the cleanse, various foods were eliminated and slowly reintroduced. After the first week, a lightbulb suddenly went on in my head: I was no longer swallowing funny to get rid of my postnasal drip, since it was now non-existent, and my dull and constant headache was totally gone. My energy levels increased, my face cleared up, and I began to lose weight.

One morning during the third week of the cleanse I went out to breakfast with friends and had two bites of a friend's cinnamon muffin. Within 10 minutes, literally, my postnasal drip came back, even though it had been gone for a couple of weeks. It was so obvious, so absolutely evident, so tied to the fact that the only change I'd made was eating the cinnamon bun, that I knew something in that roll was causing my reaction. Within an hour, my headache was back as well. It was dull, but it was still back.

Until I started the cleanse and my headaches stopped, it simply had never occurred to me they were anything but an adult annoyance. Now, after two bites of a roll I had one again. Maybe my problems *were* more than just seasonal.

I continued to "test" what the issue might be. Was it white sugar? I tried several sweets but did not have a similar reaction. In fact, the only common ingredient that caused a negative reaction was wheat/gluten. I adopted a gluten-free diet.

When I became lax and let my GFD slide, my weight gain was immediate and my symptoms returned in full force. Not only that, the symptoms built up to the point I could no longer ignore them. Recently, someone on my staff actually asked if I felt all right. My face was so puffy I didn't look well. Two weeks later, having gone off gluten once again, I lost weight and the contours of my face returned to normal.

If I inadvertently got "glutened" or just let my guard down and indulged, for the next 16 hours or so I was very irritable, off-center and "down." This pattern, more than anything, convinced me to get off gluten entirely and truly make the commitment to live gluten free. The change has been dramatic. Given the impact gluten is having on my body in ways I can see, what might it be doing to internal structures and processes I can't see?

Edema is a symptom of classic CD.[59] A link between celiac disease and hereditary angioneurotic edema was made in 2002.[60] Fluid retention also may be affected by malnutrition, and/or an unhealthy diet that could lead to low albumin levels and/or vitamin B1, B5, and B6 deficiencies.[61] One woman told me she had suspected she might be gluten sensitive due to intestinal issues. As soon as she eliminated wheat she noticed an immediate improvement. Within two weeks she'd lost 15 pounds, along with a layer of fluid (edema) in her hands, arms, legs, and feet she didn't even realize was there.

A case study of a 27-year-old man revealed "his ankle edema disappeared" after being on a GFD for three months. A liver issue from which he suffered also resolved itself during this period, and his polyneuropathy got better. Edema is an atypical symptom of CD and needs to be more on doctors' radar screens, prompting early identification and, if necessary, treatment.[62]

A new study concluded that a GFD "had a beneficial impact on BMI [body mass index]; underweight patients gained weight (66%) and overweight/obese patients (54%/47%) lost weight. The improvement in BMI adds to the impetus to diagnose celiac disease."[63]

The Highs and Lows of Celiac Disease

Vitamin and Mineral Deficiencies—A special health report from Harvard Medical School presented a clear view of the results of nutrient deficiency—low vitamins and minerals. "Over time, this [deficiency] contributes to chronic illnesses such as heart disease, osteoporosis, and cancer.... Acting in concert, these essential vitamins and minerals help keep billions of cells healthy and encourage them to grow and reproduce."[64]

CD affects your body on a cellular level. Nutrient deficiency due to malabsorption is the mainspring—along with immunological antibody reactivity—of numerous symptoms and illnesses associated with or caused by gluten. The big question is what is causing the hypo (low) status of certain vitamins or minerals? In more cases than many doctors suspect, the answer may lie in your breadbox. In her book *Recognizing Celiac Disease: Signs, Symptoms, Associated Disorders & Complications*, Cleo Libonati draws on extensive research to catalog the vitamin and/or mineral deficiency or immunological reaction of over 300 hundred CD symptoms and associated ailments.[65] And you may be shocked at what comes up when you do a little Internet research using the keywords *gluten* or *"celiac disease"* and *PubMed* (the information database sponsored by the NIH U.S. National Library of Medicine).

If you test in the *low normal* or *below* range of a vitamin or mineral and eat a healthy diet, there may be a serious reason for it—malabsorption—and you may consider testing to see if gluten could be the culprit. And if there is no known cause for your ailment, this also may be a red flag for you to get tested. After all, *something* is making you sick and tired of being sick and tired. There *is* a reason, even if your doctor doesn't know what it is. In the meantime, supplementation with gluten-free vitamins and minerals could be in order, but before taking any medicine, even supplements, be sure to talk with your doctor.

Hyper and Hypo—Are you beginning to realize that perhaps CD is not really a disease? I have never accepted the word *disease* to describe my intolerance, and I detest using the word with a child. Disease is a heavy burden for a youngster who is actually suffering from a toxicity issue. For example, if you were to roll in poison ivy, you might break out in a rash that, in time, would heal and disappear. If you rolled in it again, the rash would return. Likewise, gluten sensitivity (both CD and GI) is a condition dependent on the consumption of gluten which, to those genetically predisposed, is an irritant much like poison ivy. If you never came in contact with poison ivy, you'd never develop the rash; if you never ate gluten, you'd never develop the myriad health issues linked to it. So even though gluten sensitivity is not in itself a disease, it can certainly *lead* to myriad diseases and symptoms over time. Fortunately, if the offending protein is removed, particularly before it triggers major damage, the body has a chance to heal.

Would you eat poison? Of course not! Yet for many, gluten is a toxin that may set in motion a domino effect that damages intestinal villi, which leads to malabsorption and antibody reactivity, which may cause the body to run amok. Vitamin and mineral deficiencies can lead to physical destruction, deterioration, and degradation of any part of the body, a process that can occur over many years. In other words, a low vitamin/mineral level can trigger a bucketful of ailments you could avoid. Below are just a few examples:

- ***Vitamin B6 (pyridoxine) and B9 (folate) deficits*** were found to be "significantly and independently associated with homocysteine levels." Homocysteine levels depend on the degree of villi damage; the greater the damage, the higher the levels.[66]
- ***Vitamin B12 levels*** should be assessed in patients with "depressive disorders, dementia, psychosis or risk factors for malnutrition such as alcoholism or advancing age associated with neurological symptoms, anemia, malabsorption [all three of which can result from CD], gastrointestinal surgery, parasite infestation or [a] strict vegetarian diet."[67]
- ***Vitamin D*** is "known for its role in calcium homeostasis for optimum skeletal health" and has recently been associated with prevention of cancer and hypertension, and immune function. It may play an important role in rheumatic and other non-bone-related diseases.[68]
- ***Hyperhomocysteinemia*** (too much homocysteine in the blood; also known as HH), with or without low vitamin B12 levels, may lead to dementia. B12 deficits may also lead to unexpected gastrointestinal, hematological, neurological, and psychiatric manifestations.[69] HH has been linked to low folate and vitamin

B and is associated with cardiovascular disease, premature atherosclerosis, and venous thrombosis.[70]

- ***Hypocholesterolemia*** (low cholesterol) "can reveal a severe disease (cancer...malabsorption...)." Following an absolute GFD can improve symptoms.[71]
- ***Hypoglycemia*** (low blood sugar), when linked to CD, normalizes on a GFD.[72]
- ***Hypokalemia*** (low potassium) may also be linked to CD. "A severe acute diarrhea with metabolic and systemic complications, the so-called coeliac crisis, is a possible presenting clinical feature of a previously undiagnosed adult celiac disease." A young woman who exhibited a sudden onset of "weakness of all four limbs and a severe diarrhea" got better on a GFD with added potassium supplementation.[73]
- ***Hypokalemic rhabdomyolysis*** (low potassium levels accompanied by breakdown of muscle fiber leading to muscle fiber contents being released into the bloodstream)[74] and *tetany* (a calcium imbalance that leads to muscle spasms)[75] also may be symptomatic of CD. One paper notes the case of a 38-year-old patient with these issues. Once the patient was treated for CD, his electrolyte imbalances were completely resolved. The study concludes that "celiac disease should be considered a cause of hypokalemic rhabdomyolsis."[76]
- ***Hypoproteinaemia*** (low blood protein), along with amenorrhoea, hypoalbuminemia, psychoneurotic issues, and weight loss occurred as atypical symptoms of CD in a 38-year-old woman who was initially misdiagnosed with IBS.[77]
- ***Iron deficiency anemia and zinc deficiency*** were found to be the two most common lab results, along with "prolonged prothrombin [blood clotting] time...and elevated transaminase levels..." in a study of children with CD. "Paleness (40.4%), underweight (34.8%), and short stature (31.2%)..." are among other common findings.[78]
- ***Vitamin K*** deficits can have serious repercussions. "Overt vitamin K deficiency results in impaired blood clotting... Symptoms include easy bruising and bleeding that may be

> manifested as nosebleeds, bleeding gums, blood in the urine, blood in the stool, tarry black stools, or extremely heavy menstrual bleeding. In infants, vitamin K deficiency may result in life-threatening bleeding within the skull..."[79] Bleeding as a result of low vitamin K is "a rare complication that occurs almost exclusively in patients with typical CD manifestations." It completely resolved on a GFD for one young patient.[80]

"Coeliac disease may present with a single vitamin deficiency with potentially catastrophic results." A seemingly healthy 42-year-old man "presented in haemorrhagic shock...His duodenal biopsy and INR, a clotting measure, normalized on a gluten-free diet."[81]

The stories and citations above present just a few examples of diseases, disorders, and symptoms that have developed due to the malabsorption of essential vitamins and minerals needed to keep our bodies functioning optimally.

9 Neurological Dilemmas: The Mind-blowing Hazards of Gluten

Neurological Impairment

It was only a few years ago that a friend was experiencing a severe neurological problem. When she tried tracking down a neurologist in New England who was knowledgeable about the devastating effects of gluten, she didn't get very far. Aside from a few gluten experts, our primary care physicians, pediatricians, and gastroenterologists barely have a handle on the classic issues associated with celiac disease (CD), and these issues represent only a small part of the gluten sensitivity spectrum. Since it often takes decades for new medical research to be accepted, I fear the connection between gluten and neurological maladies may be at the bottom of the recognition list.

Nevertheless, mind-altering neurological and cerebral symptoms and maladies such as anxiety, apathy, depression, headaches, insomnia, irritability, and migraines can be associated with gluten. In *Recognizing Celiac Disease*, Cleo Libonati identifies more severe problems including ataxia (a gross lack of coordination of muscle movements), autism spectrum disorder (ASD), dementia, epilepsy, learning disabilities, multiple sclerosis (MS), peripheral neuropathy, schizophrenic disorders, and tremors.[1] As time goes on, I expect further studies will help connect the dots.

The stories represented here provide mountains of hope for millions with mild to devastating neurological and cerebral issues their neurologists and primary care physicians may know little about. For those who are gluten sensitive, many such ailments turn around on a GFD. Other diseases are very slow to mend and some cannot be reversed, but a GFD may halt their progression.

If you have an eight-syllable neurological (or any other) disease or disorder, it would behoove you to do some research, even if your doctor says your condition is *genetic* or *incurable.* Don't wait until your next appointment to begin this exploration. You have nothing to lose and may have significant health benefits to gain by sharing what you learn with your doctor. Even if you've reached the point of no return or are gravely ill, removing gluten might help! However, it is important to get tested and discuss the results with your doctor before you begin a gluten-free diet. See Appendix A—Empowerment, for research tips on how to conduct research. And remember, "neurologic manifestations of gluten sensitivity are a scientific fact, not a theological issue."[2]

Dr. Marios Hadjivassiliou and his research team remind us that gluten sensitivity presents itself in ways other than celiac disease. Although neurological ailments associated with CD were recognized back in 1966, it took 30 years before research revealed that **gluten sensitivity could "manifest solely with neurological dysfunction"**[3] (in other words, without intestinal damage). Screening with the *antigliadin antibody* test is urged so patients are not denied "a harmless but potentially effective treatment in the form of a gluten-free diet."[4] It is shocking to me that at the same time this world-renowned doctor is imploring practitioners to use the antigliaden antibody test, some of our own gluten gurus seem unaware of its value in detecting gluten sensitivity beyond CD—and I have heard this with my very own ears! Ignoring the entire range of non-celiac gluten intolerance, many seem concerned only with full-blown celiac disease.

Some of the neurologic disorders that have reared their ugly heads in association with gluten, particularly among those who are middle-aged, include cerebellar ataxia, dementia, epilepsy, myoclonic ataxia, and neuropathies. In this 2004 study, researchers found over half of the CD patients were apt to suffer from neurologic conditions such as attention deficit hyperactivity disorder (ADHD), developmental delay, headache, hypotonia, and learning disabilities, known as the "softer" disorders.[5] One study found that neurological disorders were linked more to "immunological-inflammatory processes, than to malresorptive vitamin deficiencies,"[6] Another reported that "**both vitamin depletion and immunological mechanisms may cause neurological disorder**" and stressed that physicians need to become more aware that "celiac disease can cause neurological diseases, especially polyneuropathy, cerebellar ataxia, and encephalopathy."[7] A study dating from 1991 found untreated CD patients may become apathetic, depressed, easily agitated, negativistic, sad, temperamental, uncommunicative, and withdrawn; in severe cases, researchers observed that patients exhibited a lack of thirst, appeared dazed, and were afflicted with seizures.[8] "Subtly reduced cognitive function resulting from early vitamin B12 deficiency might be the only initial symptom of these intestinal disorders, followed by megaloblastic anemia and dementia."[9]

"Neurologic complications of CD have been known for a long time as a consequence of vitamin deficiency (B12, E, D, folic acid [B9], pyridoxine [B6]),"[10] cites a 2001 study. Another study mentions vitamins B1, B3, and other nutrient deficiencies.[11] Are most neurologists aware of this connection? Sometimes I wonder. If you have any of these issues and have not been offered testing to see if you are malabsorbing, you might be wondering, too.

Memory, Dementia, and Depression

I know of two women in their early seventies and one in her mid-fifties who have a form of dementia. They've been seen by "the best" doctors, to no avail. I expect their families had no idea that gluten might be the problem. The possibility of a connection between gluten and these women's dementia weighs heavily on my mind, as each has a number of other symptoms and ailments indicative of CD. It is beyond my comprehension how families with terrible health issues will brush aside cutting-edge information; the testing is so easy—it's an open door! Many ailing folks treat their doctors as gods, expecting them to know everything, but this information is just too new, and doctors are not being educated in any comprehensive way on the subject. I discovered when discussing dementia with another woman that she wasn't at all worried because she was taking B-complex vitamins. Yet for those malabsorbing, vitamin supplements may do little good.

Dick and I met at a local CD support group. His health issues will likely strike a chord with many suffering from similar ailments. The good news is that after seven months of a strict, gluten-free (GF) lifestyle, all of his symptoms disappeared.

I Got My Life Back, by Dick Stevens

I was born in 1943. As a young child I had reactions to pollens and dust and was diagnosed with grass/tree/weed allergies by age 10. For the next seven years, until I left for college, I received desensitization serum every five days. Over the next four decades I brought other symptoms to my physician's attention with little resolution. Visually annoying, itchy, and sometimes painful eczema-like patches surfaced on my elbows, scalp, and eyebrows. Small, .5 cm flakes of dry skin would peel off, leaving bare flesh as raw as hamburger. Doctors prescribed ointments, which I applied to no avail. I also developed moderate rashes on each side of my torso below the ribs, and small pimple-type bumps appeared below my kneecaps. I know now that all of the above skin conditions were probably dermatitis herpetiformis, an atypical manifestation of CD. (For more on this condition, see Chapter 11 on skin.)

Most disturbing, at about the age of 55, I was plagued with quite serious memory loss. I frequently could not find words to complete sentences; I could visualize the word but not retrieve it. As an insurance executive, this was not good for my position. In addition, I began to suffer from a debilitating fatigue, often needing shorts naps in my car after lunch.

After a while I began to experience a deep depression; I felt disconnected and alone. Although I was never diagnosed with seasonal affective disorder (SAD), my symptoms were similar and coincided with the typical time frame for this disorder: fall through late January.

I also experienced moderately discomforting acid reflux and two episodes of heart arrhythmia (premature ventricular contractions). Because I had very frequent single extra heartbeats—a heart electrical problem—I had a number of echocardiograms and wore a Holter monitor for 24 hours. Fortunately, the results "showed no signs of previous heart attacks or valve problems." My acid reflux was relieved with a prescribed medication.

While having an annual physical at the age of 60, the nurse practitioner was disturbed by my symptoms and ordered blood tests. The results showed I was anemic and had very low iron (ferritin) stores [associated with memory issues]. She ordered a workup with a gastroenterologist who surmised bleeding in the colon, but my colonoscopy showed a healthy colon with no polyps. The doctor then performed an upper endoscopy and confirmed with a biopsy that I had very serious damage to my small intestine from celiac disease. The next step was not-very-informative nutritional counseling from a hospital-affiliated nutritionist.

I received more help from a local celiac-support group. After six months on a strict gluten-free diet—I never put anything into my mouth without examining it or asking about the ingredients to determine if it contained gluten—a repeat upper endoscopy later showed "villi not entirely back to normal—some normal/abnormal areas—patchy." Even so, during that period all of my symptoms disappeared, ***including my memory problems!*** For the first time in my life I knew what it felt like to be healthy, virile, and energetic.

After another six months, I was no longer anemic, and my iron stores had returned to normal. A third endoscopy was performed two years after beginning the gluten-free diet. This time my small intestine and villi were normal; a repeat tissue transglutaminase test was normal as well.

Dick had three endoscopies. Nowadays, if one's symptoms respond to a GF lifestyle, doctors "in the know" are unlikely to recommend a follow-up endoscopy, and certainly not months after beginning a GFD. It can take one to two years, or longer, to heal the gut.

The snippets below, excerpted from research done between 2004 and 2010, link gluten to dementia and other neurological issues:

- A high homocysteine level [an amino acid, high levels of which may be linked to increased risk of Alzheimer's disease, heart disease, osteoporosis, and stroke],[12] with or without low vitamin B12 levels, is linked to dementia. Vitamin B12 deficiency may lead to "psychiatric, neurological, gastrointestinal, and hematological findings."[13]

- Ten to fifteen percent of those with gluten sensitivity may experience "central or peripheral nervous system and psychiatric disorders." In a case study with exacerbating neuropsychiatric disorders, a GFD produced continuing remission of encephalopathy (brain disease).[14]

- A high homocysteine level and low vitamin B levels are associated with the degenerative process leading to dementia and other neuropsychiatric disorders. Although this study did not concern itself with CD, it did suggest recognizing patients with B6, B12, and folate deficiencies. Treating these deficiencies decreases the level of homocysteine.[15]

- One study concludes that transglutaminases are probably linked to the degenerative aspects of brain disease in Alzheimer's disease.[16]

- According to Dr. William Hu of the Mayo Clinic, some patients with dementia experienced "reversal or stabilization of the cognitive symptoms...when they underwent gluten withdrawal." Screening for CD was recommended if a patient had diarrhea, loss of weight or was younger than 70 years of age.[17] But what if a patient is over age 70, with or without classic CD symptoms, and has dementia coming on?

- "Abnormalities of brain perfusion [increased blood flow] seem common in coeliac disease.... and, at least in the frontal region, may be improved by a gluten-free diet."[18]
- Patients with dementia should be screened for B12 deficiency, depression, and hypothyroidism.[19] Although this study doesn't mention CD, these conditions are associated with CD as well.

Dr. Joseph Murray of the Mayo Clinic considers three theories to link cognitive deterioration to CD: immune reactivity, inflammatory cytokines, and nutritional deficiency.[20] Dr. Kenneth Fine of EnteroLab asserts that 30 to 40 percent of the U.S. population is gluten sensitive.[21] It stands to reason these numbers may be even higher in older folks, since they have been consuming gluten for longer. Those who are malabsorbing may be at risk due to low levels of B vitamins and iron, among other vital nutrients. Testing for gluten sensitivity and treating with a GFD for those who test positive could go a long way toward preventing neurological disorders caused by nutrient deficiencies.

Comprehensive studies are needed to explore the association between gluten sensitivity and cognitive decline, but few efforts are underway in this area. This lack of focus is not difficult to understand. There is little money to be made from patients who get healthy by following a GF lifestyle.

Autism and ADHD

Autism, ADHD, learning disabilities, irritability, disruptive behavior, and developmental delays are issues affecting far too many of our children. For children sensitive to gluten and dairy, removing these toxins from their diets has resulted in life-altering changes.

Too many doctors are pushing drugs and too many parents of autistic and/or ADHD children are taking the easy way out by administering them. An alternative may be a gluten-free/casein-free diet (GF/CF), but living gluten and/or casein free is a lifestyle change that takes devotion and determination. You can't just "try" these diets for a month; it takes much longer to get a complete handle on them so there are no slipups.

Angela, an extremely busy working mom, was committed to finding an answer for her children. The letter below, which she first wrote to help a friend and later forwarded to me for inclusion here, is a stunning example of

the impact parents can have on the life and future of an ailing child. I wish all challenged youngsters could have such a devoted parent.

Letter to a Friend, by Angela T., APRN, CRNA

One of my two sons has been diagnosed with autism spectrum disorder (ASD), the other with attention deficit hyperactivity disorder (ADHD). Neither has ever used meds for these conditions.

D., my youngest son, was diagnosed with ASD when he was three. We'd suspected something was wrong from the time he was about 18 months old. At 20 months he started speech therapy but made very little progress. At 26 months he was also offered occupational therapy, early intervention, and more speech therapy. He still made very little progress. At 37 months he received the formal diagnosis of ASD. He was essentially non-verbal, violent, and non-interactive, and the developmental pediatrician offered us Prozac for his behavior. I turned down the Prozac in order to have time to research and think about it. While searching for more information I found *Unraveling the Mystery of Autism,* a book by Karyn Seroussi, another mom with an ASD child. Karen talked about toxins, food allergies, and the recovery of her child. I decided to try some of her suggestions. We had nothing to lose, I figured, since there was always Prozac.

The first thing we did was remove all dairy products from D.'s diet. In less than a week he was using a letter board and saying the letters. He'd been suffering from chronic constipation, and this started to improve as well. A week after removing dairy we removed all gluten. This was much more difficult. Gluten is in everything! D. continued to show progress. Within a month of being gluten and casein free he started in a program at the elementary school called PPCD—preschool program for children with disabilities. He was the only child with dietary restrictions. He was also the only child to go on to an integrated kindergarten, followed by a "normal" first-, second-, and now third-grade class. He has received no special services since kindergarten. He has never had a one-on-one aide; he never needed it. He has not experienced 100 percent recovery, but since he's been on a GF/CF diet, enhanced with supplements, vitamins, minerals, and herbs, it's unlikely anyone would suspect he has a problem. Like any child, he occasionally has a bad moment. However, he used to be "bad" 24/7, to the point we could not go out in public with him due to his meltdowns.

His brother R., who's been diagnosed with ADHD, was five when I decided to try the diet on him. We held him in preschool for a second year because he just couldn't get the hang of the alphabet, recognize letters or settle down. Within a month of taking gluten and casein out of his diet, he was reading. With time, his behavior and sleeping habits also improved. He is still more hyper than I would like, but he is capable of learning and sitting in a classroom without disrupting it. He has never been on any meds and takes the same supplements as D.

For three years the boys also went without starches like rice, potato, corn, and cane sugar. They are back on some of them and have done all right, but they still do not do well with corn, gluten, or processed dairy. I pack two lunches and have to make special trips to stores or farms to get products they can tolerate. But they are not on mind-altering drugs that could potentially affect their growth or have other, sometimes severely negative, side effects. It would be easier and cheaper to give a single pill than what I have done, but it wouldn't have fixed their underlying biomedical problems, food intolerances, gut dysbiosis, etc. For more information, you might want to read Jenny McCarthy's book, *Louder Than Words: A Mother's Journey in Healing*. She did a very good job of presenting the issues without being too technical.

Experts on autism estimate that more than 50 percent of ASD children respond to diet and biomedical interventions, yet the average pediatrician is unlikely to mention dietary intervention. If you can find a DAN (Defeat Autism Now) doctor, he or she can help you explore all options for recovery. Some of these doctors are better than others; it is always good to ask around. Also if you can attend a DAN conference it will open your eyes to a whole new world and let you know—unfortunately—that you are not alone.

The other thing to keep in mind is that the label of "autism" is different for every kid. Each child has a unique key that will help unlock the mystery of the disorder. Diet works for a lot of kids, and the effectiveness of supplements can vary a great deal from one individual to another. We've also done chelation (getting rid of the heavy metals) with our boys, since they each had elevated levels of arsenic, mercury, tin, aluminum, and lead. They also had problems with yeast overgrowth in their guts, and the Specific Carbohydrate Diet™—no gluten and no starches—was recommended by their autism doctor. After making these changes, the boys weren't sick for years. Then, this past fall they started eating corn again and developed some respiratory issues. Once I removed the corn, their respiratory tracts cleared. Some of their food issues are allergies; others are intolerances.

I realize this is a lot of information, and at first some of it may seem "way out there." At least it did to me. I am a Certified Registered Nurse Anesthetist, and when D.'s first speech therapist suggested I take milk and wheat out of his diet when he was 20 months old, I thought she'd been in the mountains of New Hampshire too long. After all, I had a medical background; I knew what a food allergy was. I have never been so wrong in my life. Sometimes education and credentials can get in the way. I just count my blessings that, after finally reading Karyn Seroussi's book, I listened.

If your child suffers from frequent diarrhea or constipation, poor sleeping habits, or food compulsions, it's likely he or she may benefit from dietary changes. To help make these changes manageable, find Jenny McCarthy's and/or Karyn Seroussi's book, but be warned that for the first two to four weeks you may see a worsening of gastrointestinal and/or behavioral symptoms before you see significant improvements.

Asperger's Syndrome

Asperger's syndrome, one of the disorders on the autism spectrum, affects an individual's "behavior, use of language and communication, and pattern of social interactions."[22] Sarah's story shows the lengths to which a devoted and dedicated parent will go to help her child thrive. By the time Sarah's daughter, Rhilynne, was four years old, she didn't want to play with other kids and was beginning to show signs of obsessive-compulsive disorder (OCD). By the time she was nine she was out of control. When confronted with her daughter's diagnosis of Asperger's, Sarah not only poured herself into improving Rhilynne's health and avoiding the prescription drug scene, she also started a business baking delicious gluten-free delights (visit www.rsbakery.com).

I Can't Believe It's the Same Kid, by Sarah Del Soldato

Nine-year-old Rhilynne was irritable, angry, and out of control to the point the school wouldn't let her back into a regular classroom. Rhilynne was also sensitive to different textures, could not wear anything with a jeans-like feel, and had a strong sense of smell that compelled her to smell everything. When the other kids laughed it really bothered her; she knew her behavior was not normal.

After undergoing a battery of tests, she was diagnosed with Asperger's syndrome, bipolar disorder, and OCD—characterized by exhibiting tics and locking doors—and directed to a therapist who preferred natural remedies before meds, followed by a nutritionist who suggested a GFD.

If she accidentally eats gluten she is miserable and weepy for up to two weeks, and her behavior issues and tics return. In these instances, I've taught her to project herself into a sketchpad and take her mind elsewhere through art. These mind-over-matter techniques have helped her to gain control of her body and her tics and to avoid behaviors such as hissing, smelling things, and being very mean. Even without eating gluten, Rhilynne still has skin-sensitivity issues, so she lives in sweatpants or yoga pants because they don't bother her. But now that she's living a GF lifestyle and taking some herbal supplements, I can't believe she's the same kid!

Sarah also adopted a GFD. She didn't intend to give up gluten but ended up doing so because it was easier to cook family meals. After a while she noticed a positive change in her own health. Her chronic eczema disappeared, and the crippling stomach pain that often kept her awake at night was gone as well. She now "sleeps like a baby."

Kim Wilson, author of the *Everyday Wholesome Eating* series found at www.simplynaturalhealth.com, uses only whole foods when cooking for her family and in her cooking classes. Her inspiration to switch her family to a gluten-free diet came after her son responded positively to a GF lifestyle. She, too, had read Jenny McCarthy's *Louder Than Words.*

Pre-diagnosis Cleared, by Kim Wilson

Our son was about 18 months old when he was given a pre-diagnosis of Asperger's/autism. When he was about 20 months old we changed his diet cold turkey, eliminating all gluten. We were already eating whole foods and no animal products, including no dairy products. Within one week a completely non-verbal boy began making speaking sounds. Two months later he spoke his first clear words. As his "brain fog" cleared we saw him become more focused, engaging in fewer repetitive activities and being more aware of his environment. He was cleared of the Asperger's/autism diagnosis at the age of two and a half. These results were so motivating I've devoted almost exclusive attention to developing gluten-free recipes ever since.

Why is it that so many gastrointestinal maladies plague autistic children? Do they have CD, or might they have the newly recognized gluten intolerance? Do not be dissuaded if you read research that says there is not enough evidence to prove interventions like GF/CF (gluten-free/casein-free) diets work. Doors are opening for these children, but there is tremendous need for more research connecting gluten, dairy, and other substances to autism, and coaching on a GF/CF lifestyle must be very thorough. The learning curve is steep, but it is not insurmountable.

Abdominal distension, constipation, and diarrhea are symptoms found in a wide array of autistic children. Other gastrointestinal issues found in those with autism include: "inflammation (esophagitis, gastritis, duodenitis, enterocolitis)...dysbiosis with bacterial overgrowth, food intolerance or exorphin intoxication (by opioid derived from casein and gluten)."[23] Several surveys in the United States found gastrointestinal manifestations to be very common in autistic children. Respondents described issues with the colon, esophagus, intestinal permeability, liver, small intestine, and stomach,[24] a range of complaints that appear to have much in common with symptoms of CD.

In an Italian newspaper, Dr. Alessio Fasano related that "the incidence of celiac disease in these [autistic] patients is 2% while the hypersensitivity to gluten gets to 17–18%." He also states that intestinal permeability to gluten is the likely culprit for schizophrenia as well.[25] Of course, a child being screened for CD may test negative while still being gluten intolerant. For information on testing options that identify celiac disease or gluten intolerance, see Chapters 16 and 17.

In 2000, researcher Dr. Robert Cade and colleagues found autistic children had a very high concentration of IgG antibodies to gluten and casein, 87 and 90 percent respectively; 30 percent had high IgA antibody levels to both. "The presence of IgG antibodies means that gluten and casein, with their morphine-like components [that appear to affect the brain and behavior], get into the blood (where they should not be) in large amounts. ***The presence of IgA antibodies means the intestinal mucosa is sensitive to gluten or casein,"[26]*** which is perhaps the reason so many of these children have intestinal issues.

The neurotoxic effects of gluten and dairy protein, found in one 2008 study "might be explained by excessive opioid activity linked to these [gluten and casein] peptides. Research has reported abnormal levels of peptides in the urine and cerebrospinal fluid of persons with autism. If this is the case, diets free of gluten and/or casein should reduce the symptoms associated with autism." One outcome of this study found that a gluten-free and casein-free diet notably decreased the manifestations of autism.[27]

A 2009 study reported an association among autism, maternal rheumatoid arthritis, and type 1 diabetes. For the first time an important link has been detected between autism spectrum disorders and maternal CD, likely due to fetal environment, genetics, and "prenatal antibody exposure."[28] Dr. Aristo Vojdani and colleagues found some autistic patients "make antibodies against Purkinje cells [neurons in the cerebral cortex][29] and gliadin peptides." These antibodies could be causing some of the manifestations of autism.[30]

Autistic children may be affected with a newly described syndrome defined by a combination of allergies, apraxia (a movement disorder), and malabsorption. In 2009, Drs. Claudia Morris and Marilyn Agin found that coordination issues, food allergies, gastrointestinal symptoms, and low muscle tone were revealed in a group of autistic children who had high antigliadin antibodies, low carnitine, and deficiencies in vitamin D and zinc. ***All had genetic markers for gluten sensitivity.*** With supplementation these children experienced dramatic improvement in behavior, coordination, eye contact, imitation, sensory issues, speech, and development of pain sensation.[31]

One case study with an interesting title, *Celiac Disease Presenting as Autism*, tells of a five-year-old with severe autism whose "gastrointestinal symptoms rapidly resolved, and signs and symptoms suggestive of autism progressively abated" when the child was placed on a gluten-free diet. The study went on to say "…nutritional deficiency may be a determinant of developmental delay." The bottom line is this: It is vital to screen children with autism spectrum disorder issues for "nutritional deficiency and malabsorption syndromes."[32]

> ***"Out of desperation" many people are trying a gluten-free/casein-free diet as an alternative treatment for their children on the autism spectrum.[33]***

What all this means is that there is a *huge* need for more studies on the autism/gluten/casein connection. Considering the wider view of CD with its many neurological ramifications, it should be imperative to test for gluten sensitivity not just with the tTG and EMA—tests geared to recognize full-blown CD—but with the AGA: IgG and IgA antigliadin tests that may identify gluten sensitivity *before* the patient has developed celiac disease per se. Since malabsorption may be part of the process, it's also important to test for nutritional deficiencies. Knowing there is a significant learning curve to successfully implementing a GFD, it's essential to offer intense coaching on a GF/CF (gluten-free/casein-free) diet to those about to adopt one. The littlest bit of gluten can keep the disease process going; it stands to reason that the littlest bit of dairy/casein could also. (See Chapter 21 for more about dairy.)

ADD and ADHD

When Todd was building our barn he mentioned that two different schools wanted to put his daughter on Ritalin. She'd been having difficulty concentrating and focusing, her handwriting was all over the place, and she was hyperactive and not doing well in school. Irritable and always hungry, she'd also put on 10 pounds from eating too much junk food trying to "fill herself up." Todd did not consent to the use of drugs. He knew there must be a better way for his daughter. Of course, I immediately told him about the gluten factor and, being an intelligent man who wanted the best for his daughter he shared my information with her. About 18 months later, we had another conversation about his daughter, in which he said she was doing great!

Achieving Her Potential, by Todd Bartlett

"Since getting the gluten out of her diet, my daughter is performing better in school, has a more positive attitude, and has better social skills. She's also much happier. And those extra 10 pounds—well, they peeled right off. In fact, she seems 10 times healthier. For example, a bug that used to turn into a three- to four- week ordeal now lasts only a couple of days."

From the time Todd's daughter was a year old until about a year into her gluten-free/dairy-free diet, she'd used a nebulizer. She'd also used an inhaler each winter, but since getting the injurious proteins out of her diet she hasn't needed it. These days she has no health problems at all.

Perhaps, like me, you're wondering about the many millions of kids just like her—bouncing off the walls in school, unable to concentrate or sit still, dealing with asthma, bipolar disorder, allergies—and taking heavy-duty drugs so freely prescribed to control these ailments. How many of these kids might benefit from a GF lifestyle?

ADHD is a developmental disorder involving inattention and hyperactivity. One study claims it is common among undiagnosed CD patients, who, once treated with a GFD, may see their symptoms begin to disappear. This study advises that "CD should be included in the list of diseases associated with ADHD-like symptomatology."[34] Research reveals behavior and learning may be affected by diet and nutritional deficiencies, especially an omega-3 deficiency related to "behavioral food reactions" in children with ADHD.[35] In another study, **attention increased and aggression and hyperactivity markedly decreased in nearly all ADHD patients taking Mg-B6 (magnesium and vitamin B6) for two months.**[36] And a third study concluded that low ferritin levels, an indicator of iron stores, play a part in ADHD behavior, and iron supplementation (along with a GFD, if gluten sensitivity is the cause of the iron deficiency) may aid children with this condition.[37] ***Remember, never give iron without consulting a doctor; too much can be toxic.***

Drs. James Braly and Ron Hoggan, co-authors of *Dangerous Grains*, report: "About 70% of children with untreated celiac disease show exactly the same abnormalities in brain-wave patterns as those who have been diagnosed with attention deficit disorder. Another recent study, the first of its kind, reported that **food allergens, including wheat, could reproducibly cause abnormal brain waves.**" The most exciting finding of this study was that all the patients' abnormalities vanished after they followed a GFD for a year. "For these children, diet not only treats their celiac disease but also their brains and ADD."[38]

Gluten Ataxia

Ataxia is characterized as an "inability to coordinate voluntary muscular movements"[39] due to central nervous system damage, and a link between this condition and gluten has long been suspected. In 2008, Dr. Marios Hadjivassiliou and his colleagues shed light on a new form of transglutaminase (tTG) found in the brain. These "antibodies against transglutaminase 6 can serve as a marker ...to identify a subgroup of patients with gluten sensitivity who may be at risk for development of neurological disease."[40] The tTG: IgA antibodies are detected "in the gut and brain of patients with gluten ataxia with or without any enteropathy ... but not in ataxia control subjects." This finding lends credence to consideration that gluten ataxia is part of the same "spectrum as celiac disease and dermatitis herpetiformis" and that it is linked to the immune system.[41] However, as you will see in the next story, this degenerative disease, if detected early and treated with a GFD, can halt its progression and even turn around.[42] The picture of CD in the world of traditional medicine is slowly changing to embrace a much-needed, wider view of non-celiac gluten intolerance.

Gale's story below documents the potential for a rapid onset of degenerative neurological effects due to gluten sensitivity, as well as an equally rapid return to health after adopting a GF lifestyle. This incredible saga makes me wonder just how many unnecessary surgeries take place and/or how many people are wheelchair-bound or in some other way incapacitated who could be leading a normal life if they adopted a GFD. In light of the significant medical research that has been done in this area, Gale, a physician assistant, reveals great frustration at the slow pace of education among our health care professionals.

From Health to Hell and Back, by Gale Pearce, PA-C

I am a 68-year-old male who has practiced family medicine as a physician assistant for the past 35 years. In order to sustain my license I must obtain at least 100 hours of Continuing Medical Education (CME) every two years, and every six years I must pass a National Certifying Exam. To that end, I've attended multiple annual conferences at the national and local levels over the course of my career, and I've always accumulated more than enough CME hours to maintain my certification. Yet during that entire 35-year span, I rarely heard a discussion about celiac sprue, and the discussions I did hear were limited to lectures about gastrointestinal diseases in children. My daughter had major intestinal problems throughout her childhood, which made my interest in this area of medicine more acute but, still, I never had the opportunity to attend a single lecture that mentioned a more generalized form of celiac disease; or heard, in an adult, that CD caused anything other than gastrointestinal symptoms; or was privy to any discussions about the hereditary nature of the disease.

As a result, even though I am a skilled and experienced medical professional, I was totally unprepared for my own experience with celiac disease. By March of 2008 I had retired from my regular practice and was working one to two days a week at a clinic in a rather remote area of Alaska. In my free time I was in the finishing stages of building our retirement home, working rather hard physically and feeling good. In other words, I was enjoying the retirement life. True, I did have a few medical problems—slightly elevated blood pressure, controlled by medications, and mild anemia and pernicious anemia (low B12 levels), treated with monthly doses of B12. Diagnosed with polymyalgia rheumatica about eight years earlier, I also was taking a corticosteroid at low dosages of 3 to 10 mg, with an occasional burst to 30 mg for a few days when I experienced a flare-up, followed by tapering off to the lower dose. Several attempts to discontinue this medication had failed, even with extremely slow taper rates. In April of 2007 I had a rather severe bout of spondylolisthesis (a degenerative disease of the vertebrae often caused by osteoarthritis) that necessitated a spinal fusion. Once I healed from surgery, I was back to working hard on the completion of our new home.

One day in mid-March, after working a full day in the clinic, I returned home feeling tired, but no more so than usual. Prior to going to sleep that night I noted my stool was significantly darker than normal. A few hours later I awoke to use the bathroom again. This time the stool was black and I was feeling decidedly dizzy, so much so that I needed support to keep from falling. Obviously I was bleeding internally. I awakened my wife. "We need to go to the hospital," I said, as calmly as possible. It was a trip of about 50 miles over icy roads.

A little over a week later, after receiving 12 units of blood and having multiple endoscopies, a colonoscopy, and a camera endoscopy, none of which revealed the source or cause of the bleed, I was discharged. That the bleed had been somewhere in my small bowel was the only thing my doctors knew for certain.

At the time of discharge I had a lot of trouble walking with a normal gait. I felt as if I couldn't get my heels off the ground. I was very tired and could not regain my normal stamina. Because I'd lost so much blood, the doctors said it would take a while to get my strength back—approximately one week for each unit of blood I'd received. Twelve weeks came and went, however, and I was no better. I still had no strength and my gait retained its ataxic nature. I was admitted for further tests and diagnosed with normal pressure hydrocephalus (NPH).

The local neurosurgeon was convinced I needed a shunt, but he did not want to do the surgery in this rather minimally staffed hospital so he referred me to a multispecialty clinic in Seattle. The neurosurgeon there was not convinced of the NPH diagnosis. After a thorough evaluation he diagnosed me with ataxia and referred me to a neurologist to determine the source of the problem.

While in Seattle I was staying with my daughter who, four years previously, at the age of 36, had diagnosed herself as gluten intolerant. She had been unable to convince her gastroenterologist to do a complete CD panel of four blood tests, and the results of her single test came back "equivocal." So she elected to initiate a GFD on her own. Her symptoms cleared completely. When she challenged her diet with a meal containing gluten, the symptoms she'd experienced all her life, even under the intense care of a well-recommended and competent gastroenterologist, returned with renewed intensity. She went back to the GFD and her symptoms quickly resolved. Since that time she'd done a lot of incidental research on symptoms of CD and gluten intolerance.

When my daughter heard me discussing the issue of ataxia, she printed out a list of potential CD symptoms for me to review. Believe me, it was humiliating to listen to her talk about CD and its symptoms so clearly when I knew little or nothing about this disorder. After all, I was supposed to be the medical professional in the family.

I then did some research of my own. Sticking to literature from reputable medical journals and documented papers from clinics such as Mayo, Columbia Presbyterian in New York, and the Center for Celiac Disease Research at the University of Maryland, I dug as deep as I could into the symptoms of gluten sensitivity. It was all there: anemia, B12 deficiency, gastrointestinal issues, ataxia, and on and on. The literature was comprehensive and totally compelling; I was convinced I had gluten ataxia, an unusual but well-documented form of CD.

By this time I routinely walked with a cane because of my unstable gait and was on my way to being wheelchair bound. I had no time to waste trying to convince the doctors to do the appropriate tests. My daughter, who was fixing gluten-free meals for herself every day, offered to do the same for me. I started a GFD that very day, and my wife elected to do so as well so she could learn how to shop for and prepare gluten-free meals once we returned home. Three days later my ataxic gait was 90 percent better. The cane was gone completely. The next time I saw the neurologist, a little over a week after starting the GFD, I had *no evidence of ataxia* and only a little peripheral neuropathy in my toes. My energy had started to return and I felt like I had my life back. At this point the doctor ordered blood tests, but I'd already been off gluten for more than a week and the tests came back normal. [You must keep consuming gluten until you have the blood tests or the results may not be reliable. And even under ideal conditions, the tests generate a certain percentage of false negatives, which is why a growing number of people prefer stool testing to detect gluten sensitivity.]

I am now down to 3 mg/day of the corticosteroid, have been able to discontinue more than half of my medications for hypertension, and take no medications for hyperlipidemia (high cholesterol). All my tests are within normal limits without any medications, and my body aches have nearly subsided.

Based on my experiences, I am convinced CD is a very real, life-threatening, life-altering disease that can be genetically transmitted. *The largest challenge within the medical community is the lack of dissemination of CD information.* Few practitioners suspect CD as a possible cause of or contributor to numerous disorders. Still, the information is there for the taking. There is much more to learn, of course, but a huge reservoir of well-researched information already exists that is not being used by the medical profession.

For more of Gale's insights, see his encounter with contamination, *Don't Ever Go Off that GFD*, in Chapter 14; his comment on "the low level of suspicion" of CD among medical professionals in Chapter 23; read Paul's story, *The Raw Truth*, about dermatitis herpetiformis in Chapter 11; and his wife Wanda's story on type 2 diabetes, *Return to Normal*, in Chapter 10.

The outstanding research on gluten ataxia by Dr. Marios Hadjivassiliou and his team has helped to establish a link between this neurological ailment and gluten, but in our pharmaceutically dominated culture, so much more research needs to be done.

"Ataxia and peripheral neuropathy are the most common neurological manifestations of gluten sensitivity."[43]

Gluten ataxia represents up to 40 percent of idiopathic (unknown cause) sporadic ataxia, so patients with this disorder should be screened with anti-gliadin antibody (AGA) testing as soon as possible after diagnosis. Those who test positive may experience a reduction in symptoms by following a GFD.[44] Atrophy of the brain, dysarthria (speech disorder), ocular (eye) issues, and neuropathy, along with upper- and lower-limb ataxia, were found in a highly significant number of patients with gluten ataxia. Gait (walking) ataxia was discovered in *all* patients, but only a small percentage (13%) had intestinal issues.[45] A 2001 German study found bladder dysfunction, deep sensory loss, and reduced ankle reflexes were also significant features of sporadic ataxia.[46]

A 2008 study claimed it is critical to give the antigliadin antibody (AGA) test to patients with idiopathic ataxia, because a highly significant number of CD patients do not have gastrointestinal symptoms and thus will remain undiagnosed if only the tTG and EMA are given. The study also stated that for those found to be gluten sensitive, a GFD may lead to "complete resolution of neurological symptoms."[47]

Neuropathy

Peripheral neuropathy is damage to the nerves of the limbs and organs causing numbness, pain, tingling, muscle cramps, and/or weakness. It may lead to bladder dysfunction, constipation, digestive problems, heartburn, perspiration issues, sexual dysfunction, and more.[48]

I met Tamsin, who tells her story below, at the 12th International Celiac Disease Symposium in New York City in 2006. Until receiving a diagnosis of CD, she'd suffered for years with a variety of neurological issues; then she developed pancreatitis. (See more on pancreatitis in Chapter 10.)

Neurological Manifestation of Celiac Disease, by Tamsin V. Metzler

There are many faces of celiac disease. Mine was in disguise from the time I was a baby until I was 35. At the age of nine months I was introduced to Cheerios, an oat cereal, which caused a reaction that made my skin itch, weep, and ooze. From then on I continued to have issues with oats, as well as with wheat, rye, and barley.

Years ago, celiac was considered a "wasting-away disease"; if you didn't look malnourished or have typical gut manifestations, the doctors didn't pursue it as a diagnosis. Since I didn't have these symptoms, my parents and the pediatrician thought I had an allergy to the offending foods. At the age of 18 months I had a combination of chicken pox and a viral infection. Afterward I developed cerebellum ataxia and lost all motor control. I could no longer stand, walk, or sit up. Fortunately, the motor function returned, leaving me with moderate balance issues, but because I was mostly better, no further testing was done.

At the age of 34 I experienced peripheral neuropathies, paresthesias, hives, and shock-like feelings going up and down my arms whenever I ingested gluten. This frightening occurrence led me to a neurologist to rule out MS. My symptoms certainly suggested MS, but after a spinal tap and other tests, the doctor thought I might have a neurological manifestation of celiac disease. Fortunately this neurologist knew about the connection between cerebellum ataxia and CD.

I immediately started on a GFD, and my neurological symptoms went away. Three years later I developed autoimmune pancreatitis, which resulted in the removal of two inches from my pancreas. I am now participating in a research study that is examining the link between pancreatic issues and CD.

Looking back, I realize that many of the physical problems I've experienced over the course of my life might have pointed the way to testing and a much earlier diagnosis of CD, but doctors were just not aware of the potential connections. Massive migraines, osteopenia diagnosed at age 34, reflux, short stature, severe joint pain in my hands and knees, hives at my joint sites, and itchy, swollen feet, hands, and lips are just a few of the symptoms I've experienced, and every one of them can be an indicator of gluten sensitivity.

My daughter, Mackenzie, was diagnosed with celiac disease in the second grade, a year after a mononucleosis infection. Her only symptoms were anemia, occasional knee pain, on-and-off constipation, and slight eczema when she ate wheat or graham crackers. Because she was diagnosed at an early age, she will hopefully be able to avoid a lifetime of illness and decrease her chances of developing other autoimmune conditions.

Today the average person with CD is sick for about 11 years before receiving an accurate diagnosis. It is my fervent hope that awareness of gluten sensitivity in the general public and, most especially, in the medical community, will someday reduce or eliminate this agonizing wait so people can begin to heal.

CD wears many masks and thus must be assessed in patients with attention/memory loss, cerebellar ataxia, epilepsy, and peripheral neuropathy.[49] I wonder just how many folks with any form of neuropathy would test positive for gluten sensitivity. That seems like an easy study to do. Who knows, maybe the neuropathy associated with diabetes is really associated with gluten. My burning feet disappeared after being on a GFD for just a few weeks. A young artist I met had tingling and numbness in her fingers, toes, and the middle of her upper lip. Her symptoms disappeared in a few days after being on the GFD.

Neurologic issues—neuropathy and ataxia being the most common—are expressed in about 10 percent of CD patients,[50] with axonal sensorimotor neuropathy being the most prevalent neuropathy type. Dr. Hadjivassiliou and his team recently observed that 11 of 15 participants with sensory ganglionopathy stabilized on a GFD. (The other four did not comply well with the diet).[51]

Another study by Dr. Norman Latov, director of the Peripheral Neuropathy Center at Cornell University, claims that "**20–25% of the people with CD might have neuropathy.**" Both deficiencies of vitamins B1, B6, B12, and E, as well as autoimmune mechanisms, may lead to neuropathies and can be attributed to CD.[52]

Dr. Scot Lewey, a board-certified gastroenterologist and specialist in digestive diseases, states that, "the symptoms of neuropathy are paresthesia (numbness) or dysthesia (burning, tingling, heaviness, 'pins and needles' sensation)." He also refers to skin hypersensitivity and a "bug-crawling" feeling.[53]

A GFD brought substantial recovery for two CD patients who suffered from "progressive weakness of the limbs … and [other] neurophysiological abnormalities …" This 2007 Italian study stressed that patients with neuropathy of unknown cause should be screened for CD even if they have no gastrointestinal complaints.[54] Perhaps any patient with neuropathy should be screened for the wider view of gluten sensitivity as well.

Multiple Sclerosis

MS is an autoimmune disease caused by damage to the myelin sheath that surrounds the neurons. It can affect balance, bodily functions, coordination, sensation, strength, vision, and more.[55] There is no known cure, or so they say.

Ilana is a chiropractor and the daughter of an old friend. When I heard she was having MS-like symptoms, I immediately contacted her and encouraged her to get tested for CD/GI. Through the EnteroLab stool test she found she was intolerant to gluten, soy, and yeast. Eliminating these proteins along with dairy totally changed her life. It is thrilling to have a medical practitioner respond with such a strong story. "I really feel like this path has been carved out for me for a reason," Ilana wrote to me, "and I'm thankful I can help educate people every day about it. I'm so glad you're writing this book."

A Bend in the Road, by Ilana Goldberg, DC

When I was 29 years old and caring for my mother during her battle with terminal cancer, I noticed a weakness in my legs, sometimes so severe that I couldn't go down a flight of stairs without grasping tightly to the railing. I had always enjoyed running as exercise; now I couldn't walk more than 15 minutes without my legs becoming exhausted. At the time I attributed the symptoms to stress and de-conditioning. My daughter was born a year later and shortly after I began to experience another odd symptom: The vision in my right eye would become blurry, especially after exercise. As a chiropractor, I knew that a neurological symptom worsening with heat could be MS, but I dismissed it as impossible. No one in my family had MS, lupus, or any other autoimmune disease.

When my vision hadn't improved after three months—in fact, it had gotten worse—I asked a neurologist friend to send me for the MRI. The results showed "patches of demyelination in the brain, clinically correlated with MS." As a new nursing mother and a practitioner devoted to holistic care, I wanted to look into alternatives to the standard treatments of steroids and injection interferon drugs. In my research I kept coming across evidence of food sensitivities linked to MS, most often gluten, dairy, legumes, eggs, and yeast. After an ELISA (enzyme-linked immunosorbent assay) blood test used to detect antibodies showed I was sensitive to dairy, I began my elimination diet. However, it wasn't until a few months later that I finally did the stool test for food sensitivity through EnteroLab.

While gluten sensitivity had not shown up on my blood test, gluten, eggs, and soy did show up on the stool test. When I cut out the dairy I had begun to feel slightly stronger and more coordinated. Once I eliminated gluten I saw even more improvement. Finally I removed all grains (even rice) and really started to feel stronger. It has been a long process of healing but an amazing journey. Since then I have devoted my practice to the treatment of chronic disease through nutrition and holistic treatments.

I now put virtually all of my patients on a grain-free, dairy-free diet, and the change in their health is dramatic. Joint pain disappears, excess weight falls off, digestion troubles cease, blood sugar and blood pressure stabilize, neuropathies improve, and there is an overall balancing of the endocrine system including estrogen, thyroid, liver, and adrenal issues. I believe gluten sensitivity is very widespread, which is part of the reason the standard American diet does so little to prevent chronic diseases.

A vitamin B12 deficiency appears to play a role in MS, and if your vitamin B levels are low it could be due to CD-caused malabsorption. Research for maladies such as MS, Lou Gehrig's (amyotrophic lateral sclerosis or ALS), Huntington's (HD), Alzheimer's, and other neurodegenerative diseases in connection with gluten is very scarce and much more is needed. What's holding things up? Pharmaceutical companies conduct thousands of studies on drugs. Where are the GFD-related studies? Why not recruit 1,000 people with newly diagnosed MS or Parkinson's, etc., test them for antigliadin and tTG antibodies and, if the results are positive, put them on a strict GFD? And at the same time, test them for dairy antibodies and measure their vitamin B levels, since many neurological issues seem to be associated with these issues. It's true there are some studies in progress, but I expect I'll be long gone before the numerous gluten-associated ailments covered in this book are seriously addressed on a large scale in the United States. *And I plan on living to a ripe old age!*

In one 2010 study, a 29-year-old woman with MS who adhered to a GFD saw her antibodies and villi return to normal. Her brain and spinal lesions decreased, her symptoms disappeared, and she had a normal neurological follow-up.[56] Of course, it's always possible her original diagnosis was incorrect. Until enough studies have been done to prove an irrefutable link between gluten and MS, we can't know for sure. What we do know, at least in this woman's case, is she got better, and she did so by making changes in her life that—even if they hadn't worked—could do her no harm. Looking at it this way, a GFD seems like a fairly easy choice when faced with the alternative of deteriorating health for the rest of one's life.

A Norwegian study showed a notable elevation in antigliadin antibodies in MS patients compared to the controls. There was also a significant increase in casein antibodies, yet the EMA and tTG results for these patients were negative.[57] Along with elevated AGA: IgG, a high level of tTG: IgG antibodies has been found in MS patients, and those with gluten antibodies should consider a GFD.[58] Another study found that high levels of homocysteine were linked to MS.[59]

Inflammatory and degenerative neurological features are found in patients with MS *and* in patients who are vitamin B12 deficient. Distinguishing between the two may not be easy. Vitamin B12 functions in the formation of myelin, and low B12 levels have been found in MS patients. It appears there may be a causal role between low B12 and the development of MS.[60] In a 1993 study, researchers claimed that "since vitamin B12 is required for the formation of myelin and for immune mechanisms, we propose that its deficiency in MS is of critical pathogenic significance."[61]

I recently met a young woman with MS who was being wheeled through a home show by her husband, accompanied by her mother." The husband was "all ears" as I talked about gluten and MS. The mother excitedly mentioned another daughter who had recently adopted a GFD and whose issues were all clearing up. I asked the young woman if either of her neurologists had ever suggested testing to see if she was gluten sensitive. I don't need to tell you the answer. It's the reason I'm writing this book.

Alzheimer's, Huntington's, Parkinson's, and Amyotrophic Lateral Sclerosis

A 2010 study suggests that tTG found in the brains of patients may be linked to Alzheimer's, Huntington's, Parkinson's, supranuclear palsy, and other degenerative neurological diseases. In fact, researchers postulate that tTG activity could be the root cause of these debilitating diseases.[62] Another study found a "high prevalence of gluten sensitivity in genetic neurodegenerative disorders such as hereditary spinocerebellar ataxia and Huntington's disease." A wider range, not involving the intestines, may include brain stem dysfunction, chorea, encephalopathy, Guillain-Barre-like syndrome, migraine, mononeuritis multiplex myelopathy, and "neuropathy with positive antiganglioside antibodies."[63] A 2004 study detected that nearly half of the Huntington's patients had high antigliadin antibodies.[64] And two other studies report the ratio of antibodies to tissue transglutaminase may be high in patients with Huntington's[65] and Parkinson's.[66]

A very recent study of a young man exhibiting "progressive neurologic symptoms and brain MR [magnetic resonance] imaging findings," both of which may be indicative of ALS, showed improvement when he was placed on a GFD.[67] In a United Kingdom study, "celiac disease with neurological involvement, mimicking amyotrophic lateral sclerosis" was revealed in a 44-year-old male. "Management: Strict gluten-free diet."[68] Patients suffering from these debilitating diseases may want to test for dairy intolerance as well.

A rather complex abstract finds—among other factors—that vitamins B, E, and K, along with several minerals, are needed to keep the mitochondria ("the power plant of a cell" that contains enzymes needed for cell activity)[69] healthy and energized. This paper suggests that Alzheimer's and other dementias, ALS, Down syndrome, Friedreich's ataxia, MS, Parkinson's, strokes, and even aging can result from deficiencies within the cell.[70] Of course, more work is needed to determine exactly how cells break down and what can be done in terms of prevention, but one thing is certain: Your cells will not be happy if they are starved for vital nutrients because your body is malabsorbing.

Seizures

I know several people diagnosed with seizures whose neurologists never mentioned testing for CD or non-celiac gluten intolerance (GI). The connection between gluten and seizures has been known by researchers for over four decades, but somehow the information is just not getting to our doctors. This lack of education in the medical community surely keeps a lot of people deep in the depths of degenerative disorders and debilitating, chronic illness.

If you or someone you love is having seizures, tics, foot drag or, for that matter, almost any neurological issue, go out on a limb and ask to be tested for gluten sensitivity. Even if your doctor agrees, however *do not assume you will receive sufficient testing.* Be sure to take the blood testing information in Chapter 16 with you and compare it to the lab CD panel before the tests. Better yet, discuss with your doctor what tests he or she is ordering. If you have the four recommended blood tests and they are all negative, you then might want to consider stool testing (described in Chapter 17). Stool testing is more effective in detecting gluten sensitivity, since the antigliadin antibodies are produced in the intestine and show up in the stool before they ever get into the blood.[71] Many gluten-sensitive people do not test positive for full-blown CD but still may have serious neurological or other issues linked to gluten.

A 2010 study relates the case of three young girls with unmanageable seizures who exhibited low blood calcium (signs of anemia and osteomalacia) and who were diagnosed with CD. The bottom line: Low blood calcium caused by CD and resulting in seizures must be treated not just with vitamin D and calcium supplements but also with a GFD.[72]

Gluten has been newly associated in temporal lobe epilepsy with hippocampal sclerosis (HS), a hardening of tissue in the hippocampus region of the brain.[73] Thus, gluten sensitivity also should be considered in the process of finding the underlying cause of HS.[74]

The case of a young woman with difficult-to-treat seizures who responded remarkably to a GFD speaks to the importance of including CD screening in the differential diagnosis of patients with refractory epilepsy. This study notes "there is a well-documented relationship between epilepsy, occipital calcifications, and celiac disease."[75] Perhaps this information *is* well documented, but who knows about it? Which Ivy League schools are covering this connection in their courses on neurology or medical curricula? One doctor I talked with said med schools would never teach about CD/GI because there is just too much to it. Instead, he believed doctors would get this kind of training during their residencies. Maybe so, but do enough medical instructors know about the newfound connections between gluten and a wide variety of symptoms?

A Spanish study concluded that even without intestinal symptoms it is crucial to screen for CD "in patients with epilepsy and occipital cerebral calcifications."[76] Children with incorrigible seizures and weight loss should also be tested for CD.[77] Blurred vision, loss of focus, seeing colored dots, and visual hallucinations were some of the visual symptoms reported.[78]

The bottom line of one 2001 study states that **"CD should be suggested as a differential diagnosis in children with unclear white-matter [brain] lesions even without intestinal symptoms."**[79] Posterior cerebral calcifications and epilepsy also should be a red flag to screen for CD.[80] The effectiveness of a GFD appears to be "inversely related to the duration of epilepsy and the young age of the patient" (an excellent reason why children with seizures should be assessed for gluten sensitivity *as quickly as possible*). Folic-acid deficiency resulting from untreated CD may be the possible root cause of the calcifications.[81]

Neuromuscular Issues

A six-month-old child with a movement disorder that looked like paroxysmal nonkinesigenic dyskinesia (PNKD), "an episodic movement disorder" that affects muscles and nerves,[82] exhibited a full turnaround in neurological symptoms after being diagnosed with CD and placed on a GFD.[83] Chorea, another involuntary-movement disorder,[84] has also been linked to gluten. In a study of four patients with chorea, their motor issues were greatly enhanced after they began following a GFD.[85]

Research specialist Dr. Hadjivassiliou and colleagues state that, in one study, "neurological symptoms antedated the diagnosis of coeliac disease in all [study participants], and most had minimal or no gastrointestinal symptoms at the onset of the neuromuscular disorder." CD may be accompanied by a broad array of neuromuscular conditions such as inclusion body myositis (IBM), neuromyotonia, polymyositis, and various types of neuropathy. **The bottom line: It is very important to screen for antigliadin antibodies (AGA) in patients with a neuromuscular disease of unknown cause.**[86]

A link between CD and Becker muscular dystrophy (a genetic disorder with progressive muscle weakness of the legs and pelvis) was made a decade and a half ago. A nine-year-old boy who suffered from diarrhea, growth issues, and iron deficiency anemia was diagnosed with CD. Acute rhabdomyolysis (damage to skeletal muscles, which can lead to kidney damage)[87] landed him in the hospital, and for some time prior to diagnosis he had high serum creatine kinase levels,[88] which are often an indicator of muscle damage.

A 1995 study concluded that **all patients exhibiting signs of "progressive myoclonic ataxic syndrome" (twitching of muscles and loss of coordination) should be screened for CD.**[89]

Myoclonic Jerks—Tics

Joan is a young mother who reached me through my website, www.x-gluten.com. When I asked if she would be willing to share her son's success story, she said she'd be happy to do so, since she'd found so little helpful information through the medical community.

Wrongly Diagnosed with Tourette Syndrome, by Joan

My eight-year-old son, who had exhibited ADHD symptoms and had difficulty focusing, had massive digestive struggles. He was also getting red cheeks and myoclonic jerks (involuntary muscle twitches and sudden movements), along with worsening nasal allergies and lots of sniffling. And he tested positive on a nasal swab for a Bipolaris mold in his nose. His doctor, however, dismissed these peripheral symptoms and diagnosed him with Tourette syndrome.

Now that he is on a gluten-free/casein-free diet, all of these issues except his ADHD symptoms and lack of focus have completely cleared up. I am hopeful, in time, being CF/GF will remedy these issues as well.

"Rag Doll" Fatigue, Leg Drag, Eye Droop, and Lots More

I came to know Cara through her incredible website, www.theglutenfile.com, which reports the most recent research by the most forward-thinking doctors in the realm of gluten sensitivity. Research updates can also be found on Facebook under The Gluten File.

Cara's daughter's story (adapted with permission from information on Cara's website) clearly illustrates a wide array of gluten-sensitivity symptoms, even though her daughter did not test positive for CD on the traditional tTG blood test. She was a weak positive on the antigliadin antibody test, which is now being recognized for identifying non-celiac gluten intolerance. In the past, such a reading was often ignored; today it would likely signal one is sensitive to gluten. As you probably know if you've read this far, many people with neurological maladies (and numerous other ailments) may not test positive on the more traditional tTG and EMA tests, yet numerous signs and symptoms can point to the degenerative, elusive damage done by gluten.

Lesson Learned: Don't Wait—Just Do It! by Cara

J., my youngest daughter, started having diarrhea rather abruptly around age three—bright fluorescent green, foul-smelling, explosive episodes several times a day. The doctor suggested her problem might be rotavirus and, if so, it would have to run its course. It was a mighty long course. Months passed, but I was told intestinal viruses often take months to clear and I should be patient. More months passed, and we were told to try eliminating milk (which helped some) and then to eliminate juices (which she didn't drink). Whatever was going on with my daughter wasn't setting off any bells or whistles in the doctor's office.

Explosive diarrhea, as frequently as five or six times a day, became the norm for over a year. Family life changed, as we were confined to activities within minutes of a toilet. My daughter's happy-go-lucky nature soured. She had dark purple circles under her eyes. Over a two-year-period her weight dropped from the 75th percentile to the 25th percentile but nobody really noticed, even me.

Eventually she developed rough, red rashes on her hands that extended up her wrists. She had a recurring illness that included a mosquito-bite-like rash, usually accompanied by vomiting and low-grade fever. She began having fleeting neurological or neuromuscular episodes that included mild leg drag, staggering, drooping eyelid, lazy eye, and periods of limp-body, "rag-doll" fatigue. She had a couple episodes each of slurred speech, difficulty swallowing, and loss of bladder control. Initially, I'd observed something worrisome about once a month. Later, I began seeing disturbing symptoms weekly or daily.

My daughter's issues were obviously upsetting, but I wasn't a complete novice to the world of neurology. After three years of bizarre neurological and other wide-ranging complaints, I'd recently been diagnosed with a B12 deficiency.

My first thought was that J. might be having seizures. I discussed the symptoms with our neurologist, and we agreed I would keep a close watch on her, waiting for a "bigger" sign. I was in no hurry to put her through an EEG, and I dreaded having to give her potent antiseizure medication unless it became absolutely necessary.

One day nearly two years after the onset of her diarrhea, I took J. for a routine "well-child" checkup. Our appointment happened to be with a different doctor in the pediatric group, and when I lamented J.'s continuing daily episodes of diarrhea, this doctor took serious note. "That's not right!" she exclaimed. She referred us to a gastroenterologist, a step I should have taken on my own much sooner. Lesson learned: Don't wait for your doctor to suggest a referral to a specialist. Just do it.

The gastroenterologist considered celiac disease as a distinct possibility. It was the first time I had ever heard of it. She asked about our family medical history, which happens to include a very high prevalence of autoimmune thyroid disease—me, my father, both of my siblings, my grandparents, and other relatives. I also mentioned my recent diagnosis of B12 deficiency, presumably caused by pernicious anemia.

The doctor discussed the need for further tests. I went home and searched celiac disease. Based on what I read in online publications from the American Academy of Family Physicians, so many things fit. I knew we might be on to something.

J. underwent several diagnostic tests, including tests for celiac. She was negative for anti-tTG but positive for antigliadin IgG, and an IgA deficiency had not been ruled out. Based on her test results, the doctor felt it was unlikely J. had celiac disease but recommended proceeding to a biopsy anyway, since there was a weak possibility she did.

After careful consideration and discussion with one of the pediatricians, we opted to skip the biopsy. We realized J.'s blood results were a weak indicator that a biopsy would reveal damage. And while intestinal biopsies are a relatively safe procedure, they are not without risk. From my reading, I also knew that several medical experts in the field believed there was a possibility gluten sensitivity could manifest neurologically without showing *any* gut damage on a biopsy. For these reasons, we opted for a GFD trial. J. was five years old.

Within a week we saw a significant reduction in the frequency of her diarrhea. Five or six daily episodes dropped down to one or two. Eventually the diarrhea stopped altogether, although even today occasional loose stools are not uncommon due to additional food sensitivities. Her neurological symptoms were never diagnosed, but over several months they completely resolved themselves and have never returned. My guess is they were closer to gluten ataxia than seizures. (She's also had no further episodes of the mysterious "rash-and-vomit" illness.)

Over time J.'s happy-go-lucky demeanor returned. Her general health improved. She had strep throat four times the year before going gluten free. In the years since she's had it only once. School absences due to illness dropped considerably. She stopped visiting the school nurse every afternoon after lunch, something I was not even aware she'd been doing. Ultimately we discovered she had problems with other foods, most notably dairy and corn. As of this writing J. has been on a GFD for eleven years; she also avoids all major sources of dairy but can tolerate corn on occasion. And we have the total support of her pediatrician, who believes gluten was the culprit despite the lack of a concrete diagnosis.

Read Cara's comments in Chapter 23 regarding the challenges for diagnosis and treatment of nutritional issues within our health care system.

Schizophrenia

Schizophrenia, "one of the top 10 causes of disability worldwide," affects approximately one percent of the population at a huge expense to mankind, and many researchers are actively working on identifying causes and finding a cure. The first of four studies executed at John's Hopkins University referenced here found a subset of patients with this disorder experienced a substantial reduction of symptoms and, in some cases, a full recovery when following a GFD.[90] The most recent, in 2011, found that even though CD and schizophrenia have nearly the same prevalence in the general population, CD is more common among those with schizophrenia, who have "higher than expected titers of antibodies related to CD and gluten sensitivity."[91] Patients with "multi-episode schizophrenia had significantly increased levels of IgG antibodies to gliadin...." Compared to controls, increased levels were also found in those with recent-onset psychosis. The study concluded that these two conditions "may share some immunologic features of celiac disease, but their immune response to gliadin differs from that of celiac disease."[92] The last study found patients with "a history of any autoimmune disease" have a 45 percent greater chance of developing schizophrenia.[93] Here's yet another instance where large-scale studies are sorely needed.

In 1984, Dr. F. Curtis Dohan and colleagues found that "grain glutens are harmful to schizophrenics."[94] Dr. Dohan suggested that the opioid peptides of gluten and very likely the dairy protein casein could "go from gut to brain and cause symptoms of schizophrenia." As expected, he found gluten-free diets had a crucial effect on patients with schizophrenia and that "where grains and milk are rare," so is schizophrenia.[95] As far back as 1976, patients were found to reverse their schizophrenic symptoms on a grain-free diet.[96]

In a case study of schizophrenic patients, IgG antibodies to gliadin and casein were found to be 86 and 90 percent, respectively, and IgA antibodies to gliadin and casein were 86 and 67 percent, respectively. All five of the patients given a chance for dialysis along with a GFD showed notable improvement or a return to wellness. Interestingly, nearly 40 percent of the patients given dialysis only with no changes to their diet also became well or revealed noteworthy amelioration.[97] (During dialysis, the blood is cleansed of gluten and casein peptides.)

It is studies like these that have led researchers to conclude that the ***"resolution of longstanding schizophrenic symptoms" attributed to a GFD results from changes on the cellular level.***[98]

I met M. while traveling west. She shared with me that her daughter, who'd been diagnosed with schizophrenia, had had tremendous success with a GFD. As her psychotic symptoms subsided on the GFD—they would reappear within 30 minutes of accidental gluten ingestion—M., who is a huge asset to the gluten-free community, came to know the real child. Eventually her daughter no longer needed psychotropic drugs, and today she is doing well. ***Caution: Never adjust the dosage or stop taking any drug without consulting your doctor. Doctors knowledgeable about the role of gluten in neurological symptoms are of great value when dealing with issues of this type.***

This mother's willingness to explore solutions beyond conventional treatments drastically changed her daughter's life. The sheer belief so many have in the god-like role of traditional medicine continues to amaze me, especially when a simple change in diet could be the answer.

An Old Friend

I first read about schizophrenia being connected to gluten in Danna Korn's *Wheat-Free, Worry-Free*. The book went on to describe studies that showed that schizophrenic symptoms subsided on a gluten-free diet. I immediately put the book down and called an old and dear friend. One of her brothers, now deceased, had suffered from the mental anguish of schizophrenia for decades, and her son had committed suicide a few years earlier due to a difficult schizophrenic teenage life. When I told her what I'd been reading she said, "Annie, my mother was very sensitive to wheat and diagnosed herself as having celiac disease." Does this mean my friend's brother and son may also have had CD? Sadly, we'll never know.

I then had a flashback to the same friend's younger brother, who had died of leukemia at age 12. My wheels started to spin. From all the reading I'd done, I knew gluten was associated with many blood disorders and that it could cause osteoporosis, osteopenia, and other degenerative bone ailments. I also knew bone and blood were intimately connected. Is it possible that multiple vitamin deficiencies due to malabsorption caused by gluten sensitivity could compromise one's immune system to the point where it is less able to fight against cancer, invasive viruses, etc. I doubt I'll see answers in my lifetime, but the words leukemia, lymphoproliferative disorder, tumor, and other cancer-related terms are cropping up in CD studies. (See Chapter 13 for more information about possible links between CD and cancer.)

Do I want to corral a group of parents with children suffering from leukemia—and their doctors? Yes. Do I have that kind of energy? No. Would they pay any attention to me? Definitely not! Why? Because most parents expect the doctor to know about any possible issue related to their child's illness. If only this were the case. The human body is an intricate, multifaceted machine, and no matter how well-educated or experienced, every skilled medical professional will continue to expand his or her knowledge over the course of a career.

In today's world of specialization, many medical professionals operate in their own small sphere of influence, with doctors at one end of the continuum and researchers at the other. In the middle there appears to be a huge lack of crossover about what is really making some people sick. No one can know it all, and if your doctor doesn't know enough to even *suspect* gluten sensitivity, then you certainly aren't going to get tested. Even if you are tested, you may not receive *enough testing* to get to the bottom of the problem. This is why it's important for each of us to be his or her own advocate, working in partnership with doctors to be certain we get the very best care available.

Depression

What Bridget describes in her story below may well have been the weight of depression, with highs and lows caused by the neurotoxic effects of gluten and dairy on the brain and central nervous system.

Nothing Short of a Miracle, by Bridget Skjordahl

A few months after adopting a gluten-free diet, I happened to catch an episode of "The Oprah Winfrey Show" on which Jenny McCarthy was a guest. They were talking about autism and a gluten-free/casein-free diet. As they described the signs of autism, it was all horrifyingly familiar. *The only difference between these children and me, I thought, is that I have 40 years of rote/learned behavior to fall back on when I must engage in social interactions.* I realized after watching the program that part of what distinguished a "good" day for me (fewer symptoms) from a "bad" day was the level of my desire to engage socially. Engagement on a "bad" day, though painfully difficult, was often required of me in my business. On good days, such interaction was effortless and pleasurable.

I never knew when the good days would hit, or how long they would last. When I had a day where I really felt sociable, I often felt compelled to get in touch with everyone I'd been avoiding since my last good day, sometimes people I hadn't been able to bring myself to contact in months or years. I would set up lunch and coffee meetings to catch up, only to have the day of a scheduled meeting dawn as a "bad" day. When such a day hit I often couldn't bring myself to get showered and dressed, let alone leave the house. I cancelled a lot of lunch and coffee dates at the last minute.

In light of my experience, Jenny's explanation of the effects of gluten and casein on those with autism made a lot of sense. I decided to start eliminating casein from my diet. Within a week I began to see a dramatic improvement in my neurological symptoms, along with a degree of mental clarity I hadn't felt since I'd been in a severe car accident in 1992. It was nothing short of a miracle, and another answer to my prayers.

I continued to see improvement in my health, and after about eight months I felt as if I'd finally turned the corner.

For Bridget's story about her accident and the resulting changes in her health, see *A Healing Journey* in Chapter 6. Also see her story, *Living Well without Gluten and Dairy* in Chapter 19.

A 2010 German study reports that "interestingly, **35% of [the] patients with CD reported of a history of psychiatric disease including depression, personality changes, or even psychosis.**" Twenty-eight percent suffered from migraines.[99] The research described below relates to depression as well as to bipolar, behavioral, and panic disorders and makes a connection to irritable bowel disorder. The gut and brain are intimately interwoven, and both are highly susceptible to devastating affects of gluten sensitivity.

The 2009 clinical guideline from the National Institute for Health and Clinical Excellence in the United Kingdom suggests screening patients with depression and bipolar disorder for CD.[100] Patients with CD who participated in an Italian study expressed notably increased manifestations of dysthymia (depression), headaches, and symptoms of peripheral neuropathy on an unrestricted diet than the control group. Sticking to a GFD can help reduce many neurological symptoms.[101]

In a group of 29 adolescents with CD, nearly a third exhibited major depressive disorder and more than a fourth had a disruptive behavior disorder compared to controls.[102] Children with CD may exhibit behavior disorders due to "significantly decreased plasma concentrations of tryptophan" that may affect serotonin levels.[103] The occurrence of panic disorder and major depressive disorder is also increased among CD patients,[104] and among children with demyelinating disease, "depressive and anxiety disorders are common."[105] Since these types of issues may resolve fairly quickly on a GFD for those who are gluten sensitive, **patients with "behavioral and depressive disorders" should be screened for CD.**[106]

Researchers estimate that between 10 and 20 percent of the U.S. adult population has irritable bowel syndrome (IBS), and IBS appears to be linked to gluten (see Chapter 7 for more about this connection). Between 70 and 90 percent of IBS patients seeking medical care also suffer from anxiety and mood disorders. Patients with major depression, panic disorder, and schizophrenia also reveal a high prevalence of IBS.[107] Other disorders frequently accompanied by IBS include post-traumatic stress disorder (PTSD) and social phobia.[108] Nailing down every nuance of cause and effect between gluten and numerous psychiatric maladies will continue to be a convoluted undertaking, but the effects of gluten on many sufferers of these illnesses seems straightforward enough to warrant serious and continued consideration by the medical profession and patients alike.

When one study found a combination of high levels of homocysteine and low levels of vitamins B9 (folate) and B12 to be linked to depression, the study concluded with a recommendation for supplementation with these B vitamins.[109] Could gluten be playing a part here as well?

A 2003 study "recommend[s] consideration of B12 deficiency...in all patients with organic mental disorders, atypical psychiatric symptoms and fluctuation of symptomatology. B12 levels should be evaluated with treatment resistant depressive disorders, dementia, psychosis or risk factors for malnutrition such as alcoholism or advancing age associated with neurological symptoms, anemia, malabsorption,..." Such recommendations are admirable, but aside from alcoholism, gastrointestinal surgery, parasitic infection, and/or a strict vegetarian diet, what is *causing* B12 deficiency?[110] Fifteen percent of elderly folks have a B12 deficiency.[111] How many of them are malabsorbing due to the gluten in "healthy" whole wheat?

Even though the Italians are way ahead of the U.S. in CD research (and detection), a 2001 Italian study by G. Addolorato and his team stated: "At present, the role of a gluten-free diet (GFD) on psychological disorders is still poorly known."[112] More than a decade later, the psychological impact of gluten continues to be "poorly known" among many U.S. neurologists, primary care physicians, and other health care professionals. If this were not the case, imagine this "a-b-c" scenario—and the implications it could have on improving patient outcomes and reducing health care costs:

a. Having psychological problems? Gee, let's check your vitamin B12 level.

b. Oh, you have a B12 deficiency. Let's screen you for CD/GI.

c. Oh, you are gluten sensitive. Try eating a 100 percent GFD and see if you improve.

I grant you, it's not as good for big pharma's bottom line as "Here are three prescriptions. Let me know if you're having any deleterious side effects," but it sure seems worth a try.

Migraines, Headaches, Tics, and Restless Legs Syndrome

When her son's tests for gluten sensitivity were inconclusive, this mom followed her instincts. Then she wrote a book, *Bagels, Buddy, and Me* (www.bagelsbuddyandme.com), to help explain celiac disease to children.

Even the Dog, by Melanie Krumrey

About five years ago my middle son, Cooper, began having chronic headaches. They worsened over the course of a year, and instead of just having them every night at bedtime, he began having them all day and sometimes waking up in pain with them at night. He also complained of stomachaches, developed nervous tics (eye-blinking, chewing on clothing and fingernails), and had some sensory issues: gripping things, floppy body, and occasional clumsiness. He complained of fuzzy vision, had circles under his eyes, and began to look sort of grey. "Mom, I don't feel good," he'd say, again and again. The doctor ordered an MRI to check for a tumor. Fortunately, none was found. The pediatric neurologist (a doctor with a very big ego) diagnosed Cooper with migraines and Tourette syndrome. I just knew that wasn't the problem, but we tried the migraine diet of no nuts, chocolate, strawberries, cheese, etc. Nothing changed.

Then a friend mentioned celiac disease. Her son was in the process of being diagnosed and our boys had a lot of similar symptoms. I got online and did some research, then asked my pediatrician to do a blood test. He said he doubted this was my son's problem, but he didn't mind testing. Cooper's results showed he is IgA deficient. Unfortunately, this deficiency throws the results of other testing off, so the overall test results were inconclusive. His endoscopy was also negative. One antibody, however, was elevated enough to convince me to try him on a GFD. After two weeks of being gluten free, his symptoms were almost completely gone.

As I did more research I realized I, too, had common symptoms of gluten sensitivity—fatigue, restless legs syndrome, diarrhea, bloating, indigestion, and stomachaches—and I'd been slowly losing weight without trying, by that point about 25 pounds. Before all my reading I'd thought these things were just "normal" for me. Now I wasn't so sure, so I decided to get tested. Based on Cooper's experience with blood tests and the endoscopy, I elected to have a stool test. The results revealed very elevated antibodies, indicating gluten intolerance. They also showed I was malabsorbing fats with off-the-chart numbers. Of course, I immediately started a GFD, but it's taken five years for me to achieve a full recovery. In the meantime, my other two children have also tested positive for gluten sensitivity.

Whenever my kids are introduced to a new concept, I always look for a book to help explain things to them, but at the time we were being diagnosed there was nothing out there. So I wrote and self-published a children's book about celiac disease. I got the story idea when Buddy, our new golden retriever, needed to go out several times a night because of diarrhea. A friend told us their retriever could not tolerate wheat and we should try different food. We switched from a wheat-based to a rice-based dog food and Buddy was never sick again. We couldn't believe it. The dog was gluten intolerant, too? How weird is that—the whole family except for dad.

Migraines

"More than 45 million Americans have headaches severe enough to require the help of a health care professional."[113] Migraine and tension headaches are also common in patients with CD. In one study, 28 percent of CD patients were migraine-sufferers.[114] More than 75 percent of children following a GFD had an improvement in their headaches. A poor response could be due to issues with compliance.[115] The cause of the migraines may be a low level of serotonin found in patients with CD.[116]

A woman "who had occipital cerebral calcifications" with unmanageable migraines was diagnosed with CD. After following a GFD, her migraines vanished.[117] An increased number of headaches among CD patients were revealed, and CD was found in a higher percentage of headache patients than among the public. This 2009 Italian study concluded that patients with headaches should be tested for CD and that for those who test positive, following a GFD has an effective outcome.[118]

Restless Legs Syndrome

People with restless legs syndrome (RLS) have an irresistible urge to move their body due to "uncomfortable sensations that may involve involuntary movements."[119] **In a 2010 study of CD patients, more than a third had RLS, a very high percentage had neuromuscular issues, and 40 percent suffered from iron deficiency**. When these patients were placed on a GFD, half reported improvement. The study concluded that testing RLS patients for CD is most important.[120]

The title of this study spells it out: *Celiac disease as a possible cause for low serum ferritin in patients with restless legs syndrome.* Since CD can cause iron deficiency, patients with low blood ferritin and RLS should be tested for CD as well.[121] (See Chapter 8 for information on the association between CD and anemia.) A 1998 study found that RLS patients with "ferritin levels greater than 50 mcg/l" will experience fewer RLS symptoms.[122] If you have RLS, consider asking your doctor to check your ferritin levels. The results may be surprising.

"Increasing evidence suggests that iron deficiency may underlie common pathophysiological mechanisms in subjects with ADHD and [in those] with RLS."[123] This study was not about CD, but since we know CD can cause iron deficiency, one could assume CD might be a contributor to ADHD as well as to RLS.

There are, of course, many more neurological diseases than those I've listed here, and research on potential connections between them and celiac disease and/or non-celiac gluten intolerance (CD/GI) is in its infancy—most studies have been done within the past 10 years. In the fast-moving field of medicine, many medical professionals are simply not aware of this cutting-edge information, which is why it's so important to do your own research and bring copies of it to your doctor. (See Appendix A for research tips.) No matter what your ailment, even if you've been told it is *genetic or incurable*, becoming an active partner in managing your health—learning all you can about your body and the maladies affecting it—can lead to information and insights that can drastically improve your quality of life.

Autoimmune Disease 10

THE IMMUNE SYSTEM is designed to keep your body healthy. When it malfunctions it can attack your brain, blood vessels, digestive tract, eyes, glands, heart, joints, kidneys, lungs, muscles, nerves, and skin.[1] The result of such an attack is known as an autoimmune disease or AID. (AIDs are not to be confused with the specific autoimmune disease of acquired immune deficiency syndrome [AIDS]). AIDs, including celiac disease (CD), the only autoimmune disease with a known cause, can ravage the body in a variety of ways. They frequently lead to disability and are a significant cause of death. ***Approximately 50 million Americans***[2] ***suffer from one or more of the 80 autoimmune diseases identified so far.***[3] However, since many of these disorders have overlapping symptoms, they are often difficult to diagnose.

More and more, autoimmune diseases are being associated with gluten consumption. Celiac disease may be silent, with no obvious symptoms, but the chances of it occurring in individuals with certain autoimmune disorders are 10 to 30 times greater than in the general public. For example, gluten may act as a predisposing trigger for developing type 1 diabetes, autoimmune thyroid, and other autoimmune endocrinological disorders.[4]

In 1999, Italian researchers led by Dr. A. Ventura found that "**the prevalence of autoimmune disorders in celiac disease is related to the duration of exposure to gluten.**"[5] In other words, if you are sensitive to gluten and remain either undiagnosed (a far-too-common occurrence) or fail to adhere to a gluten-free diet (GFD), you have a greater chance of developing additional autoimmune diseases. The incidence of autoimmune disease appears to increase as one ages. Ventura's study found that patients diagnosed with CD in the age groups 2–4, 4–12, 12–20, and over age 20 had a greater chance of developing a second autoimmune disease the older they got. For example, patients ages 2–4 had a 10.5 percent chance of developing another AID; for those 21 or older, the odds jumped to 34 percent.[6] I wonder how this type of progressive increase would relate to a group of 60-year-olds with newly diagnosed CD. Significant research substantiates the connection between gluten and a variety of autoimmune disorders, including Addison's, cardiomyopathy, colitis, Crohn's, dermatomyositis, liver disease, lupus, scleroderma, and thyroid disease, to name a few.

A significant study by Aristo Vojdani, an immunologist and chief scientific advisor for Cyrex Laboratories, showed that "***predictive antibodies***" (immune proteins produced in response to an antigen or irritant—such as gluten or dairy—that lead to an immune response) ***could be present up to 10 years before signs of disease materialize*** and that "neurotransmitters and hormonal imbalances" in the body are signs of pending illness. If these factors are recognized and treated early enough, the disease process may be halted or even reversed.[7] As described in a 2008 Italian study, examples of autoimmune diseases that may exhibit these types of early antibodies include Addison's, celiac, Crohn's, Hashimoto's thyroiditis, primary biliary cirrhosis, and type 1 diabetes.[8]

A 2009 study from the Netherlands points to more and more research suggesting intestinal permeability—sometimes called leaky gut or permeable gut—is involved in the development of autoimmune diseases, including CD and type 1 diabetes.[9] When the barrier between the intestine and the blood system becomes damaged from too many antibiotics or other medications or from toxins, infections, poor diet, gluten, etc., particles that don't belong in the bloodstream find their way through the intestinal wall. The intrusion of these "foreign bodies" causes the immune system to work overtime and begin attacking various organs and tissues. Vojdani's work reveals that when the "barriers are broken, food intolerances and sensitivities develop. If this leaky gut condition is not addressed, the end result is autoimmunity and in many cases 'leaky brain.'"[10]

If you have an autoimmune disease, has your doctor suggested getting screened for celiac disease? If someone turns out to have both CD and another AID, an early CD or gluten intolerance (GI) diagnosis, followed by a gluten-free lifestyle, could help to normalize the second AID, particularly if these changes are made before major damage occurs. For those who are gluten sensitive, eliminating the substance could potentially keep them from developing additional AIDs.

For me it was too late. I have fairly extensive damage from a thyroid disorder (hypothyroid) diagnosed 15 years or so before I learned about gluten sensitivity, though I suspect I'd been gluten intolerant for years prior to my thyroid diagnosis. Others have been more fortunate. I know of two women with hypothyroid whose levels returned to normal when they realized they were gluten sensitive and removed the toxin from their diet.

A huge amount of pain and suffering related to these disorders—not to mention the cost of dealing with complications—could be avoided by early screening with specific antibody tests. Since celiac is the only autoimmune disease with a known cause, could it be that gluten is a common denominator among other AIDs? Much more research is needed to fully explore this connection, and it may be years before it's conclusively proven or disproven, but it's interesting how many people with AIDs begin to get better on a gluten-free diet. In the meantime, prevention is the name of the game. If you're having autoimmune health issues, consider getting tested for CD and other auto-antibodies *before* your health takes a deeper dive.

Diabetes

When we talk about diabetes it's important to realize there are two distinct flavors: type 1 and type 2. Type 1 diabetics cannot produce insulin; thus, in order to live they must receive it externally through shots or a pump. Type 2 diabetics either don't produce enough insulin, or their cells can't utilize the available insulin. It's this second flavor of diabetes that has become an American epidemic. According to data from the 2011 National Diabetes Fact Sheet, 79 million adults in the U.S. are prediabetic—in other words, at risk or borderline for developing type 2 diabetes. Nearly 8.3 percent of the U.S. population (26 million people) already has the disease, more than 10 million of them over age 65. The complications are staggering: amputation, blindness, heart disease, high blood pressure, kidney disease, neuropathy, and stroke. The financial implications are equally depressing. In 2007 alone, costs in the U.S. associated with diabetes-related medical expenses, loss of work, disability, and early death totaled $174 billion.[11]

For those with type 1 diabetes (T1D), the damage is already done. There is no cure, at least not yet, although some exciting research is on the horizon. The majority of those with this disease manage it well through a combination of medication, diet, and exercise, but perhaps we can do more.

A 2002 study found CD to be 20 times more prevalent in those with type 1 diabetes than among members of the general public. In a significant number of T1D patients, CD is "already present at diabetes onset, mostly undetected" and another remarkable percentage "develop celiac disease a few years after diabetes onset," even though most T1D patients diagnosed with CD exhibited no symptoms of the disorder prior to diagnosis. Not surprisingly, screening for CD was recommended for those with type 1 diabetes.[12]

The correlation in this study is impressive; however, the only blood test given was the endomysial antibody (EMA: IgA). Since one test may not be enough to identify everyone on the continuum of gluten sensitivity, how many with type 1 diabetes might have been gluten sensitive years before being diagnosed with CD (perhaps even before being diagnosed with diabetes)? As one can imagine, the numbers might have been quite higher. Because T1D is also linked to Addison's, autoimmune thyroid, CD, and other autoimmune diseases, it's important that T1D patients be screened for antibodies to these conditions as well.[13]

A 2008 Spanish study found that 8 percent of those with T1D also had CD and 19 percent had another autoimmune disease. The outcome of **this study recommends screening type 1 diabetic patients for celiac disease, "especially in the first 5 years after diagnosis" to help prevent "long-term complications, such as lymphoma and osteoporosis."**[14] Although this study provides additional insight to the connection, the two blood tests used for CD screening did not include the more recently recognized anti-gliadin antibody test (AGA). Is it possible that if those with autoimmune diseases had been given this test as well, an even greater percentage would have been indentified as gluten sensitive? And if those so identified followed a gluten-free lifestyle, would it help to reduce their existing symptoms, or perhaps prevent them from developing other autoimmune disorders altogether? Studies such as this one certainly point in that direction. This study is just one of many that relied on only one or two tests and did not include the AGA or the total serum IgA. For information on the full range of blood tests recommended for accurate diagnosis, see Chapter 16.

A is for Attitude: Ilyena Kozain's Story

The first day I saw Ilyena Kozain she was a teenager, riding her bike in our neighborhood. I stopped the car, introduced myself, and asked if she lived nearby and if she did any babysitting or housework. Since then our families have become close friends.

Ilyena's story conjures up a deep concern about the inadequacies of testing, the lack of expertise and sensitivity among certain members of the medical profession, and the real need for expert coaching on a gluten-free lifestyle. Ilyena was diagnosed with type 1 diabetes at the age of 15. At my urging (by this time she was 17), she was tested for celiac disease. Her blood test results were negative and the stool test, one of the most sensitive tests for discerning gluten sensitivity, was not on the radar screen of her doctor. Because her tests were unremarkable, Ilyena was offered no nutritional counseling, despite studies that show a strong association between the two conditions. (Since CD can be developing for years or decades without symptoms, the inevitable question is: Which came first, the disease or the gluten causing the disease?)

About a year later, Ilyena, who'd grown up in Germany, went back to visit old friends. When she returned she informed me she was embracing a gluten-free lifestyle. Drinking beer and eating hearty German bread had not agreed with her. In fact, after indulging, she said she'd felt awful.

Subsequently, Ilyena's mother, Nina, who had no obvious symptoms, wanted to support her daughter by following the GFD too. When both mother and daughter submitted samples for Dr. Fine's stool test (see Chapter 17), both tested positive.

Nina dropped some weight after beginning a GFD but, more importantly, her seasonal allergies are much better. And Ilyena, in addition to alleviating her digestive troubles, has seen her nasty case of acne basically disappear. Of course, she was also taking medicine for this condition, but I can't help but think that healing her body on the inside has had a positive effect on her skin. (See Chapter 11 for information on the link between gluten and skin disorders.)

Ilyena has one of the most positive, dynamic, A+ attitudes I've ever seen, regardless of age. She is very strong, always smiling, and deals with life as it comes. I expect one day she'll be practicing preventive medicine.

Long before Ilyena's run-in with German bread and beer, Nina reported that her daughter always became bloated after eating a pasta meal. Ilyena referred to this condition as her swollen "food baby." Perhaps the description wasn't too far from the mark. One study found that children who were fed gluten at less than three months of age were at greater risk of generating islet antibodies (organ-specific antibodies that destroy insulin-producing cells in the pancreas). Those given gluten for the first time after six months of age had no increased risk of generating these antibodies or of developing celiac disease.[15] Another study showed that in individuals with type 1 diabetes, early detection of CD is important because it may result in fewer insulin reactions and better diabetic stability.[16] Type 1 diabetics may have greater glycemic control on a gluten-free diet, and those who also have hypothyroid and osteoporosis may be able to absorb medications for these conditions more effectively.[17]

Over a decade ago, one review suggested that initiating a GFD early in the life of a genetically predisposed child could be a preventive measure against developing type 1 diabetes. This same study found there is as much chance for celiac disease to develop *before* the diabetes as after.[18] But because of how long it can take for CD to be recognized, the question of "Which came first ...?" remains intriguing.

A well-executed review by Dr. Geoffrey Holmes, who is affiliated with the Derbyshire Royal Infirmary in the United Kingdom, reveals 52 different references regarding the association between type 1 diabetes and celiac disease, some from as far back as 1969.[19] Considering some of these questions were raised over *four decades ago*, it's more than frustrating that in this second decade of the 21st century many doctors are unaware of the extensive body of research exploring the diabetes-gluten connection.

Type 2 diabetes (T2D) has always been considered a metabolic disorder, but new research by Dr. Daniel Winer, an endocrine pathologist at the University Health Network of the University of Toronto, claims that T2D is in the process of being redefined as an autoimmune disease. Cutting-edge research postulates that insulin resistance (a sign of T2D in which cells cannot properly use insulin to regulate blood sugar levels) is the consequence of "B cells and other immune cells attacking the body's own tissues."[20] Of course, should this theory be proven true, pharmaceutical companies will jump on the bandwagon with a plethora of new drug therapies, but is it also possible that for some, treatment (or even prevention) could be significantly enhanced by simply adopting a gluten-free lifestyle?

In Chapter 9 Gale Pearce tells the story of how he adopted a gluten-free lifestyle to gain control of his gluten ataxia and numerous other conditions, but Gale was not the only member of the Pearce household with health issues. His wife, Wanda, was a type 2 diabetic.

To receive treatment for his condition, Gale had been referred to a multispecialty clinic in Seattle. Wanda, who accompanied him from their home in Alaska, inadvertently left her own meds behind.

Return to Normal: Wanda's Story, by Gale Pearce, PA-C

When I adopted a gluten-free lifestyle seven months ago in Seattle, Wanda, my wife of 47 years, decided to join me in this endeavor, both as a gesture of support and because it would make life easier for her in the kitchen. Wanda has since learned to cook all over again, and we both agree we eat at least as well now as we did before the GFD.

Wanda had been on medicine for type 2 diabetes when I got sick, but in the confusion of medical appointments, testing, and travelling to Seattle, she left her medications at home in Alaska. Even though she didn't have her meds she continued to monitor her blood sugar, and after we started on the GFD her readings improved. She went in for her routine checkup when we finally got home, only to find her glycosolated hemoglobin (A1C or HbA1c, a measure of glucose levels over time) was at its lowest level in two years. It has since returned to normal. Based on these results and with her doctor's concurrence, Wanda was able to eliminate her medication.

Wow! This compelling account begs the question as to whether type 2 diabetes is caused by a sheer overload of carbohydrates or by a sheer overload of the gluten-saturated "all-American diet"? Could gluten be a factor in the development and/or treatment of type 2 diabetes along with sugar consumption, obesity, and lack of exercise?

The title of one study done a decade ago poses this provocative question: *Is Type 2 diabetes a chronic inflammatory/autoimmune disease?*[21] A more recent study reveals that "latent autoimmune diabetes in adults (LADA) shares genetic features with both Type 1 … and Type 2 diabetes, …" LADA is "a slowly progressing subtype of Type 1 diabetes" with features similar to type 2.[22] Obviously, a huge opportunity exists for more research on the elusive role of gluten and its relationship to both type 1 and type 2 diabetes and even hypoglycemia, which in one study responded positively to a GFD.[23]

Thyroid Disease

Thyroid hormones affect the functioning (or malfunctioning) of many parts of the body. Two major types of thyroid malfunction, Hashimoto's disease (hypothyroid) and Graves' disease (hyperthyroid), can result in serious health issues if not addressed. A lengthy list of symptoms exists for these conditions, many of which overlap symptoms of CD.

Autoimmune thyroid disease is common as one ages; it also is much more prevalent among women. The other day I noticed a woman eating a great salad and made a comment about how good it looked, even without the croutons. She told me she was having thyroid problems and couldn't tolerate the medications her doctor had prescribed. She had been reading about how bad wheat and gluten can be for some people, so she took herself off gluten and life turned around for her. I wish I'd gotten her contact information; I could certainly identify with her story.

I'd probably had hypothyroid issues for years before I was diagnosed, yet I had many of the classic symptoms: dry skin, hair loss, fatigue, weight gain, and brittle nails. Many of these symptoms are also common in those who are gluten sensitive, and when gluten is removed from the diet, their symptoms are lessened or disappear, especially if the disorder is caught early enough. For me it wasn't early enough; the damage was done.

Gastrointestinal symptoms of a malfunctioning thyroid may affect any part of the GI tract. "The liver is the most affected organ in both hypo- and hyperthyroidism. Specific digestive diseases may be associated with autoimmune thyroid processes, such as Hashimoto's thyroiditis and Grave's disease. Among them, celiac sprue and primary biliary cirrhosis [also linked to CD] are the most frequent…."[24]

TPO (thyroid peroxidase) is an enzyme needed for the production of thyroid hormones.[25] One study suggests that since there is a greater incidence of CD among autoimmune thyroid patients "all subjects with TPO [antibodies] should be routinely screened for CD."[26] Another recommends that patients with Graves' disease (overactive thyroid) be tested for CD, since the occurrence of CD in participants with Graves' was significantly higher in comparison to the controls.[27] Addressing CD with a GFD increases the absorption of medications needed for hypothyroidism as well as those needed for osteoporosis.[28]

One study reported that polyendocrine syndromes (conditions that affect many glands, and thus hormones) are likely to occur in patients with autoimmune thyroid diseases (AITDs). Those with AITDs also exhibited a greater incidence of CD (and vice versa) and have also been shown to have a high rate of IgA deficiency. It's easy to see why it's vital to test for CD in those with autoimmune thyroid diseases[29] and prudent to screen for IgA deficiency as well.

Thyroid, Vitiligo, and CD

Having suffered numerous symptoms since high school, Judy was diagnosed with CD at the age of 45. Since then she's also been diagnosed with osteopenia and osteoporosis, and she still has unresolved abdominal pain.

A Long and Arduous Journey, by Judith E. Houston

I'd had stomach ailments since high school. They were never very bad, but I remember not being able to eat a lot without feeling very full and bloated, and

I weighed less than 100 pounds until my late 30s. I developed knee trouble during adolescence. Sometimes it was so bad my knees would just lock up and I'd tumble down the stairs. Eventually I "outgrew" it. Occasional lower back muscle spasms plagued me, and right before my senior year I was diagnosed with hyperthyroidism and vitiligo (skin pigment deficiency). When my thyroid levels got out of whack, I took medication to regulate them.

During my college years I continued to have stomach issues, including pain and gas; I couldn't seem to eat more than a few bites without feeling nauseous. My knees no longer locked up, but knee pain made skiing difficult. A sports medicine orthopedist said I had some sort of joint displacement in both knees that would likely require knee replacement surgery when I got older. Yahoo, another thing to look forward to!

For 10 years after college the pain and discomfort when eating continued. I was given upper- and lower-GI series and CAT scans, and I tried several anti-inflammatory and anti-gas medications, plus something for ulcers. Nothing worked. Finally I went to a doctor at a prestigious New Hampshire hospital who diagnosed me with "irritable bowel syndrome." By this time I was disgusted with the medical community. I stopped trying to figure out what was causing my IBS and just endured the almost-daily discomfort.

In 1995 I was married and shortly thereafter I suffered an early miscarriage. (I learned later that spontaneous abortions can be linked to CD.) Subsequently I was diagnosed with depression, another symptom of CD, and I've been on mild antidepressants off and on ever since. About a year after our oldest daughter was born, my stomach pain was bad enough to warrant another batch of tests. This time my gallbladder was proclaimed the culprit. It was removed and some of my symptoms went away.

Even with meds, my thyroid levels never returned to normal. They would spike and recede, then spike again. So I wouldn't have to endure this rollercoaster ride for the rest of my life, my endocrinologist recommended I have my thyroid ablated with radioactive iodine. A relatively standard-sized capsule, taken from a lead cabinet and handed to me by a lab technician in lead gloves, took care of it—a very odd experience, to say the least. I've been on thyroid meds ever since.

My vitiligo also had started to go nuts, spreading to my hands extending rapidly to every part of my body. Even the blond streak in my hair, something I'd admired since childhood, turned totally white. The "skunk lady" had arrived! Once a self-proclaimed "sun worshipper" of the North Shore, I was now relegated to wearing SPF 1000 sunscreen, ducking under shady trees, and wearing hats, long pants, and long-sleeved shirts to keep from frying in the sun.

My iron levels had been low for as long as I could remember, and throughout my second pregnancy I'd been taking "horse pill" iron supplements. "Nothing to be alarmed about," said my doctor, "just take an extra iron." After the birth, however, my iron levels never really rose. I was constantly fatigued and never felt clear-minded—definitely not a good thing when you're a professional engineer.

A new doctor was the most persistent in trying to figure out the cause of my anemia. Several tests, including another round of upper and lower GIs and more CAT scans, didn't find anything except "more than the usual number of polyps" in my lower abdomen. However, in the spring of 2007 an endoscopic biopsy confirmed I had celiac disease.

A hospital dietician who admitted she knew nothing about the disease—only what she'd quickly reviewed on the Internet while I recovered from the procedure—relayed the basics of a life-long gluten-free diet. Since then I've joined a support group, where I've met many others with similar stories. A nutritionist who gave a presentation at one of our meetings on the relationship between CD and osteoporosis suggested I have a bone scan. I was then diagnosed with osteoporosis in my left hip and osteopenia in my lower back. I took calcium supplements as prescribed by my doctor for many months. A re-scan showed the additional calcium is no longer necessary, although I sometimes have pain in my hip as well as occasionally painful fingers, toes, and neck from osteoarthritis. Fortunately, my knees seem to be okay.

Within about six weeks of being on a GFD, along with taking anti-reflux meds, I no longer felt nauseous after eating. My acid reflux and the pain and gas I'd felt after almost every meal had totally dissipated. After years of stomach ailments, this was amazing! I also put on some unwanted weight, no doubt due to finally absorbing nutrients and calories, but since joining a gym and walking a couple times a week, I'm trying to shed the weight and tone up.

I also suffer once or twice a month from the same sharp pains in my upper abdomen that occurred during the later trimester of each of my pregnancies. These pains have slowly subsided but otherwise I feel better than I have in years. It's been a long and arduous journey.

Thyroid—Have you been seeing an endocrinologist for thyroid problems? Has your doctor mentioned screening for CD? Unfortunately it takes years if not decades for new research to reach home plate. Here's some of the significant CD/thyroid research done between 1999 and 2002.

In one study, the incidence of antibodies for diabetes and autoimmune thyroid issues in patients before they were diagnosed with CD was more than 11 and 14 percent, respectively. These antibodies, which are directed toward specific organs, appear to be "gluten-dependent and tend to disappear during a gluten-free diet."[30]

Gluten also may play a part in creating high levels of thyroid and pancreatic antibodies and, in some cases, the ensuing malfunction of related organs.[31] ***Conversely there are instances where a GFD may "single-handedly reverse" a problematic thyroid.***[32]

A young woman with autoimmune Addison's disease as well as hypothyroidism and premature ovarian failure made great progress on a GFD, eventually needing less and less thyroid and adrenal medication. This study urged an early diagnosis of CD to avoid the risk of lymphoma and other complications and suggested that, if not addressed, CD could be a cause of hormonal thyroid medication not being assimilated into the body.[33] Patients with Hashimoto's and Graves' also may be in jeopardy of developing brain disease called Hashimoto's encephalopathy.[34]

A 2005 study reports that autoimmune thyroid disease is linked to celiac disease, lupus, myasthenia gravis, pernicious anemia, primary adrenal autoimmune disease, rheumatoid arthritis, and vitiligo.[35] (For information on fetal and neonatal thyroid disorders, see Chapter 12.)

Vitiligo—Vitiligo, an autoimmune pigmentation condition linked to thyroid and Addison's disease, causes "areas of the skin [and hair] to lose their pigment and become white because of a reduction in the body's production of melanin."[36] "Actual onset of vitiligo in genetically susceptible individuals seems to require exposure to environmental triggers."[37] Genes involved with the condition may be shared with autoimmune thyroid disease and other AIDs, thus substantiating a genetic association.[38]

One study identified 9.1 percent of CD patients as having vitiligo suggesting a genetic link.[39] The appearance of other autoimmune conditions such as Addison's disease, autoimmune thyroid disease, lupus, and pernicious anemia is notably increased in patients with vitiligo as well as in their first-degree relatives; this connection also suggests a genetic link.[40] More autoimmune diseases that may share this genetic predisposition are adult-onset, insulin-dependent diabetes mellitus, psoriasis, and rheumatoid arthritis.[41] Is gluten the provocative agent among these multiple autoimmune complex diseases?

Arthritis

Numerous types of arthritis can cause enormous pain, disability, and reduced quality of life. As of now osteoarthritis is not considered an autoimmune disease. Regardless of how it's qualified, however, if you've spent years malabsorbing the vitamins and minerals crucial to keeping your cartilage, bones, and joints healthy, what shape do you suppose they could be in?

Rheumatoid Arthritis—"Rheumatoid arthritis (RA) and coeliac disease (CD) are two autoimmune disorders which have commonalities in their pathogenesis."[42] In other words, there are a lot of similarities in the way these two diseases develop. Fourteen new genetic associations between CD and RA have been revealed in a 2011 study from the Netherlands suggesting T-cell and antigen activity.[43]

A 2001 study titled *A vegan diet free of gluten improves the signs and symptoms of rheumatoid arthritis: the effects on arthritis correlate with a reduction in antibodies to food antigens*, lends credence to the ill effects of gluten. The study concludes that immune reactions to food may be decreased by eliminating antigens (gluten, dairy, etc.) found in the diet.[44]

Nearly a half century ago Dr. R. Shatin had great success with a protein diet containing no meat and no gluten but supplemented with vitamins. Incredible arthritic remissions occurred in 20 of the 30 patients he studied.[45] He noticed that "the worldwide distribution of rheumatoid arthritis corresponds to the distribution of wheat ingestion."[46] I find this information both exciting—because I think he's "right on," even though his initial study didn't establish a clear correlation—and disturbing because so little research has been executed over the ensuing decades to prove the point one way or the other.

Juvenile Idiopathic Arthritis—Attention parents and grandparents! Your child's doctors may be unaware of this little-studied arthritis/gluten association, so the ball is in your court. Over 40 percent of the children with arthritis in a 2003 study were found to have serologic markers for CD. Only one of these children had a positive biopsy for CD, yet over 75 percent had high antigliadin IgG and many had other elevated CD/GI markers. When the children were placed on a GFD, their growth levels improved and their arthritic symptoms were reduced. The researchers recommended screening children with juvenile idiopathic arthritis (JIA) for *silent* CD.[47] Children with JIA also have a heightened incidence of autoimmune thyroiditis, CD, and subclinical hypothyroidism and should be screened for these ailments.[48]

An 11-year-old boy with a recurring type of arthritis and silent CD went into remission after adhering to a GFD. This 1999 study stressed that doctors need to be attentive to CD-associated arthritis, since the treatment lies in the diet.[49]

CD/GI, as well as other common irritants such as dairy and/or soy, can be very easy for parents of children with JIA to recognize. Tests for gluten and other intolerances can detect antigens that may be raising havoc in the body.

Psoriatic Arthritis—An increased occurrence of CD and elevated anti-gliadin IgA antibodies is found in patients with psoriasis. And inflammation and stiffness are more intense in those with higher AGA: IgA levels.[50]

Whether a diagnosis is "psoriatic arthritis with CD" or "juvenile rheumatoid arthritis with celiac disease and psoriasis" doesn't really matter. What matters is that eliminating gluten for these children can be a big step toward better health. One study showed complete remission of joint issues, along with healthy growth, in a young girl being treated with non-steroidal drugs while following a GF lifestyle.[51]

The complex case of a young boy impacted with celiac disease, enthesitis (inflammation of places where ligaments and tendons attach to the bones), juvenile psoriatic arthritis, and psoriasis led authors of a 2010 Italian study to stress the importance of rheumatologists and dermatologists (not to mention other specialists) working together to identify the multiple diseases that can co-exist with CD.[52]

Tin Man Needs Oil, by S. M.

In my 40s life changed for me in ways I didn't expect. Always nimble, I suddenly found myself more like the "Tin Man" in need of oil as my joints became increasingly intolerant of movement. It was especially noticeable in my hands, which could no longer hold a glass without the use of hand braces. No one seemed able to identify my malady save for calling it "arthritis."

At a visit to an alternative doctor about another matter, I happened to mention my stiff, achy joints, and he suggested my problems might be due to wheat intolerance. Sure enough, after I stopped eating wheat (nothing else in my diet shifted) for three weeks, I had the full use of my hands and no stiff, achy joints. Based on these results, I now stay away from all things containing wheat. The myriad of gluten-free/wheat-free products on the market means I can eat just fine, and with more restaurants accommodating those with food sensitivities, eating out continues to get easier as well.

A few studies support the connection between arthritis and CD. In one, a 42-year-old woman who was nearly incapacitated due to swelling and joint pain in her knee was hugely helped by a GF lifestyle. This woman had also had dermatitis herpetiformis (DH), a manifestation of CD, for 12 years. This study lends credence to the "more than coincidental" association of joint issues and CD/DH.[53]

Atheroprotective and anti-inflammatory characteristics were observed in patients with rheumatoid arthritis who followed a gluten-free vegan diet.[54] And in another study, patients responded favorably to an elemental diet, supporting the idea that rheumatoid arthritis begins in the intestine and may be in response to an ingested antigen.[55]

Low vitamin D was also found among patients with inflamed arthritic joints and persistent pain. An association of low vitamin D in the development of inflammatory and autoimmune diseases is surfacing, and new guidelines are needed.[56] The association of CD and RA is another huge area in need of research, but don't hold your breath. Think of the lost revenue in painkillers alone!

Osteoarthritis, Red Skin Tone, and Edema—Have you noticed how many people have red faces? In many cases it's not sunburn! This red skin tone, along with edema (holding fluid in tissues), seems to be a growing trend. Check out your ankles. Do you have a layer of fluid there? Surely you've heard that older folks absorb fewer nutrients. Why do you suppose this is? Many of these chronic symptoms have been associated with gluten sensitivity. If you suspect gluten may be your problem, see Chapters 16 and 17 for testing options.

Feeling Better and Better, by Judy Logan

When I was in my 40s, I was frequently troubled by some vague intestinal discomfort, which I tried to treat with remedies from the pharmacy or health food store. In my 50s, symptoms increased and I tried eliminating various food groups like dairy, sugars, etc., with no results. By age 60 I was spending too much time in the bathroom and using too many anti-diarrheal meds. I asked my doctor about being tested for celiac disease and even brought him an article on the topic, but he didn't think I fit the profile.

Last year I read a book by Shari Lieberman called *The Gluten Connection: How Gluten Sensitivity May Be Sabotaging Your Health—And What You Can Do to Take Control Now* and realized there are many people with gluten sensitivity who don't necessarily have full-blown CD. So, even though my doctor wouldn't order the tests, I decided to put myself on a gluten-free diet. Wow! Not only did my digestion improve, in less than a week I had significantly less joint pain and stiffness in my lower back and knees, a problem I'd been living with since osteoarthritis with edema had been confirmed in my knees two years before.

I've been off gluten for 10 months and continue to feel better and better. I've also experienced another, unexpected benefit: In recent years my skin tone had been getting redder, not just my face, but my arms and hands as well. As a physical therapist I work closely with many different people. I could see how red I looked in comparison to them, but on a GFD my skin tone has improved noticeably.

These days I'm not even tempted to eat anything with gluten. When I go out to eat I make a game of finding something gluten-free yet interesting and satisfying, and I continue to explore and learn as much as I can.

Sobering thoughts:

- ***"More than 46 million people in the United States have arthritis or other rheumatic conditions. By the year 2020, this number is expected to reach 60 million."***[57]
- ***"About 435,000 Americans have a hip or knee replaced each year."***[58]

A new study from Germany concludes: "Both genetic and environmental factors contribute to rheumatoid arthritis (RA) as well as osteoarthritis (OA)."[59]

A 2010 study found back pain and sacroiliitis may be linked to undiagnosed CD. After following a GFD for 11 years, most patients had no apparent symptoms, although some sacroiliac joint involvement could still be detected. Thus, CD patients with rheumatic issues should continue to be evaluated.[60] There are few studies on musculoskeletal pain associated with CD, but many storytellers in this book speak of back, pelvic, shoulder, muscle, joint, bone, and other pain that subsided once they started following a GFD. When your gut heals enough to absorb nutrients, every cell in your body has a chance to heal and become better. The fact that both OA and RA become worse as people age could be a factor of one's genetic predisposition and the length of time one has consumed gluten, rather than age alone.

A 1998 study claimed there was *no known cause* for the deterioration of cartilage and the disfigurement of OA, but it went on to say, "It is clear now that this constellation of events [leading to arthritis] is not associated with aging, and traumatic, hormonal, environmental [something we consume], and genetic factors are the obvious culprits in the pathogenesis of OA."[61] Hallelujah! The older I get, the more comforting it is to learn that old age has little to do with the vast majority of illnesses plaguing our population.

Arthritis need not necessarily be a part of the aging process and, surely, it should not be a factor in any child's life. Gluten and dairy appear to be antagonists for much joint and muscular pain. For example, dairy makes my body stiff; life for me is better without it. Perhaps a great many arthritic symptoms would become less troublesome or disappear altogether if one could remove the offending irritant.

If you're suffering from arthritic pain, determining whether or not you're gluten sensitive might just put you on a path toward better health.

Cardiomyopathy

"Cardiomyopathy associated with celiac disease is a serious and potentially lethal condition. However, with early diagnosis and treatment with a gluten-free diet, cardiomyopathy in patients with celiac disease may be completely reversible."[62] Is the phrase "deadly effects of gluten" too strong a term to use when applied to cardiomyopathy? More and more research says no, it is not!

"If only I'd known then what I know now," as the saying goes, when the son of distant friends landed a job in our town. I bumped into him once, and he explained how tired he felt. Eventually he dragged himself to his doctor, who found nothing wrong. His symptoms progressed and he was finally diagnosed with cardiomyopathy; his enlarged heart was working overtime to keep his body functioning. What he needed, according to his doctors at a prestigious Boston hospital, was a new heart. Unfortunately, one did not arrive in time to save his life.

Looking back, I highly suspect this young man was gluten sensitive. We'll never know for sure, but studies associating cardiomyopathy with gluten have shown that when the noxious protein is removed from the diet, the patient gets better. You may have one of the best doctors in the country, but if s/he is not up on gluten and its devastating effects, you could be in trouble. The information is too new and it is not being taught. I know you expect your doctors at the very best hospitals would know if gluten were associated with your health issues. If only this were true. In reality, much of this information is brand new, and much more research needs to be done. Even information that's been around for a while can be hard for doctors to keep up with; after all, there aren't many crash courses in "Gluten 101" available to medical professionals in this country.

A 2002 study reported an increased incidence of CD among participants with idiopathic dilated cardiomyopathy. Results indicate that cardiac function in these patients may be enhanced by a GF lifestyle.[63]

A 2009 Chilean study showed a heightened occurrence of CD among those with cardiomyopathy. A middle-aged woman whose heart failure had been due to "dilated cardiomyopathy of unknown etiology ..." revealed "a normal left ventricle and systolic function" after a month on a GFD.[64] A 2010 study from Turkey suggested that carnitine deficiency in CD patients was the cause of dilated cardiomyopathy.[65]

Perhaps a red flag should pop up when we're confronted with *any* condition for which the cause is labeled idiopathic or unknown. Whether known or not, *something* is causing the illness, and nutrient deficiencies can lead to a plethora of ailments. Not surprisingly, those with CD may be very deficient due to malabsorption.

Idiopathic Thrombocytopenia Purpura

A mutual friend put me in touch with Maureen, whose health issues brought her perilously close to seeing the other side of the grass. Her story is a good example of developing multiple autoimmune diseases (AIDs) once you have the first one. Luckily, she was able to turn her health around.

A Strong Correlation, by Maureen

Other than being anemic for many years, I had never had any serious health issues, but at the age of 40 it seemed my body started rebelling against me. It started in November 2006 when I was diagnosed with Graves' disease, an autoimmune hyperthyroid disorder. By February, my period was heavier than usual. This heavy bleeding continued for a week or so before I called my primary care physician (PCP). After blood tests determined my platelet count was 2,000 (normal is between 250,000 and 400,000), I was told to get to the hospital immediately. I drove myself to the emergency room and was rushed through registration and brought to a room where a bunch of people started working on me, asking questions, taking blood, etc. It was a little scary, but I really didn't know enough to be worried. I had a couple of blood and platelet transfusions, but after the transfusions the doctors determined my body was destroying the platelets, so I was admitted.

To make a long story short, three days in the hospital and many tests later I was diagnosed with idiopathic thrombocytopenia purpura (ITP), an autoimmune disease where the body destroys its own platelets. I was put on a steroid that caused me to gain weight, have trouble sleeping, and become a raging bitch. I dealt with ITP for about a year, being weaned off the steroid once but put back on it when my platelets crashed again. My last dose was in January 2008. Since then my platelets have remained at a normal level, but I worry every month that the ITP might return. I was never given a reason as to what caused this condition.

When in the process of weaning off the steroid I was given radioactive iodine to destroy my thyroid, with the predicted result that I'm now hypothyroid and must take drugs for this condition every day.

I also had a bone density scan during this period and was subsequently diagnosed with osteopenia. The doctors said this condition was probably a result of the Graves' disease, but they didn't want to put me on medication because I was too young. We agreed we'd just repeat bone density scans every year and watch it.

In November of 2008, just after Thanksgiving, I began having episodes of diarrhea and bad cramping every five days or so. After the third episode I went to my PCP. She did several tests, all with negative results. She then had me schedule a colonoscopy; she thought it might be irritable bowel syndrome. I also had an appointment with my endocrinologist during this period who, upon seeing how much weight I had lost and listening to my symptoms, asked if I'd been tested for celiac disease. When I said no the doctor ordered blood tests and the results were positive and later confirmed by an endoscopy.

I count myself lucky that I was diagnosed fairly quickly. After reading the book *Dangerous Grains* by James Braly and Ron Hoggan, I learned there is a strong correlation between celiac and anemia, Graves', ITP, and osteopenia.[66] I still don't understand it all, but after nearly three months on a gluten-free diet, I feel fantastic and my platelet level has remained normal.

Two years after Maureen told me her story her bone density has significantly improved and her platelets remain normal, with no signs of ITP.

Written in Blood

A 2010 German study found that not only is iron deficiency anemia frequent in patients with CD, but thrombocytopenia (low blood platelets) and thrombocytosis (high blood platelets) can be factors as well. With the aid of folic acid and a GFD, the patient's thrombocytopenia normalized and he recovered from co-existing conditions of macrocytic anemia and malnutrition. CD must be taken into account when blood counts linked to gastrointestinal signs stray from the norm.[67] A 2010 study states that "idiopathic thrombocytopenic purpura (ITP) is a common acquired bleeding disorder of childhood." The authors stressed that patients with this bleeding disorder should be checked for autoimmune thyroditis and CD.[68] In addition to thrombocytosis and thrombocytopenia, reports a team at the Mayo Clinic, CD may also be linked to hyposplenism, IgA deficiency, leukopenia (decreased white blood cells), and venous thromboembolism.[69] Two different studies of CD in conjunction with ITP, accompanied by either inclusion body myositis (an inflammatory muscle disease)[70] or hepatic granulomatous, suggest an autoimmune mechanism linking the three conditions.[71]

If you have any of these multisyllabic health issues, especially those related to blood cell count, color, size or shape—even if you don't have intestinal problems—you may want to consider getting properly screened for CD and, if positive, adopting a GF lifestyle.

Liver Disease: Autoimmune Hepatitis and Primary Sclerosing Cholangitis

An Australian study concludes that "primary biliary cirrhosis is clearly linked to coeliac disease. The full story of these linkages is yet to be written." Individuals who are gluten sensitive and not treated with a GFD can develop end-stage liver disease as a result of hepatitis linked to CD.[72] An Italian study noted: "Two main forms of liver damage namely, cryptogenic and autoimmune, appear to be strictly related to gluten-sensitive enteropathy." This study, which included patients with non-specific reactive hepatitis (celiac hepatitis), detected a high level of liver enzymes (hypertransaminasemia) in nearly half of them. After the affected patients adopted a GF lifestyle, this milder liver damage normalized over a period of six to twelve months. More acute liver damage, such as "chronic hepatitis or liver cirrhosis," may also get better on a GFD.[73] Hepatic T-cell lymphoma may be a resultant complication of CD.[74] An exacting exam for *latent* or *silent* CD is recommended for any patients with a liver condition of unknown origin.[75]

Father to Daughter: Grampy Nick's Story

My father, Nick Coniaris, should have lived a longer and much healthier life. Had I known then, back in 1975, what I know now, he could have. His parents lived in good health to their mid-90s. Grandpa made his daily walk up the hill to visit the "Greek boys" who owned the donut shop, and Grandma did well until her last couple of years, when she slipped into dementia.

For 14 years before his death my father suffered from what his doctor said began as autoimmune hepatitis and in the end appeared to be a liver disease called sclerosing cholangitis. Eventually he died from liver cancer. There are now studies that show some liver ailments can reverse course in those on a GFD. The fact my father couldn't venture too far from the "john" for many years could very well have been symptomatic of classic celiac disease—or was it a symptom of autoimmune hepatitis being caused by CD? My guess is that he had CD, which led to liver complications and an early demise at the age of 72. I've read and seen too much to think otherwise.

After learning of gluten-related research on autoimmune hepatitis and sclerosing cholangitis, I wrote to my father's doctor, a close friend, to see if Dad might have had either of these conditions. Below is his answer.

> June 6, 2006
>
> Dear Mrs. Sarkisian,
>
> I remember Nick fondly every time I go by his old house. We all miss him in Hollis.
>
> I was sorry to hear about your grandson having celiac disease. Primary care doctors are less up-to-date about how common it is than we in gastroenterology. Even for us, this information is only about ten years old in being accepted as true.
>
> Nick had a complicated liver disease that behaved in the end like sclerosing cholangitis. However, he had components that looked in the early stage more like autoimmune hepatitis and we know that there are crossover and combinations that can occur in any given person.
>
> Celiac is so common now; it is one cause of liver disease. Sclerosing cholangitis and other chronic liver diseases can result in cancers. To know if Nick might have carried the gene, it would be clear if one of his siblings or children tested positive. Even if that were the case it is not possible to tell if the gene came from Nick or your mother without testing her side as well.
>
> Best wishes to you all,
> David Golden, MD

I have two genes, which means that I got one from my father and one from my mother. See Chapter 18 for more information on this topic.

Some of the liver diseases associated with CD are autoimmune hepatitis, non-specific reactive hepatitis ("the most common"), primary biliary cirrhosis, and primary sclerosing cholangitis.[76] Liver disease can occur in people of any age, including children. A 2009 Swedish study of children with CD concluded that "severe hepatic damage or failure" could evolve and that children with CD should be assessed for "liver function and vice versa, children with severe liver damage should be investigated for untreated celiac disease."[77] The link is obvious! **Nearly 40 percent of children and adults with "fatty liver 'transaminitis' or hepatitis" who have barely any symptoms have liver issues that improve or resolve themselves on a GFD.**[78]

Has someone in your family had no response to a hepatitis B vaccine? CD could be the reason, but when the patient adheres to a GFD and the gut heals, his/her reaction matches that of the general, healthy population.[79]

The liver research above, much of it from other countries, is a strong indicator that for many, gluten is toxic and may cause disastrous consequences if the GF lifestyle is ignored. Gluten sensitivity is a worldwide problem.

At a gluten-related conference I heard the story of a man who needed a liver transplant who was diagnosed with CD. When his doctors put him on a GFD his liver began to mend; ultimately, he no longer needed the transplant. This story was undocumented, but there is a formal study proclaiming that **patients with critical liver dysfunction who adopt a strict GFD may preclude liver failure, even when a liver transplant is being contemplated**. Of the four patients in this study who had acute liver disease, "hepatic dysfunction reversed in all cases when a gluten-free diet was adopted."[80] Seems to me this should be headline news, but I wonder how many folks with severe or even mild liver ailments have ever heard the words *gluten* or *celiac disease* uttered by their doctors.

Pancreatitis

New connections to CD will be on the horizon for a long time to come. Others have been around for decades. Research in the last 15 years or so has linked pancreatic disorders to gluten. If you're in pain from issues relating to your pancreas, the research below could point the way to relief. Share these studies with your doctors and ask that they test you for CD/GI. (For more information on the connections between pancreatitis and neuropathy, see Tamsin Metzler's story on the neurological manifestations of celiac disease in Chapter 9.)

Autoimmune Pancreatitis—A 2007 Swedish study concluded that adult patients diagnosed with "CD are at increased risk of pancreatitis."[81] An Italian study found pancreatic enzymes to be elevated in about 25 percent of CD patients. Testing for CD is recommended in the case of elevated amylase or lipase blood levels, especially if no signs of pancreatic disease exist; even though patients may exhibit no symptoms.[82] CD can surface as acute pancreatitis, as it did in a young child who suffered from sporadic stomach pain and vomiting. His amylase and lipase enzymes were elevated and, when tested, he was found to have CD.[83] **Patients with "papillary stenosis or idiopathic recurrent pancreatitis" also should be screened for CD.**[84]

A 2001 Italian study reported the case of a young girl with autoimmune thyroiditis, CD, and macroamylasemia. The child was referred due to "chronic abdominal pain and growth retardation associated with persistent hyperamylasemia and suspected chronic pancreatitis," and the "CD-related antibodies to amylase and to exocrine pancreas tissue resolved with a gluten-free diet."[85]

Recurring acute pancreatitis is frequently associated with CD and is difficult to distinguish from other forms of pancreatitis. A new protocol is called for in diagnosing cases of pancreatitis associated with intestinal damage, since the only beneficial step is a GF lifestyle.[86] See the section on *Exocrine Pancreatic Insufficiency* in Chapter 13 for more information.

Addison's Disease

A 1999 medical history by R. B. Tattersall on adrenal disease suggests that hypoadrenia (low adrenal hormone) may be "a bit of Addison's disease,"[87] a much more serious adrenal disorder. Hypoadrenia appears to have a boatload of symptoms similar to those of gluten sensitivity. If you have hypoadrenia your adrenal glands are not working up to snuff and this can lead to serious endocrinological health problems.

Patients with Addison's disease (AD), alopecia (hair-loss condition), hypophysitis (inflammation of the pituitary gland), or multiple endocrine ailments may simultaneously have CD. A GFD may be helpful in dealing with the endocrine issues and is a *must* in the *prevention* of anemia, infertility, and osteoporosis. This 2002 Finnish study suggests "prolonged gluten exposure may even contribute to the development of autoimmune diseases."[88]

A 2007 Swedish study suggests that due to "a highly increased risk of AD in individuals with CD … **individuals with AD should be screened for CD**."[89] It is vital to test for IgA deficiency as well, as there is also a high incidence of this deficiency in patients with autoimmune Addison's.[90] In one case, a patient had Addison's disease, ovarian failure, and thyroid disease. After CD was diagnosed as well, she showed notable improvement on a GFD and was able to lessen adrenal and thyroid meds. Villous atrophy had reversed in 12 months. Early detection is vital to reduce complications such as lymphoma.[91]

For more on adrenal (and pituitary) dysfunction, see *A Healing Journey*, Bridget Skjordahl's story in Chapter 6.

The Pituitary Gland—Hypophysitis

Hypophysitis is an autoimmune condition wherein the pituitary gland does not produce enough hormones, a lack that can negatively affect the adrenal and thyroid glands. A 2010 study relates a "strong association of CD with other autoimmune disease" and reveals a high level of antipituitary antibodies (APA) in patients recently diagnosed with CD. High levels of APA correspond to poor growth in children.[92]

A recent Italian study also showed a high prevalence of these antibodies in newly diagnosed CD patients. "**High APA titers are associated with height impairment, ... suggesting that [the] autoimmune pituitary process could induce a linear-growth impairment.**"[93] In children and adults who continue to have growth issues, autoimmune damage to the pituitary may result in growth hormone deficiency.[94] Following a GFD usually "leads to a rapid catch-up in growth and to normalization of the pituitary function." Children not showing this catch-up gain may have a growth-hormone deficiency and may benefit from treatment with growth hormones.[95]

Fibromyalgia

Fibromyalgia is a chronic syndrome that "engulfs patients in a downward, reinforcing cycle of unrestorative sleep, chronic pain, fatigue, inactivity, and depression."[96] Sufferers may experience stiffness, headaches, and muscle/connective tissue tenderness.

Research ties fibromyalgia to IBS (see Chapter 7) as well as to depression, and these ailments are both strongly associated with CD. No matter what disease you look up, many of the signs and symptoms seem interwoven and overlapping; and once you have one autoimmune disease you have a greater probability of developing others, especially if you're gluten sensitive and don't adopt a GFD.

Drs. Vikki and Richard Petersen, coauthors of *The Gluten Effect*, state, "**There is no question as to the link between fibromyalgia and gluten sensitivity**.... In the United States, between four to eight million people suffer from fibromyalgia, which is roughly two percent of the population... . Ninety percent are women."[97]

A survey among celiac-support-group patients found the prevalence of fibromyalgia (FM) to be nine percent.[98] CD patients commonly have FM or irritable bowel syndrome. Dyspepsia, non- cardiac chest pain, and reflux are frequent in FM patients, and 30 to 70 percent of them also have IBS.[99] Forty percent of FM patients suffer from depression.[100] Since a high percentage of FM patients have IBS and vice versa, they may share a common genetic mechanism for how the disease develops.[101] (For more on the links between IBS and CD, see Chapter 7.)

Certainly the doors are wide open for research linking fibromyalgia to celiac disease. Meanwhile those with FM seem to get better when the toxic protein is eliminated from their diet.

Stiff-Person Syndrome

Once again little research exists for this debilitating disorder, which is characterized by muscle rigidity, spasms, and stiffness.[102] Inroads are being made connecting stiff-person syndrome (SPS) to CD and glutamic acid decarboxylase (GAD) antibodies, but is your primary care physician, rheumatologist, or neurologist seeing this research? If you have SPS or any other debilitating autoimmune disease and have not been offered testing for gluten sensitivity, you know the answer.

In 2011, "the high prevalence of gluten sensitivity in patients with stiff-person syndrome" prompted Dr. Marios Hadjivassiliou and colleagues to explore the connection between "gluten sensitivity and GAD-antibody-associated disease." A very high percentage of patients with SPS were positive on the GAD antibody test—86 percent; these numbers decreased after patients initiated a GFD. The same was true for those with gluten ataxia. It appears there is a connection between "gluten sensitivity and GAD antibody-associated diseases."[103]

"Antibodies against glutamic acid decarboxylase (GAD) are involved in the pathophysiology of stiff-person syndrome (SPS) and type 1 diabetes." This case study of a man with SPS and T1D, along with CD and dermatitis herpetiformis, led researchers to surmise an association among the four diseases.[104]

GAD antibodies are also linked to epilepsy, sporadic cerebellar ataxia, and type 1 diabetes, an association that some medical professionals believe suggests an autoimmune root.[105] *Just a coincidence or an additional shared pathophysiological mechanism?* is the subtitle of one article that begs to question whether CD, copper deficiency, dermatitis herpetiformis, microcytic anemia, and type 1 diabetes are linked to stiff-person syndrome.[106]

Scleroderma and Lupus

Scleroderma is an autoimmune, systemic, connective-tissue disorder (CTD) that causes hardening of the skin and clawing of the hands. It also may affect organs. Lupus, another systemic autoimmune CTD, is a chronic condition causing severe inflammation that can affect the skin and organs.[107] There is *no known cause* for these devastating diseases. Research on the association between gluten and CTD is not plentiful, but there is enough being done that word should be getting out. Still, mainstream medicine is barely getting a handle on classic CD and associated anemia and osteoporotic conditions, so if you have a connective tissue disorder it's understandable—though not acceptable—if you haven't been offered testing for CD.

As you read the research, keep in mind that many of these studies have not included the antigliadin antibody tests (AGA) or the IgA deficiency test. If they had, the numbers of those sensitive to gluten might be significantly higher.

Holly and I met at the first New England Celiac Conference in 2009. She has at least four autoimmune diseases, including CD, not to mention cancer. Her story is one of incredible courage.

A Sense of Humor to Survive, by Holly Malinowski

At age 28, I lost a baby close to my due date. The placenta had hardened, preventing nutrition from reaching the fetus, which consequently suffocated. The doctor had no idea what caused this to happen. A year later my legs went blue and the doctors thought I had Raynaud's disease; they gave me some meds and life got better. At age 30 I was pregnant again. The doctors said the tragedy of my previous pregnancy could never happen again, but this fetus also died of suffocation due to hardening of the placenta. This time they studied the placental tissue and found I had scleroderma, an autoimmune disease that was attacking the placenta.

For quite some time I took experimental drugs to try to keep my organs soft and pliable as long as possible. Life was pretty good; I was stiff and a little sore but otherwise okay. At about age 39 my lung function crashed. I turned blue, but after I was brought back I was okay.

I have asthma, and I seem to be allergic to everything on the planet but a horse and a hickory tree. I was getting bi-weekly allergy shots and using puffers three to four times a day just to exist.

Slowly I lost intestinal function and was living on a lot of liquid supplements. By age 42 I couldn't swallow; my throat was sore, my belly hurt, I hated food and I lived in the bathroom. Finally the doctors did an endoscopy and found I had celiac disease. No gluten allowed! I've been on a GFD diet for eight years now. Once in a while I have a gluten disaster, but it's never on purpose.

I developed rheumatoid arthritis at age 26 (my dad and my grandmother had it). I also have lupus and have had a bout with multiple myeloma [bone marrow tumors]; now my doctors feel each of these ailments has been ***caused by CD***. When gluten is in my system, my arthritis goes south with swollen joints, pain, and stiffness; my belly swells; I need to eat soft foods (six small meals and lots of water); and it takes two to three weeks to regulate again. Gluten makes my asthma act up, too. I was already dairy-free before being diagnosed with CD. Dairy makes me stiff and bloated and brings on intestinal issues, so I try diligently to keep both gluten and dairy out of my diet.

At the time of my CD diagnosis my immune system had totally crashed. This, too, the doctors thought, was caused by celiac disease. Most scleroderma patients die within 10 years. I've had the condition for 21 years and have learned to have a sense of humor about it. I continue to run a full daycare center every day and am now raising my ninetieth baby from the age of four to six weeks to about the third grade. So I fight on!

After reading Holly's story, how could you not surmise that gluten is the root cause of much devastating illness? Even her doctors thought CD caused her multiple degenerative diseases.

A 2009 Italian study found a "high incidence of celiac disease in patients with systemic sclerosis"—in other words, scleroderma.[108] Systemic sclerosis (SS) is often linked to other autoimmune conditions, and half of SS patients have digestive issues. CD diagnosis in those with SS is crucial to improving their quality of life.[109] "Coeliac disease may account for malabsorption in scleroderma patients even when test[s] suggest bacterial overgrowth."[110]

Does gluten sensitivity sometimes masquerade as systemic lupus erythematosus (SLE)? Dr. Hadjivassiliou and colleagues found three patients who were wrongly diagnosed with SLE. Back in 2004 they stressed that people with gluten sensitivity can experience diverse symptoms and disorders without having enteropathy (damaged villi). Physicians need to become aware of manifestations associated with gluten intolerance that do not fall within the realm of CD with damaged villi.[111]

Sjögren's Syndrome

Dry eyes and mouth are features of Sjögren's syndrome (SS), a chronic autoimmune disease with links to rheumatoid arthritis (RA). About half of all patients with primary Sjögren's syndrome (pSS) develop disease that affects the kidney, liver, or lungs or that may surface as peripheral neuropathy, skin vasculitis, and more. The risk for lymphoma is also increased with some of these diseases.[112]

Patients with pSS may exhibit a "rectal mucosal inflammatory response after [a] gluten challenge." Such a response may denote gluten sensitivity that has not yet damaged the villi—in other words, the person may be gluten intolerant but not have full-blown CD.[113] If this is the case, it is most important that the AGA (antigliadin) tests be included with the more commonly administered tTG (tissue transglutaminase) and EMA (endomysial antibody) tests.

"B-cell lymphoproliferation is a characteristic feature of this syndrome [SS] and the lesion may range from benign to malignant.... **Patients with Sjögren's syndrome have over [a] 40-fold increased risk of the development [of] B-cell non-Hodgkin's lymphoma.**"[114]

About 20 percent of pSS patients exhibit neurological disorders; thus screening for SS is suggested in patients with axonal sensorimotor neuropathy, cranial nerve involvement, or myelopathy (spinal cord issues).[115]

In a 1999 Finnish study, a close link was detected between SS and CD; inflammation is commonly found in the intestinal tissue, even in non-celiac (latent) SS patients.[116] Gliadin and gluten antibodies in patients with SS indicate that intestinal damage may be a frequent happening in those with this condition.[117]

Getting Healthy: Gloria Davison's Story

When I heard Gloria had been hospitalized for the inability to make saliva, I immediately got in touch with her and urged her to get tested for gluten sensitivity.

Even though she tested negative for Sjögren's, her doctor still thought she had it and put her on a course of treatment, including a steroid. After being released from the hospital she wanted to lose some of the weight she had gained due to the steroids. She also wanted to get as healthy as possible, since she was adopting a baby very soon. She decided to be tested for CD but was given only one test (an all-too-common scenario), and the results came back negative. She decided to do the GFD anyway, along with getting some exercise. Within a few weeks she began to feel better. Not only that, she'd lost 14 lbs. Within 90 days of beginning a GFD she felt so much better she was able to stop her medication for dry mouth. Eventually she was able to get off the steroids as well, and she lost 50 pounds.

Since the baby has arrived, Gloria admits she has had difficulty maintaining a totally GF lifestyle. "At times I cheat," she confesses, "and, of course, those are the times I feel icky." The proof is in the pudding!

Dermatomyositis and Polymyositis

Dermatomyositis (DM) and polymyositis (PM) are inflammatory muscle diseases often accompanied by a general feeling of weakness. DM is often accompanied by a skin rash; PM by joint pain.

Several times I have tried to get through to an acquaintance whose child has been diagnosed with dermatomyositis, but to no avail. They were taking him to doctors in Boston, but even in some of our finest medical facilities, many skilled, experienced doctors don't have a clue about the potential association between connective tissue disorders and CD. We, as parents, need to do backflips for our children if they have some terrible degenerative disease. A gluten-free lifestyle may be an answer for many.

A 2006 Canadian study states: "The association between dermatomyositis and celiac disease in children has been well documented." (I'd bet fewer than one percent of PCPs or skin docs know that!) This study reported that DM and nutrient deficiencies resolved in an adult woman who followed an absolute GFD. She had the DQ2 and DR3 genes that have been linked to DM and CD. **The bottom line is that patients with DM should be screened for CD, even if they do not have intestinal issues.**[118]

In 1996 a woman with arthritis, diarrhea, PM, and proteinuria (excess protein in the urine) was diagnosed with CD. All symptoms resolved on a GFD.[119] In 2002, a report noted exceptional improvement in a woman with DM and numerous malabsorption issues who'd also been diagnosed with CD. "Both diseases remitted completely in response to gluten withdrawal alone."[120]

One study suggested that screening PM/DM patients for celiac could lessen the effects of malnutrition and malignancy resulting from misdiagnosed CD.[121] About half of those with DM also have breast, lung, gastrointestinal, and ovarian cancers.[122] Obviously much more research is needed, but these few studies stress the importance of testing for CD in children or adults who've been diagnosed with DM or PM.

Inclusion Body Myositis

"Celiac disease is more prevalent in patients with inflammatory myopathies than in the general population," and patients with inclusion body myositis (IBM)—an inflammatory muscle disease—can display a high antigliadin antibody count.[123]

Dr. Marios Hadjvassiliou and colleagues found in a 2007 study that IBM got better as the level of creatine kinase went down. These researchers suggest that "myopathy may be another manifestation of gluten sensitivity" and that patients may benefit from a GFD.[124]

In one CD patient who suffered from ataxia, myopathy, and polyneuropathy, a muscle biopsy was suggestive of IBM. Vitamin E supplements resolved a severe vitamin E deficiency, and the patient's antigliadin antibodies disappeared and neurological symptoms and muscular irregularities were reversed on a GFD.[125]

Back in 1997, Dr. Hadjivassiliou and colleagues reported a new link between IBM, neuromyotonia (uncontrolled muscle activity), and CD, further stating that "**a wide range of neuromuscular disease may be the presenting feature of coeliac disease.**"[126] Should *all* cases of neuromuscular disease be screened for CD?

Alopecia

Although we often don't think of hair loss as a sign of gluten sensitivity, ***alopecia areata (patchy hair loss) may be the only sign of CD for some people.***[127]

In 2010 Dr. Angela Christiano, an associate professor of dermatology and genetics at Columbia University Medical Center, found alopecia can be associated with arthritis, CD, and type 1 diabetes.[128] In 2009, alopecia areata was linked to CD, lupus, myasthenia gravis, pernicious anemia, thyroid disease, and vitiligo—all autoimmune disorders.[129] Lichen planus (a skin disorder) and autoimmune polyendocrine syndrome type 1 (a condition involving the endocrine glands) have also been linked to alopecia areata, with thyroid disorders and vitiligo exhibiting the most notable link.[130]

Two young children with alopecia areata were diagnosed with CD. The GFD brought "complete hair growth and improved the gastrointestinal symptoms."[131] A child with alopecia areata, CD, and Down syndrome manifested normal hair growth after following a GFD. This study recommends testing for CD in patients with Down syndrome and especially in those with alopecia areata.[132] In a study of three children with alopecia and CD who were put on a GFD, one child had partial hair regrowth and the other two experienced complete hair growth.[133] Full "regrowth of scalp and body hair" resulted in an adolescent boy after he began following a GFD.[134]

If you or someone you love has alopecia, these connections are worth considering. Not all cases respond to a GFD, but if your loved one is one of those who does, it could be a life-altering decision.

Lichen Sclerosus

I got to know Shirley through her husband, who is a friend of my sister. It took her a long time to realize that gluten and dairy were huge irritants to her health. She wanted to share her story in hopes someone else might avoid the same fate.

Major Aggravation, by Shirley

I have a history of migraine headaches related to stress and allergies, both food and environmental. Four years ago I underwent a severe traumatic shock. Within a few months I started having diarrhea and lost weight rapidly, and my migraines got worse. My naturopath had me tested for a number of things, celiac disease being one of them. The CD test came back positive, and within a very short time of being on a gluten-free diet my digestive track returned to normal. By controlling my diet, I'm also reasonably able to control my migraines.

In spite of being on such a controlled diet I've developed another autoimmune disease, lichen sclerosus (LS) or vulvar dystrophy. I've learned that both gluten and dairy will aggravate this condition, which causes my skin to crack and bleed. The naturopaths do not know how to cure LS, so I must use a steroid topical cream to stop the advancement.

Now that I know CD is a genetic disease, I'm almost sure my mother had it. She had many of the generally accepted symptoms as well as several other autoimmune disorders, rheumatoid arthritis being the most severe. She eventually died from an abdominal aneurism caused by the drugs she took to control the pain, infections, and swelling resulting from rheumatoid arthritis and from the bowel dysfunction probably caused by celiac disease.

There is very little research connecting lichen sclerosus (LS) to gluten, but one study "confirms the autoimmune associations of vulval LS" and links lichen planus of the vulva to autoimmune activity.[135] And some of the forums talk positively about a GFD alleviating the symptoms. Since CD is the only autoimmune disease with a known cause and reverses itself on a gluten-free diet, is it possible that gluten could be the driving force behind the boatload of other autoimmune diseases? Why is it that so many disorders improve or clear up entirely when this toxic entity is removed? Traditional medicine has a long way to go in solving the autoimmune enigma. If only the profession could step away from the traditional "let's-treat-it" mentality and embrace a more holistic "let's-solve-it" mindset. The need for research continues.

Cystic Fibrosis

Cystic fibrosis (CF) is a recessive genetic disease (it is not an autoimmune disease) involving a "functional disorder of the exocrine glands, and is marked especially by faulty digestion due to a deficiency of pancreatic enzymes, by difficulty in breathing due to mucus accumulation in airways, and by excessive loss of salt in the sweat...."[136] Some of the symptoms of CF—abdominal pain, fatigue, irritability, loose and/or fatty stools, and poor weight gain—are similar to those of CD. Interestingly, a 2009 study found a higher incidence of CD among patients with CF than in the general public and consequently suggested CD testing for CF patients.[137]

In a 2010 study, the prevalence of CD was again found to be significantly more common among cystic fibrosis patients than in the general population. "Cystic fibrosis is a risk factor for celiac disease development," the study concluded.[138] Since this particular study used only the EMA blood test as a diagnostic tool, the "risk factor" may have been even greater than noted.

A child with intestinal issues and failure to thrive was diagnosed with both CD and CF. Addressing both ailments "resolved intestinal alterations and caused diminution of the acute bronchitis" that was common in the first two years of the patient's life.[139] A link between CF and CD was also found in a "14-month-old female infant with chronic diarrhea, recurrent respiratory infections and stunted growth... "[140]

One mom told me her young twins functioned so much better on a GFD and one of them also needed to be dairy free.

In today's reality, the list of autoimmune diseases is long (and perhaps getting longer), and while much of the research being done is cutting-edge, it often takes decades for new findings to be generally accepted. Imagine a continuum with all researchers at one end and all doctors at the other. In the middle are a mass of people who are sick and tired of being sick and tired, and sick to death of the side effects of prescription drugs. The researchers are doing a great job and the doctors are trying to do their job as well, but the gap between them is just too wide. There is a lack of formal education available to medical professionals on many research findings, and big pharma plays a significant role in promoting pharmaceuticals over dietary or environmental changes in treating disease. At the 2006 International Celiac Conference in

New York City I grabbed an annual publication called *Gastroenterology*,[141] a thick tome—printed on very thin paper—which is geared toward procedures and prescriptive medicines for treating gastrointestinal disorders. Although I plowed through the whole thing, I did not find one article on CD. I did find an ad for a CD test, but absolutely nothing about how gluten is affecting people, how to test for it, or the benefits of a GFD.

I understand only too well that no one wants to believe wheat/gluten could be contributing to his or her ailments, but there is a good deal of research supporting the fact that for many people it does. I can't tell you how many times I've heard, "I don't *think* I have it," or "My doctor doesn't *think* I have it." There is absolutely no *thinking* about it. The only way to know is to have adequate testing (see Chapters 16 and 17—I think the testing is important) or one could initiate a strict gluten-free diet for a month or more to see how their body responds.

11 The Skin You're In

THE SKIN—A TOPIC for another book that someday, someone else will write—is very much a mirror of health. Before I realized I was gluten sensitive, my skin was very dry and in winter I had cracks in my thumbs and the ball of one foot. I also had dandruff, rough elbows, and pebbly back arms—all due to vitamin and mineral deficiencies. I've since chatted with two moms whose sons had terrible acne. After they were diagnosed with celiac disease (CD) and adopted a gluten-free (GF) lifestyle, their acne disappeared. A veterinarian (and several pet owners) told me that an atopic skin condition in a dog cleared up when wheat was removed from its diet.

After reading the stories below you may want to do further research on the relationship between your skin condition and gluten sensitivity. The long list of skin conditions with links to gluten, included at the end of this chapter, can help you get started.

Skin: A Barometer of Your Health, by Wendy Cohan, RN

The liver, the body's largest internal organ, is responsible for detoxification. Once the liver is stressed and overtaxed, however, other parts of the body take on some of its toxicity-management functions. The skin can be an adjunct to the liver, which has the effect of creating skin disturbances such as rashes, hot spots, itchy spots, scaliness, redness, weeping eczema, and boils. Four months after going on a gluten-free diet, I noticed the skin rashes on my legs had healed. Afterward, even a tiny amount of gluten in something I ate would cause my leg to begin itching. This reaction was actually helpful, since it made it fairly easy to know which foods were safe for me to eat and which were not.

Dermatitis Herpetiformis

Dermatitis herpetiformis (DH), also known as Duhring's disease, is a manifestation of CD. Sufferers normally have itchy blisters or eruptions on both elbows, knees, feet, buttocks, scalp, etc. **A genetic link between DH and CD has been known for nearly four decades,**[1] so if you have a blistery, itchy skin condition that's driving you nuts, you might be wondering why your doctor hasn't mentioned CD testing. It's the same old story: a lack of information to help put the relationship between skin conditions and gluten on the specialist's radar screen.

The Raw Truth, by Gale Pearce, PA-C

Paul, (not his real name) an acquaintance of mine, has had a rather severe rash for the past 20 years, though he's never had any of the gut issues normally associated with CD. His job keeps him on the road a lot so he's been to doctors in many states, all of whom prescribed the standard fare—steroids and a corticosteroid cream/ointment. Each time this treatment would tame things down for a few weeks, but the rash always came back. About four years ago Paul finally retired and has been seeing various providers in his area. These docs followed the same pattern.

It got to the point where he was sleeping with a sheet wrapped around him to protect the linen from the weeping/oozing lesions he had from his neck to below his knees. He was taking up to six showers a day to just relieve the itch, but the doctors had no answers.

When I started researching my own problem I became aware of dermatitis herpetiformis and sent photos of the lesions from the medical literature to him by e-mail. "That's my rash!" he wrote back. Within a week he took the information to his doctors, but they would not refer him for a biopsy or dermatology consultation. I had not yet become aware of Dr. Fine's work [see www.EnteroLab.com for more information], so I suggested he just start on a gluten-free diet [GFD]. As I write this, Paul has been fairly (though not absolutely) compliant with the diet for six months, and his condition has improved more than 50 percent. He is off steroids, leading a relatively normal life, and enjoying his leisure time more.

Dermatitis herpetiformis is a skin manifestation of celiac disease that affects about 25 percent of CD patients. All DH patients have "at least some degree of mucosal inflammation or lesion consistent with celiac disease,"[2] says one study. Another, this one from Finland, found that even though 70 percent of DH patients have CD (damaged villi), fewer than 10 percent of these folks have any gastrointestinal issues.[3] Symptoms of DH may vary widely, explains a 2006 German study, but *all* DH patients are advised to follow a strict GFD.[4]

Gastrointestinal symptoms are infrequent in patients with DH; the tTG: IgA is the most sensitive diagnostic test,[5] and biopsies should be taken from uninvolved skin *surrounding* the blisters (not the blisters themselves). Dapsone, a prescriptive drug, may be used to alleviate skin lesions.

Autoimmune diseases also are more prevalent among people who have DH, but following a GFD can diminish the chance of lymphoma and other serious complications.[6] The chances of developing non-Hodgkin's lymphoma are notably enhanced in those with DH, but DH patients following an absolute GFD do not have an increase in mortality.[7] As with CD, DH patients may have "associated endocrine or connective tissue disorders."[8]

The case of an 11-year-old boy with urticaria, a skin rash similar to hives with itchy, pale red, and raised bumps, illustrates how DH in children can manifest itself as urticaria.[9] "Childhood DH may appear with clinical signs different from the adult version and misdiagnosis can occur if immunofluorescence, a testing technique, is not requested on skin biopsy."[10] For more information about the connection between DH and gluten, see Lee Tobin's story in Chapter 22 and Dick Steven's story, *I Got My Life Back*, in Chapter 9.

Multiple Symptoms on a Medical Treadmill, by Katie

Before the age of 18 I had been diagnosed with ADHD, hypertension, dyslexia, migraines, and what I thought were bad periods. I just assumed everyone felt the same way I did. Now I'm 35 years old and just starting my healing journey.

In the last eight years I have seen an increase in my weight and skin irritations—almost like little blisters or burns over my face and chest. "I just don't feel good," I explained to my doctor. I had extreme pain on my right side near what I thought were my ovaries. I would crave cheese and pizza and have migraines so bad I vomited every month. I had surgery for several "women's issues," including a partial hysterectomy, but the pains and migraines persisted.

My doctor, who didn't have a clue, sent me to four different specialists for allergies, skin rashes, hypertension, and migraines. It took months to get an appointment only to find I was allergic to about everything and was then handed a handful of prescriptions for what ailed me. At no time during this ordeal was I tested for gluten/wheat allergies or intolerance.

The dermatologist discovered I was allergic to my blood pressure meds. This scared me more than anything. My blood pressure was out of control and I needed those meds to keep me regulated. The next step was to change meds. About that time I was planning to search for a new doctor, but a light finally went off and my doctor suggested I cut out dairy and gluten. I stopped immediately and felt better within a day; within two weeks my skin had healed and the gas and pain had stopped. I did flirt with the idea that it wasn't gluten and would eat a cracker or piece of bread. Each time I regretted it almost immediately. After two weeks I went in for a blood test but it came back negative [remember, for an accurate reading you must keep eating gluten until you have *all four* blood tests]. I watch what I eat very carefully, and I'm doing really well. My blood pressure has even dropped 20 points.

Now that I've taken my life back I don't look for answers exclusively through my doctor. I know what makes me feel good or bad; I just keep it simple. It's just a shame it took eight years and thousands of dollars to figure out I can't eat gluten or dairy.

Your skin, a part of the integumentary system that also includes hair and nails, covers a wide territory. Along with it may come a wide variety of diseases. The list of numerous 10-syllable disorders shown below is extracted from an important Italian review of CD-associated skin manifestations by Dr. Ludovico Abenavoli and his colleagues in 2006.[11]

- Acquired hypertrichosis lanuginosa (excessive hair growth)
- Alopecia areata (patchy hair loss)
- Atypical mole syndrome and congenital giant nevi (birthmarks)
- Behçet's disease
- Cutaneous vasculitis
- Dermatitis herpetiformis
- Dermatomyositis
- Erythema elevatum diutinum
- Erythema nodosum
- Generalized acquired cutis laxa (yet another connective-tissue disorder–see Chapter 10)
- Hereditary angioneurotic edema
- Ichthyosiform dermatoses

- Linear IgA bullous dermatosis
- Necrolytic migratory erythema
- Oral lichen planus
- Pellagra
- Porphyria
- Psoriasis (see Chapter 21)
- Urticaria (hives)
- Vitiligo (depigmentation)

In one recent study, psoriasis patients exhibited "latent CD or CD associated antibodies,"[12] and a large number of psoriatic patients who tested positive for antigliadin antibodies "showed a highly significant decrease" in the severity of psoriasis after adopting a GFD. Moreover, "AGA values were lower in 82% of those who improved."[13] In an Italian study, when a participant on a GFD started to recover rapidly from skin lesions, researchers were able to establish a link between CD and psoriasis.[14]

Additional tongue-twisting skin diseases that may be linked to CD include: bullous pemphigoid, cutaneous sarcoidosic granuloma, ichthyosis, primary cutaneous amyloidosis, and sclero-atrophic lichen.[15] As far back as 1981, a study reported a case of cutaneous vasculitis that fully healed on an absolute GFD.[16] Blue rubber bleb nevus syndrome, a rare disease of rubbery skin lesions associated with critical iron deficiency, can be successfully treated with a GF lifestyle and iron supplements. If diagnosed early enough, many patients with this condition who are also gluten sensitive can achieve full recovery without undergoing "unnecessary procedures and invasive surgery."[17] If this very rare disorder can be healed with a strict GFD and iron (the essential missing nutrient that led to it), how expansive might a GFD be in healing and preventing many of the ailments of mankind? The screen appears to be very wide. (*Remember, however, it's important to always consult your doctor before taking iron.*)

Many of the 174 references noted by Dr. Abenavoli and colleagues in their review of medical literature for skin conditions associated with CD are of recent origin (since 1990). A couple, however, are nearly half a century old.[18] If you have a skin condition, has your dermatologist ever offered testing for celiac disease or non-celiac gluten intolerance (GI/CD)? If not, it might behoove you to read Dr. Abenavoli's research and make a copy for your doctor. Many of these skin diseases respond positively to a GF lifestyle; some may disappear altogether. Certainly huge studies are needed to solidify the causative effect of gluten on the skin, hair, and nails. But who will do them? Certainly not pharmaceutical companies; there's little profit in a gluten-free lifestyle or the good health it brings to many. Meanwhile you have valuable CD/GI screening information at your fingertips.

A dynamic elderly woman, a friend of my parents, had suffered with mycosis fungoides (a rare, non-Hodgkins lymphoma of fungal-like tumors of the skin) for years. She decided to do Dr. Fine's stool test and tested positive, but she received no encouragement from her own doctor to begin a GFD. Her list of ailments was long, and many of them were making life difficult for her, though she still managed to do volunteer work at a local hospital. I offered to help her with a GFD, but I think she felt it was just too great a lifestyle change to take on at her age.

If you are gluten sensitive, adopting a GFD can help at any age, but the sooner you begin the easier it is to do and the more your health will benefit. For information on comprehensive testing options, see Chapters 16 and 17.

Our Children Are Our Future 12

Are our children being done-in by the all-American, gluten-filled diet? Some researchers think so. In fact, one study reports that "up to 50% of the women with untreated celiac disease experience miscarriage or an unfavorable outcome of pregnancy."[1] Infertility and sterility, spontaneous abortions, menstrual and hypogonadal issues, early births, low birth weight, birth defects, and learning disabilities are some of the many issues that can be related to gluten. I've talked with a number of women who were unable to conceive before being diagnosed with celiac disease (CD). Once they began following a gluten-free diet (GFD) and the body replenished itself—usually within six months or so—they became pregnant.

"Coeliac disease is considerably more common than most of the diseases for which pregnant women are routinely screened,"[2] yet far too few doctors are aware of the correlation between gluten sensitivity and so many fertility- and pregnancy-related issues. And women are not alone in having fertility problems related to CD. For more on the role of gluten sensitivity in male reproductive function, see the section in this chapter on *Male Infertility, Loss of Libido, and Impotence.*

Spontaneous Abortions

We've all heard how common it is to have a spontaneous abortion (miscarriage), so common in fact that many women wait until they're three months pregnant before making the big announcement. CD is far from being the only reason a woman is unable to carry a pregnancy to term, but it is definitely a factor. In fact, ***"untreated celiac disease increases the risk of miscarriage 800–900%."***[3]

A Child is Born: Sarah Matus's Story

I met Sarah in Taos, New Mexico, in 2006 while eating at a restaurant she owned along with her husband, Antonio. As we chatted I found we had something in common—you guessed it: gluten sensitivity. A year later I ran across her name and gave her a call to renew our acquaintance. She hadn't been absolute with her GFD, she 'fessed up, but she felt fine except for one thing: she'd had several miscarriages. I shared some of the research about how important a GF lifestyle is for pregnant women who are gluten sensitive, and for their unborn children, and wished her well.

Back in Taos for a conference in 2008, I discovered Sarah and Antonio had opened a new restaurant (Antonio's "A Taste of Mexico"), this one with a "gluten-free" sign in the window. They'd just been talking about me the night before, Antonio told me, when I went over to reintroduce myself. After our phone conversation of the previous year, Sarah had become much more stringent in following a GF lifestyle, and she was due soon with their first child.

Two more years went by before I ran across Sarah's name again and sent her an e-mail. The good news was that she'd given birth to a healthy son. The bad news was that after he was born she became lax in following the GFD. She'd suffered four-and-a-half months with postpartum blues. Now she had an irritated gut, was so bloated after eating she felt like a balloon, was dealing with chronic constipation, and had elevated liver enzymes. She was also having memory issues, and that extra 10 pounds she was trying to drop just wouldn't come off. Her son was having problems with runny stools.

Through the good advice of a friend, Sarah took advantage of Dr. Fine's stool testing at EnteroLab for herself and her child. Unfortunately, she has intolerances to gluten, soy, dairy, eggs, and yeast; and her son tested positive for gluten sensitivity. This is not the kind of news any of us wants to hear, but at least she has an answer for her symptoms and maladies.

Infertility and Pregnancy Issues

A 2007 Italian study reports that unexplained infertility, in association with CD, has been described since the 1970s. "It is widely accepted that untreated CD represents a risk for abortion, low birth weight babies and short-breast feeding period." Researchers speculate that the malabsorption of folic acid and other vital nutrients caused by CD leads to poor pregnancy outcomes and thus "each woman with unexplained infertility should be screened for CD."[4]

According to a 2009 study from the United Kingdom, "Celiac disease (CD) occurs in as many as 1 in 80 pregnant women and is associated with poor pregnancy outcome.... direct immune effects in untreated CD women may compromise placental function."[5]

As the medical community becomes more aware of the role of gluten sensitivity in the problem of women's reproductive issues, more research is being done. In the year 2010 alone studies have found:

- Pregnancy complications are four times more likely to occur in women who have CD.[6]
- There is a greater incidence of menstrual-cycle irregularities—dysmenorrhea, hypomenorrhea, metrorrhagia, and oligomenorrhea—among women with CD.[7]
- "Autoimmunity and macro- and/or micronutrient deficiency" have been suggested as the probable cause of such reproductive issues as amenorrhea, early menopause, hypogonadism, impotence, infertility, low birth weight, preterm births, and recurrent abortions.[8]
- Delayed menarche and early menopause can also be related to gluten sensitivity. Women with menstrual and reproductive difficulties should be screened for CD.[9]
- Celiac disease has been linked to gestational hypertension, intrauterine growth restriction, placental abruption, severe anemia, threatened abortion, and uterine hyperkinesia.[10]
- Tissue transglutaminase antibodies (tTG: IgG) may damage trophoblastic cells (specialized cells within the placenta), thus leading to impairment of "embryo implantation and pregnancy outcome. . . . healthy trophoblast development is essential for placental and fetal development."[11]

Conclusion: the "significant correlation between celiac disease and reproductive disorders" could advise CD screening among women with these issues.[12] In my opinion "*should advise*" is more like it! Since so many pregnancy issues are related to gluten, it seems like a "no brainer" to recommend that all pregnant women, as well as those hoping to conceive, be screened for both CD and non-celiac gluten intolerance (GI). Given the direction of these studies, fertility clinics could embrace another whole new area of inquiry. The question is, "Are they willing to delve into the role of gluten as a contributor to fertility and pregnancy problems when the solution can often be addressed, simply and *inexpensively*, with a GFD diet? Or is it more profitable (and thus more tempting) to concentrate resources on investigating other, more costly fertility options? For more on the role of gluten in fertility, see Cecile's story, *A Typical American Family*, in Chapter 18.

Male Infertility, Loss of Libido, and Impotence

For men who are gluten sensitive, the male reproductive organs may also be attacked.[13] Gonadal dysfunction is found in many men with "acute and chronic systemic diseases"[14] and, make no bones about it, CD is a systemic disease. Untreated celiac disease can lead to "hypogonadism [decreased function of the gonads], immature secondary sex characteristics and reduce[d] semen quality." Hyperprolactinaemia, a disorder that "causes impotence and loss of libido," is found in a significant number of CD patients. A GFD diet supplemented with folate, iron, and zinc, the implicated nutrient deficiencies, can correct infertility in both men and women.[15]

During the normal age range at which puberty occurs, a highly significant number of boys and a significant number of girls with gluten sensitivity had "no maturity features." Body weight and height were also deficient in more than a third of this group.[16] Later in life, "the male CD patient has a greater risk of infertility and other reproductive disturbances, as well as a greater incidence of hypoandrogenism [low testosterone levels]."[17] Fortunately, when those with CD are treated with a GFD, hormonal irregularities can turn around. That's why early detection is so important.

Preeclampsia, Toxemia, and Severe Cramps

My good friend and storyteller, Kay Dunn, saw Suzanne giving a gluten-free cooking demo at a fair in Maine and thought she would be a good contact for me. When we talked, Suzanne readily agreed to share her story. Since then she has opened a dedicated gluten-free commercial kitchen in a newly built maple sugar house that offers classes, GF baked goods and mixes, other GF products, and local honey.

Years of Suffering, by Suzanne Jane

I believe I've been gluten intolerant all my life. As a child I had severe allergies every spring. I also had several food allergies, though I was never tested for an allergy to gluten. Over the years I went to many doctors for my bad, doubled-over stomachaches and other complaints such as a rash on my elbows and recurrent diarrhea. Each time I got the same answer: "There's nothing wrong with you; it's all in your head."

It wasn't until I was in my mid-thirties that I went to an MD who practiced integrative medicine—a doctor who looks at the whole body as an interconnected system—hoping against hope she could help me deal with my stomach problems, rashes, and anxiety. When (prompted by a yeast overgrowth) she suggested a blood test for gluten sensitivity, it was the first time I'd ever heard these words. Even today, more than 30 years later, there's not nearly enough information about how to handle a GFD. Back then there was practically nothing. When the results of my test came back positive I began shopping at health food stores, learning and practicing relaxation techniques such as meditation, and making other lifestyle changes. I started integrating whole foods and herbs into my diet. But I was still in denial about the effects of gluten. For example, I'd eat "just a little pizza." The fact that I'd suffer for a week afterward didn't seem to sink in.

In 1978 I lost a full-term baby at birth due to preeclampsia and toxemia. I also had an ectopic pregnancy, debilitating menstrual cramps, severe bouts of diarrhea, a yeast overgrowth in my gut, weight gain, weight loss, and, finally, a hysterectomy because of fibroid tumors and endometriosis. I never had any children of my own, but happily adopted a nephew when he was a baby.

In 1984 I was diagnosed with celiac sprue with a blood test, but it wasn't until about 10 years later that I took the GFD more seriously and went totally off gluten. Miraculously, my food sensitivities disappeared, and the next spring my seasonal allergies were gone as well. The muscle pain also went away and I had more stamina than I'd had in years.

Even while on a strict GFD, for years I still had digestive issues, cramping, and diarrhea, but not nearly as bad as they used to be. About five years ago I had more testing: (colonoscopy, endoscopy, ultrasound, allergy tests, etc.) and discovered I have a sluggish gallbladder. Along the way I also eliminated or reduced environmental toxins and cosmetics with additives and/or preservatives and got reacquainted with relaxation techniques.

In 2005, I started giving gluten-free lectures and food demos. While managing a health food store I discovered that many people with symptoms of gluten sensitivity or those who have just learned they are gluten intolerant have no idea where to turn. My first classes drew a few people, then a few more, and before I knew it I was being invited to speak in other parts of the state. At the Common Ground Country Fair in Unity, Maine, an event that draws thousands of people each September, I gave a country-kitchen cooking demo of gluten-free foods. About 100 people showed up—standing room only! The fact that I suffered so much over the years with nowhere to turn for guidance really motivates me to help others.

My mother died of a heart attack at the age of 63. Looking back, I truly believe she had undiagnosed CD. In the years before her death she developed diabetes, severe intestinal issues, and numbness in her face. She also experienced rapid weight loss and suffered from extreme anxiety. The doctors said it was all in her head. If she had been tested for gluten sensitivity, she may have had the chance for a longer and better-quality life.

As for me, I feel better today than I have ever felt. I still have some food sensitivities (mostly eggs and dairy), which I've come to learn is not uncommon. Most people attending my classes also have food sensitivities apart from CD. I now take the natural enzyme cholestyramine to aid my gallbladder, which has made yet another improvement in my digestive process. The cramping and diarrhea have disappeared. These days it's wonderful to go on a road trip without having to plan bathroom stops along the way.

Suzanne's story echoes that of many women with fertility and/or pregnancy problems. Preeclampsia, which can lead to toxemia, is a serious complication of late pregnancy typified by edema, excess protein in the urine, headache, high blood pressure, weight gain, and more.[18] That both Suzanne and her mother were told "it was all in their head" is common when one is plagued with symptoms that appear to have no cause. If your doctors can't find what ails you and are suggesting you see a shrink, and your family thinks you're a hypochondriac, perhaps the real cause is the insidious, toxic effect of gluten. You may have a chance to educate them all.

Menstrual difficulties also plague many women who are gluten sensitive. My own periods, though never painful, got so heavy that I couldn't even walk to the end of the driveway without the need to rush back. One day in my late forties I called my doc and said, "I can't deal with this anymore." Like Suzanne, I had a total hysterectomy, during which the surgeon removed a tumor the size of a grapefruit. See *From Night to Day*, B. B. J.'s story about preeclampsia, early births, and miscarriage in Chapter 6.

Another young woman I know suffered terrible pain during intercourse. Her doctor put her on steroids, but she soon had to stop taking them because of chest pain. She was lucky to find a doctor who traced her problem to gluten. Six to eight months after beginning a GFD, the inflammation and swelling causing her pain had subsided.

Another connection between gluten and pregnancy-related issues may be found in women with antiphospholipid syndrome (APS). APS is an autoimmune disease that creates "antibodies that attack platelets in blood, causing them to stick together and form clots."[19] In pregnant women the disease is characterized by "arterial and venous thrombosis, and spontaneous fetal death...Celiac disease is also associated with spontaneous fetal death; consequently, we hypothesize that antiphospholipid syndrome may be one of the causes for this event."[20] To avoid such tragedies, **women who suffer repeated miscarriages should be screened for APS.**

Endometriosis

The internal lining of the uterus is called the endometrium. When cells from this lining grow elsewhere in the body, it is called endometriosis. Although often painful, the condition is not, by definition, cancerous. However, it can cause infertility, and the "endometrial hyperplasia [increased cell production] of the uterus" must be watched and treated so it doesn't evolve into cancer.[21]

A 2011 Swedish study concluded: "Endometriosis seems to be associated with prior CD. Potential explanations include shared etiological [causal] factors and CD-mediated inflammation."[22] A Brazilian study done in 2009 found CD was common "among women with endometriosis."[23]

Nutritionist Dian Shepperson Mills offers good news for endometriosis sufferers. "When I've taken wheat out of the diet," she said, "in 80% of the women with endometriosis, the pain subsides.... And when they reintroduce the wheat the pain comes back."[24]

One study concluded that allergies, asthma, autoimmune diseases, chronic fatigue syndrome, fibromyalgia, and hypothyroidism were "significantly more common in women with endometriosis than in women in the general USA population."[25] It's not surprising. Again and again we see the interconnections among ailments associated with CD.

Miraculous, by Gina White

I was diagnosed with endometriosis at a very young age and told that due to extensive damage I would not be able to conceive children. The pain I experienced every month as my cycle began was so intense it warranted bed rest. Along with the lower cramping, I experienced substantial upper abdominal pain and burning plus extreme abdominal swelling. In my twenties these symptoms subsided somewhat and, miraculously, I did conceive two healthy sons who have since grown into fine young men.

When I turned 40, my endometriosis symptoms worsened. Bedridden for several weeks, I spent a lot of time researching my symptoms and discovered I had another autoimmune disorder as well. As a result, I had a test for celiac disease. The results were positive and I immediately went gluten free. Once I was on a GFD, I noticed my monthly menstrual symptoms became drastically reduced. Perhaps my issues with endometriosis are also linked to celiac disease.

Many women have terrible monthly issues and infertility problems, just as Gina once had. Based on studies such as those cited here, it appears gluten could be the culprit for some of those women, and removing it could resolve much pain and discomfort. I know of two other women with endometriosis who also had a positive, life-changing experience by removing gluten from their lives. Again, more studies need to be done, but if you had endometriosis and there was a possibility you could improve by simply changing your diet, wouldn't it be worth investigating? (Be sure to read Jess M.'s story, *Profound Results*, in Chapter 8.)

Birth Defects, Learning Disabilities, and Developmental Delay

At the beginning of this book I quoted researchers who believe that 1 in every 100 Americans has CD, with 97 percent of these folks remaining undiagnosed. (These numbers are slowly changing and may be about 80 percent.) Dr. Alessio Fasano has proven that 6 of every 100 Americans are gluten intolerant, and Dr. Kenneth Fine asserts that between 30 and 40 percent of the population is gluten sensitive. Even if these numbers are adjusted over time (though ongoing research, unfortunately, tends to raise rather than lower them), the inevitable conclusion is that many women who become pregnant suffer from issues related to malabsorption. Is it possible that some mothers who give birth to children later diagnosed with autism, ADD, learning disabilities, etc., may have been unable to optimally nourish their children in the womb because the mothers had subclinical celiac disease and were malnourished themselves? A sobering thought indeed.

Thyroid hormones also play a role during pregnancy. In fact, these hormones "have been shown to be absolutely necessary for early brain development." Pregnant women with thyroid disease who do not receive hormone therapy can expect a troublesome outcome.[26]

Folic acid, iron, and vitamin K are other nutrients crucial to the development of the fetus, and CD may lead to their deficiency. Some researchers surmise that "endocrine imbalances and immune disturbances" play a part as well.[27] Babies born to women with CD had "a three-fold higher risk of intrauterine growth retardation…" if the mother's CD was recognized after the birth. The bottom line is that "**treatment of celiac women is important in the prevention of fetal growth retardation.**"[28]

Once children are born, nutritional deficiencies continue to be a source of concern. For example, iron deficiency anemia in children from 6 to 24 months of age increases the risk for cognitive, motor, neurophysiologic, and social-emotional developmental issues. These problems "can be prevented and/or reversed with iron...before the deficiency becomes chronic or acute."[29]

Before we realized gluten was a problem for her, Aly, my sweet little granddaughter, was quite delayed on a number of developmental milestones: standing, crawling, walking, and talking. In addition, my daughter's breast milk supply didn't seem adequate; later, she learned she was malabsorbing herself. Since being on a GFD Aly has blossomed, but I expect she would have had a tough time in life if we had not known about the deleterious effects of gluten to her system.

13 Gluten Indicted: An "Enhancer to Cancer"

EACH OF US has known someone—a loved one, a friend, a neighbor—who passed away from cancer, a dreaded and complex disease. Over the past 20 years great progress has been made in treatment, but much more needs to be done to determine cancer's many causes. Some risk factors are well-publicized, the most common being cigarette smoking. For years tobacco companies and many medical professionals denied the connection between smoking and cancer, but eventually science caught up with them. The truth could no longer be ignored, and today most people who choose to smoke do so with full access to information about the risks to their health.

Like tar and nicotine, gluten plays a role in the cancer equation, and for those who are gluten-sensitive, this connection can be significant: ***"Untreated celiac disease increases the risk of cancer 200–300%"***[1] A wide range of cancers, including non-Hodgkin's lymphoma, throat/esophageal, stomach/intestinal/colon, and others are now being connected to gluten consumption. In addition, liver and throat ailments that can turn into cancer can clear up or improve on a gluten-free diet (GFD).

All of this information about gluten came 35 years too late for my father (see *Father to Daughter: Grampy Nick's Story* in Chapter 10). Mark Krcmaric, who tells his story below, was far luckier. His doctor, at a large university hospital, knew of the connection between gluten and non-Hodgkin's lymphoma. Because of his knowledge, Mark's story has a happy outcome.

Gluten Free, Cancer Free, and Living Free, by Mark Krcmaric

I am a type 1 diabetic with celiac disease (CD). I am also a cancer survivor. I tell my story to inform and educate those who may have CD and not know it, and to inspire those who live daily with the celiac condition.

As a child I was always "as thin as a rail." I never seemed to be able to gain weight and people were amazed at how much food I could eat and remain so thin. In 1981, at age 21, I was diagnosed with type 1 diabetes. The disease ran in my family, but I was the only member who had type 1, insulin-dependent diabetes. Fortunately, I've been able to manage my diabetes well all of my life, but this story is not about this aspect of my medical history.

In 1987 routine blood tests revealed I was anemic. Anemia is a rare condition in males, so my diabetes doctor took stool-sample tests. He was convinced I was bleeding internally, yet the tests came back negative. The anemic condition, however, did not go away. The doctor then ordered a colonoscopy and upper GI. Once again, all tests came back negative. Unable to find a cause, the doctor prescribed iron pills that eliminated the anemia.

A different diabetes doctor took me off the iron pills in 1989, after which I dropped five pounds to 145. I'm 5 foot 10 inches tall, so I was pretty thin, but my weight stabilized and I continued to eat *lots of food*, somewhere between 3,200 and 3,500 calories per day.

By 1993 my weight had dropped another five pounds, even though I was still eating a ton of food. Blood tests revealed the anemia had returned. By now I was seeing a third diabetes doctor, who ordered the same procedures I'd gone through in 1987. Stool-sample tests, an upper GI, and a colonoscopy were performed over a six-month period. Just as before, all the results were negative. [Note: The lab/hospital tests referred to here are different from those conducted by EnteroLab.] My doctor was perplexed. How could I be anemic and not be losing any blood? Why wasn't I gaining weight given the number of calories I was consuming? He referred me to a gastroenterologist for further testing. By now I was feeling like a gerbil running in a wheel. Would I ever get out of the cage?

The gastroenterologist ordered a CAT scan of the abdomen and chest. "I'm very sorry," he said when we met to discuss the results, "but we've found a mass alongside your small intestine. I need to refer you to an oncologist."

Man, nothing hits as hard as the "C" word. I was 35 years old, my life was going along nicely, and all of the sudden the reality of my mortality hit me right between the eyes. Do I have days, months—or maybe years? Cancer affects everyone around you; it was even harder for my wife, Charlotte, than it was for me. All of a sudden I realized how big the gift of life really is. It is truly a gift from God. Why did it take me so long to realize how we all take life for granted instead of appreciating the gift it is and living each day to its fullest. We worry too much about the future or regret what we've done in the past instead of taking each moment and day to live as best we can.

The oncologist said the growth was a lymphoma. He was almost certain the mass was cancerous but needed to test the cells to be absolutely sure. The tests would also determine the growth rate and thus the type of treatment needed. More than likely, I would need chemotherapy to kill the cancer. The bad part was that to get to the mass, I needed exploratory abdominal surgery, giving the surgeon an opportunity to obtain necessary cell samples and remove anything that looked bad.

During the operation the surgeon removed my appendix and took cells for testing. Two days later the doctors told me the mass was not cancerous. I couldn't believe it. What a relief! All I needed was to recuperate from the surgery. They still didn't know what the mass was, they said, but it really didn't matter. The important thing was, it wasn't cancer.

When I left the hospital two days later, I was down to 135 pounds. At home my friends told me I looked like I'd just been released from a concentration camp. The doctors told me to consume nutritional supplements in addition to my normal diet to help gain weight.

The following week I received a call from the oncologist. After further testing of the mass cells, the lab determined I had a low-grade, B-cell, non-Hodgkin's lymphoma. It *was* cancer after all. I needed to get my strength back, the doctor explained, after which I would need chemotherapy to try to kill the cancer.

My recovery was not going well. Dazed and very confused, I talked to a friend who had been through a bad cancer experience. She insisted I get a second opinion at a teaching university before going forward with the chemo. I didn't know it at the time, but her advice helped change my life forever.

I went to the University of Chicago for a second opinion. There I met with a team of four doctors who were remarkable. I spent an afternoon with them, during which I gave them my entire story and they asked a lot of questions. They confirmed the low-grade, B-cell lymphoma. However, they were much more concerned that I could not gain weight—in fact, was continuing to lose weight—despite eating large quantities of food.

Without diagnosing and treating this condition first, they explained, I would not be strong enough to undergo chemotherapy. Fortunately, my cancer was growing very slowly so there was no immediate need to treat it. Moreover, they felt that *whatever was causing my problems with weight loss and anemia might also be the cause of the cancer.* We agreed they would continue to monitor the cancer via CAT scans while simultaneously trying to determine the reason for my other problems.

Next I met with a gastroenterologist, a doctor I credit with saving my life. He told me about a condition called celiac disease and we began testing for it. Even before the test results came back, he felt 99.9 percent sure this was my problem. If it was, he explained, I'd have to adopt a gluten-free diet, but once I did so I would see *profound changes* within a short period of time. In all likelihood I would gain weight and my anemia would vanish. Because I would actually be absorbing nutrients I would get stronger. I should see changes in stool composition, he explained and, possibly, the cancer could stop growing. On the other hand, he warned, if I did not adhere to the gluten-free diet, none of the aforementioned would occur and the cancer could get worse.

Since we were in Chicago, he recommended I take my wife, Charlotte, to the best Italian restaurant in town and order my favorite pasta dish, because it would be the last time I'd ever have it [gluten-free pasta did not exist then].

Once the doctor confirmed my condition, Charlotte and I received some training on what constitutes a gluten-free diet. Back home, we rummaged through our cabinets, reading the ingredients on every box and can. Ninety-five percent of it contained gluten in one form or another. We gave that food away, and from that day to this I've adhered to a strict, gluten-free diet.

Sometimes I view my doctor as a prophet. After going gluten free I gained 20 pounds in two weeks. My anemia vanished and I got stronger. The doctors monitored me for about eight years via CAT scans and blood tests. All of my blood counts were perfect and I never needed chemotherapy. My cancer had gone into a natural remission. Just to be sure, my oncologist ordered a nuclear test designed to find cancerous masses and lymph nodes. The test took a lot longer than I was told it would and I was growing concerned. Once it was finally over the radiologist asked me to stay; he wanted to speak to me. Now I was really nervous. Radiologists *never* talk to patients. He emerged from behind the wall and asked why I was there for this particular test. I told him about my cancer history. Then he told me what took so long: He couldn't find *anything*—no sign of cancer at all. He'd spent the extra time looking hard to make sure he hadn't missed anything.

Today, I am a happy and healthy 50-year-old. I weigh 176 pounds and have to watch what I eat so I don't become overweight. I take in between 1,500 and 2,000 calories per day. I have been cancer free for twenty years and go for yearly office visits with my oncologist. I adhere strictly to a GFD. When I stray from the diet by accident my body tells me so, so I try to be as careful as I can.

Through my experience I've learned a lot about what is and is not important in this life. Live and love each day to its fullest, and let those you love know it. *Carpe Diem!* Seize the day!

Cancer and Celiac Disease

The mortality rate among adult CD patients is about twice that of the general population, "mostly due to cancer...Deaths are greatest within the first year of diagnosis."[2] In fact, a 1989 study reports that ***"malignancy may be the first manifestation of subclinical [silent] celiac disease."***[3] For these folks, as for many other cancer victims, by the time the disease is finally detected it has ravaged and weakened the body for a long time.

Research studies linking celiac disease to cancer go back more than half a century. A 1976 review by G. K. Holmes and colleagues reveals two patients with "reticulum cell sarcoma...and one with acute myeloid leukemia" had a total reversal of damaged villi once they were placed on a GFD. This same review quotes studies as far back as 1936 linking steatorrhoea (excess fat in the stool) and intestinal lymphoma, even though the cause of CD was not known back then.[4] Additional research prior to 1991 found:

- The chance of CD patients developing cancer if they'd been following a GFD for five or more years "was not increased when compared to the general population." However, CD patients who ate a "reduced gluten or normal diet" *were* found to have an increased risk, especially for "cancers of the mouth, pharynx, and oesophagus . . . and also of lymphoma . . ." Thus, following an absolute GFD can have a protective effect.[5]
- CD should be thought of as a "premalignant condition not only for lymphoma and gastrointestinal tumors, but also for adenocarcinoma of the small intestine." The conclusion: Patients with adenocarcinoma should be screened for CD.[6]
- Patients suffering a return of symptoms after reacting positively to a strict GFD should be checked for "evidence of a small bowel malignancy."[7]

Research between 2001 and 2011 found:

- Compared to the general population, CD patients have an increased level of risk for developing certain kinds of cancers (2011 study):[8]

    - Melanoma—5 times greater
    - Non-Hodgkin's lymphoma—6 to 9 times greater
    - Esophageal—12 times greater
    - Primary gastrointestinal lymphoma—24 to 34 times greater
- In one 2001 survey, 22 children with CD also had various types of cancer, including malignancies of the adrenal glands, brain, larynx, liver, lymphoreticular system, and musculoskeletal system. Many small-bowel and thyroid malignancies indicated a possible link to CD.[9]
- The older an individual at the time of his/her CD diagnosis, the greater the risk the individual will develop cancer. Thus, adults and seniors with CD should be vigorously screened for tumors.[10]
- There is an "increased risk and mortality, especially for B- and T-cell lymphoma…outside the gut." This risk is most noticeable in the first few years after CD is diagnosed. CD "is not an innocent condition."[11]
- The causes of increased tumor development are not well understood, but the following factors may play a part: chronic antigenic stimulation, environmental carcinogens (gluten is toxic for those genetically predisposed), inflammation, malnutrition, permeable gut, and proinflammatory cytokines.[12] *Note: All these factors are associated with CD as well.*
- Chromosomal irregularities in lymphocytes (white blood cells including B-, T-, and NK [natural killer] cells) may put children with CD at risk for cancer. After following a GFD for two years, children in one study had blood levels similar to the healthy controls; participants not on the diet had increased chromosomal deviations. The study concluded that chronic intestinal inflammation could be the cause of these genetic irregularities.[13]
- A new hypothesis suggests T-cells can play a key part in the obliteration of healthy tissue. The intestinal inflammation of CD—brought on by gluten or other infectious means—can be the trigger that turns on and initiates the detrimental impact of T-cells (2009 study).[14]

- IgA antibodies produced in the gut can be found on tissue transglutaminase (tTG) in the kidney, liver, lymph nodes, and muscles of CD patients, and these antibodies play a role in the disease process.[15] A disturbance in the normal, positive activity of tTG can lead to "chronic neurodegeneration, neoplastic diseases, autoimmune diseases, diseases involving progressive tissue fibrosis and diseases related to the epidermis of the skin."[16]

Lymphoma

Imagine an irritant—a piece of rough clothing, say, or a tight shoe—rubbing the same spot on your skin for hours on end. At first the skin would turn pink. Then it would become tender and red with inflammation. Finally it would begin to ooze. If the irritant weren't removed, the spot would eventually become an open sore that would never get better. Once the irritant was eliminated, however, the spot could begin to heal. The malabsorption and immune reactivity leading to inflammation is just such an irritant. With healthy cells already compromised, it's not hard to understand why people with CD are more susceptible to lymphomas and so many other ailments.

As a matter of fact, ***the link between CD and lymphoma has been known for about 50 years.***[17] A 2005 study notes that "most lymphomas complicating celiac disease are indeed related to the disease..."[18] Other research reports that CD "significantly increases [the] risk of developing small bowel lymphomas by 30 to 40 percent and other gut malignancies by 83-fold."[19] Genetic factors linked to CD "may influence the development of malignant lymphoma within pre-existing celiac disease." Malignant melanoma, prostate, and other cancers may be diet related.[20] An increased risk of developing a lymphoproliferative cancer depends on the villi damage, "with no increased risk in latent celiac disease..." [21] In other words, the greater the villi damage, the greater the risk of developing lymphomas.

Enteropathy-associated T-cell lymphoma (EATL), in particular, has been cited as "the most frequent, aggressive and fatal complication" of CD.[22] EATL can be found in the brain, nasal sinus, liver/spleen, skin, and thyroid.[23] And for even more bad news, in a 1995 review the author reports that EATL patients have a genetic link to CD.[24] The good news, however, is that results from a 2008 Italian study revealed that an absolute GFD has a *protective* effect against developing EATL.[25] Here's yet another reason to be *strict* with a GFD.

In a study led by Dr. Peter H. R. Green and colleagues, researchers found the chances of developing esophageal cancer, melanoma, and non-Hodgkin's lymphoma were heightened in those with CD. Even CD patients following a GFD had a risk of developing non-Hodgkin's lymphoma.[26] As mentioned in Chapter 10, patients with Sjögren's syndrome, another CD-linked disorder, also have a greater chance of developing this form of lymphoma—the risk has a 40-fold increase.[27]

Dermatitis herpetiformis [DH] is a skin condition with strong links to CD (see Chapter 11). DH patients with CD who do not follow a GFD also have markedly heightened chances of developing non-Hodgkin's lymphoma. DH patients who lead a GF lifestyle, on the other hand, have "no increased general mortality."[28] This is all sobering news, but as illustrated by Mark's story above, sometimes the benefits of a GFD can be startlingly positive.

Refractory sprue (discussed later in this chapter) and ulcerative jejunitis also are included in the span of lymphomas.[29] And CD may be linked to cancers associated with "rare hepatic complications, such as hepatic T-cell lymphoma."[30] Just based on my own experience, I know someone who was diagnosed with chronic lymphocytic leukemia (CLL) not long after being diagnosed with gluten sensitivity. So far, his numbers seem to be holding their own; in fact, they're lower than when he was first diagnosed. Recently he was told he only needed to have his blood checked once a year. Could gluten be a contributing factor to CLL as well?

Myeloproliferative Disease

Individuals with autoimmune disorders have a higher chance of developing diseases related to bone marrow such as acute myeloid leukemia and myelodysplastic syndrome.[31] And from reading previous chapters of this book, you know that autoimmune diseases have a strong association with CD.

Two other conditions regarded as "typical of myeloproliferative disorders or neoplastic conditions" are extreme thrombocytosis (high blood platelet levels) and acute anemia. These conditions can be caused by CD (see Chapter 8). In one case study, an 83-year-old woman with fatigue, anemia, and extreme thrombocytosis saw all her blood test and biopsy results return to normal after being diagnosed with CD and following a GFD for two months.[32]

Adenocarcinoma

"A 10- to 280-fold increased risk of small bowel adenocarcinoma" was found in CD patients compared to the population at large, noted a study done in 2004. The study concluded that patients with abdominal pain, signs of obstruction or weight loss should be assessed for cancer.[33]

CD patients also may have a heightened chance of developing carcinoma of the esophagus and pharynx, as well as adenocarcinoma of the small intestine.[34]

Multiple Myeloma

Multiple myeloma (MM) is a type of blood cancer that develops in the bone marrow. One study noted that an immunological reaction to "gliadin and to tissue transglutaminase is present in some patients with MM" and postulated that such a reaction could contribute to the disease process.[35] Another study went so far as to question whether multiple myeloma is a "more severe form of gluten intolerance than celiac."[36]

Refractory Celiac Disease

The story below is suggestive of refractory sprue—difficult to treat and nonresponsive to a GF lifestyle. When I asked if she used gluten-free lipstick, toothpaste, medicines, vitamins, etc., she said she hadn't realized lipstick needed to be GF. Yet the littlest bit of gluten in her lipstick could be enough to keep the malabsorption and immunological processes happening. With refractory sprue you *must* clean up your diet; then other issues need to be ruled out before the body can begin to heal.

There is some fairly recent research connecting atrial fibrillation to gluten—the fibrillation clears up when gluten is removed from the diet (see Chapter 14). If you have atrial fibrillation and/or what appears to be refractory sprue, help your specialists to help you by making sure your GF lifestyle is absolute, down to lipstick, lotions (your hands touch food), cutting boards, the toaster, the peanut butter jar, etc. Once you have gluten under control, it makes it that much easier to rule out any other causes.

For the Rest of Your Life, by N. G.

I am 65 years old and have always been a stay-at-home mom; I love gardening, sports, reading, volunteer work, and traveling with my husband of 40 years. Yet despite my contentment with life, I've had a number of nagging medical issues. Even as a child I remember frequent bouts of stomach pain and constipation. As a young adult I suffered with headaches, leg cramps, canker sores in my mouth, and continual stomach discomfort that only ceased after spending time in the bathroom.

The stomach pains seem to lessen during my 20s and 30s, or maybe the responsibilities of caring for three children, dogs, a home, and a husband kept me so busy I overlooked them. I did have migraine headaches, however, each preceded by an aura and then horrible vomiting. These occurred several times a year and still do, though eating candied ginger at the onset has eliminated the vomiting.

Sometime in 1985, at the age of 42, I began to have chronic "stomach problems" ranging from mild discomfort to intense aches, along with gastrointestinal issues that ran the gamut from constipation to severe diarrhea. On many days, the discomfort was enough to cause me to make last-minute changes in my activities. A gastroenterologist diagnosed my problems as irritable bowel syndrome and said I should "give my intestinal tract a break" and stay off vegetables and fruits for a while. He scheduled me for a sigmoidoscopy; the results looked normal. I took his advice and ate fewer fruits and veggies. What did I eat instead? Breads and pastas! I suffered terribly!

He then sent me for an ultrasound, which unexpectedly detected a growth on my left ovary; my gynecologist did a laparoscopy and D&C, the results of which indicated I had hyperplasia, a precancerous condition of the uterus. He put me on a hormonal medication for three months. Retesting showed it had spread, and he recommended a total hysterectomy and oophorectomy (removal of both ovaries), surgery which I had in 1989.

I dealt with my stomach ailment over the next couple of years as best I could. Mornings were the worst; the diarrhea had become more severe. I was tired, I was losing weight, and I looked awful. I'd also lost strength in my hands, arms, and legs. It was obvious I was losing muscle mass.

At a yearly checkup with my gynecologist in early 1991, he inquired about my noticeable weight loss, poor color, and overall soreness and said he wanted to run some blood work. That evening he called me at home, asking if I was "honestly" eating properly. My lab results were all dangerously low, he reported, and I was extremely anemic. He said that if things weren't turned around I was going to *die of malnutrition*. He'd even taken the prerogative to show the lab results, anonymously, to my gastroenterologist, who replied that if it were his patient, she would be hospitalized. The next day I was back at the gastroenterologist, who started me on monthly B12 shots and potassium supplements.

The doctor believed, based on the lab tests, that something was very wrong with my small intestine, most probably celiac sprue or cancer. A few days later, he did an endoscopy. "Good News!" he said excitedly, when he called with the results. "You don't have cancer. You have sprue!" He then went on to explain this meant I couldn't eat anything with wheat flour. "For how long?" I asked. His reply was shocking: "For the rest of your life!"

That was 15 years ago. I am very strict about maintaining a gluten-free lifestyle and I feel much better, though some days are still difficult. I suspect some permanent damage was done in the seven years it took to be diagnosed, and that as a result my system doesn't always work properly. A repeat endoscopy showed part of my small intestine still had flattened villi. The doctor explained there was something called refractory sprue that doesn't respond to a gluten-free diet. He suggested a steroid; I opted not to try it.

I was recently hospitalized with a life-altering episode of atrial flutter, a heart arrhythmia. When we arrived at the emergency room my heart rate was 237. Now I must remain on daily heart medication forever.

As I've learned more about the genetic component of celiac disease, I'm fairly certain my mother suffered from this condition. She was very sickly and looked wasted away. She died of viral pneumonia when I was 7 and she was 39. Other family members also have undiagnosed stomach issues, migraines, and dental enamel problems, but have not been tested as yet.

Refractory celiac disease (RCD), sometimes referred to as refractory sprue, is a condition in which the villi are resistant to the healing effects of a GFD. Several things can contribute to RCD, including failure of the pancreas to produce digestive enzymes and excessive bacterial growth in the small intestine (both discussed below). On the other hand, continued damage may simply be caused by mini hits of gluten, intentional or unintentional. If you are on a GFD and your body is not responding positively, it's important to scrutinize everything that goes into your mouth to make sure you are being absolutely compliant.

Since non-compliance with a GFD can be a contributor to CD progressing to RCD, it's important to do all you can to avoid this slippery slope. One study notes that between 50 and 60 percent of patients with RCD II, the more severe form of the disorder, progress to an enteropathy-associated T-cell lymphoma (ETAL).[37] This type of cancer is relatively rare, but for those who contract it, the prognosis is poor. Fortunately, there is a great deal of information available to those choosing a GF lifestyle. For help in successfully removing gluten from your life, see Chapters 19 and 20.

Exocrine Pancreatic Insufficiency—One of the functions of the pancreas is to produce enzymes that help digest our food. When the pancreas fails to do so, or fails to do so sufficiently, the result is exocrine pancreatic insufficiency (EPI). At one time this condition was thought to appear only in the elderly. However, in one CD study, an adolescent with chronic diarrhea, late pubertal development, and stature issues began to mend with the aid of pancreatic enzyme supplements. Researchers conclude that "pancreatic failure can occur with celiac disease at any age."[38] If CD patients fail to have a favorable outcome by following a GFD, the cause could be a severe case of pancreatic insufficiency.[39]

A 2010 study from the United Kingdom found that EPI was the root cause of continuing diarrhea in 30 percent of CD patients. Nineteen of twenty participants got better when given pancreatic enzyme supplements. As they healed, many were able to give up the supplements.[40] For more on the link between gluten and pancreatic issues, see Chapter 10.

Small Intestinal Bacterial Overgrowth—"Small intestinal bacterial overgrowth [SIBO] is a condition…[of] excessive levels of bacteria"[41] that may cause lingering gastrointestinal symptoms in many patients with CD, even after the elimination of gluten,[42] and may also lead to enhanced intestinal permeability.[43] Symptoms of SIBO include bloating, diarrhea, malabsorption, malnutrition, and weight loss.[44]

There may also be a link between SIBO and irritable bowel syndrome (IBS),[45] a condition that has already been linked to CD (see the section on *Irritable Bowel Syndrome* in Chapter 7).

If patients are responding poorly or not at all to a GFD, they should rule out SIBO and lactose intolerance[46] (possibly due to CD), as well as pancreatic insufficiency. In some cases, dairy, egg, soy, yeast, and other proteins may also be causing intestinal havoc, so CD patients should rule out these intolerances, too. Fructose intolerance may also hamper healing,[47] and it's important to keep testing for giardia (an intestinal parasite) in difficult-to-diagnose patients suspected of having CD.[48] Once all of these issues are addressed, full recuperation may result with an absolute GFD.

Recently my husband and I settled in to watch a TV program on stomach cancer. I said to him, "What do you bet they don't mention the word gluten or celiac disease?" Of course, they didn't. The companies who buy ads to make such programs possible realize little profit from patients who get better by simply changing their diets. On the other hand, Dr. William Davis, cardiologist and author of *Wheat Belly: Lose the Wheat, Lose the Weight, and Find Your Path Back to Health*[49]—a must-read—brought to light a study that found "noticeably increased risks of some malignancies such as gastrointestinal cancers and lymphoma" associated with celiac disease.[50] Such a contrast!

The answer to cancer may lie in the positive, protective response of a gluten-free lifestyle. Has your oncologist mentioned testing for gluten sensitivity? If not, if you have most any kind of cancer, especially if it has not advanced too far (or even if it has) you might consider getting tested for CD/GI. If the tests detect a sensitivity to gluten, you might find life-enhancing results by eliminating a substance that could be weakening your body's ability to fight malignant cells.

There is no question that cancer research in the gluten arena is in its infancy. It is also a fact that cancer treatment is an enormous industry. Many of us give generously to organizations in this country seeking a cure for cancer, but of the numerous (but not nearly enough) studies I found researching a possible link between cancer and gluten, three-quarters of them were done in other countries. Moreover, all but four studies were conducted in the last decade. Despite the medical advances of the twenty-first century, a veil of darkness shrouds the link between cancer and gluten. We have a long, long way to go.

14 Organ Malfunction: A Medical Masquerade

The "Heart" of the Matter

Parents and grandparents, observe the children in your family. Are they lethargic, clingy, and/or irritable? Are they reluctant to participate in activities? Is their skin color off? By now you have read enough to understand that the degenerative assault of gluten can affect *any* organ or part of your body. So if you have *any* concerns about your child's health you may want to consider having your child tested for gluten sensitivity before a more serious condition develops.

Skin Tone Tip-Off, by Annie Fields

I'd noticed that my daughter, Carolyn [not her real name] had a yellowish tint to her skin. At her six-year-old checkup I asked our doctor about it. "Her skin tone seems normal to me," she responded. "In fact, Carolyn's skin is the same color as yours."

That spring Carolyn started to experience frequent breakdowns, especially toward the end of the day. She was too tired to take a bath after dinner. By summer she was having a breakdown every night. She hated swimming lessons and spent most of the summer sitting on my lap while my other children laughed and splashed in the lake all day long.

I took her to doctors a couple of times that summer, but other than swimmer's ear they could find nothing wrong with her. Since she'd had some trouble adjusting to kindergarten, one doctor thought she was just nervous about starting first grade in the fall.

By the end of the summer she was driving me crazy. *Maybe she has mono*, I thought. It would certainly explain her lack of energy. I shared my observations, along with details of her almost-daily breakdowns, with our physician. I also explained that when she did run or engage in other strenuous exercise, her heart raced so hard it felt like it was going to jump out of her chest. Something was drastically wrong.

The doctor didn't think mono was the problem, but she ordered basic blood tests. A few days later her office called. Carolyn was severely anemic, they explained. She must be losing blood and we needed to bring her in right away. Fortunately, the doctor determined she wasn't losing blood, but her anemia was still a cause for concern. Starting right away, the doctor prescribed liquid iron three times a day.

At first we took her in for iron checks every other day; then it progressed to once a week. Her iron levels began to slowly rise. A hematologist the doctor consulted said a virus could bring on this condition. Carolyn had had a very bad viral infection over the winter, so this seemed to fit.

After about six weeks, even though she was still on the liquid iron, her iron levels started to drop. Whatever was going on was obviously more than the residual effects of a virus. We were referred to a gastroenterologist at Children's Hospital. After an initial exam, the doctor was pretty convinced our daughter had celiac disease. He wasn't ready to completely rule out more serious conditions such as cancer, but he was calm. He talked about her distended tummy, her un-muscular buttocks, her yellow skin tone, and the physical struggles she was currently having, all of which pointed toward celiac disease (CD).

The results of a celiac panel of blood tests were convincingly positive for CD. The next step was an endoscopy, the results of which, according to the doctor, showed Carolyn had "one of the most obvious cases of celiac disease" he'd ever seen. He asked us to start a gluten-free diet (GFD) right away, gave us the names of a couple brands of cereal, and told us to have her eat simply.

For the first couple of weeks after diagnosis, she woke up screaming that her throat and insides hurt—we think as a result of the endoscopy. For the first month or so, she ate rice and corn every other night (it took us a bit to get up-to-speed on the GFD), but within 48 hours of not eating gluten we began to see a change.

After the holidays, the entire family was tested. I tested positive, as did Carolyn's twin sister. The reasons for our similar yellow skin tones now made sense.

These days both girls are thriving sixth graders full of energy and enthusiasm. After our experience, our physician's office held a staff meeting outlining the many atypical signs of celiac disease.

The Heart and Vitamin and Mineral Deficiencies

Many vitamins and minerals can affect heart and lung function. For example, patients with heart failure who are thiamin-deficient may benefit from supplements of this vitamin. And magnesium may be of value for patients with arrhythmias and heart failure. Studies have also shown a relationship between vitamin D levels and heart failure: The lower the levels of vitamin D, the higher the rate of mortality from heart disease.[1]

Hypocalcemia, or a low calcium level, can also be a factor in heart-related problems. A 2010 study reports that chronically low calcium may lead to "electrocardiographic (ECG) changes and mimic acute myocardial infarction." In this study, a very low blood-calcium level, linked to CD and hypoparathyroidism, was found to be the cause of irreversible, end-stage heart failure in a young man.[2] Perhaps if the link had been discovered sooner, he might have had a chance.

If low calcium levels are addressed and treated, cardiac failure may be reversible. Thus, symptoms of tingling and numbness (paresthesia) in heart-failure patients, as well as a longer-than-usual time for the heart's electrical cycle, should trigger a check of calcium levels.[3]

The blood disorder hyperhomocysteinemia is reported to be "an established risk factor for cardiovascular diseases and premature atherosclerosis" and is linked to folate and vitamin B deficiencies, kidney and thyroid disease, malignancies, and more.[4] In turn, these disorders can be linked to CD.

The Heart and CD

A 2011 study asserts that CD patients are at "increased risk of atrial fibrillation," and earlier studies concluded that increased inflammation is a predictor of this condition.[5] A 2001 study lead by Dr. A. Vojdani reported that patients with signs of heart failure and myocarditis (an inflammation of the heart muscle) showed significant improvement on a GFD, sometimes aided by immunosuppressants. Before adopting a GFD, these patients had failed to respond to treatment.[6]

Other important CD/heart findings:

- Having CD or intestinal inflammation increased the odds of developing ischemic heart disease,[7] characterized by a reduced blood supply of the heart muscle, which can contribute to a fatal heart attack.

- "Subclinical systolic dysfunction of the left ventricle" was detected in children who tested positive for EMA, the endomysial antibody.[8] EMA is one of the antibodies strongly associated with CD.
- In a study done in 1998, a woman with persistent anemia, "cardiomyopathy and complete heart block" was found to have CD with no intestinal issues. People with chronic anemia, myocardiopathies, and rhythm abnormalities should be screened for CD.[9]
- Dr. Andrew Weil notes that antiphospholipid syndrome (APS), a coagulation disorder, can induce deep-vein thrombosis leading to heart attacks and strokes.[10] A 2010 study on deep vein thrombosis linked to CD suggests that CD may also be linked to APS.[11] (See *Stroke* below.)

Cardio/Thyroid

The heart and thyroid are intimately linked. Fluctuations in thyroid hormone can speed up heart rate, increase the risk of atrial fibrillation, and lessen vascular stability.[12] Subclinical hyperthyroidism can also contribute to atrial fibrillation as well as atrial flutter.[13] Other cardio/thyroid associations linked to thyroid hormone (either too much or not enough) include atherosclerosis, congestive heart failure, ischemic heart disease, and tachycardia.[14]

Abnormal lipid metabolism, cardiac dysfunction, diastolic hypertension conferring an elevated risk of atherosclerosis, and ischemic heart disease are also features of subclinical hypothyroidism. And for patients with subclinical hyperthyroidism, the risk of developing atrial fibrillation is nearly three times greater than for members of the general population. In patients 60 years of age and older, having a low-serum TSH (thyroid-stimulating hormone)—an indicator of hyperthyroidism—has been connected with "increased mortality from all causes and in particular from circulatory and cardiovascular disorders."[15] In other words, when your thyroid levels are out of whack, your cardiovascular system has a greater chance of being out of whack as well. And *autoimmune thyroid issues are strongly linked to CD.*

High Blood Pressure

About 30 percent of adults in the U.S. suffer from high blood pressure,[16] which is "one of the most common risk factors for cardiovascular disease and stroke."[17]

Symptoms of a severe type of high blood pressure (HBP) include brutal headaches, confusion, nausea or vomiting, nosebleeds or visual disturbances.[18] Often, however, those who have HBP experience no symptoms at all, which means they can develop related heart and kidney issues before they even know they have a problem. Whatever could be causing this disorder in so many people?

High blood pressure can result from the condition of the blood vessels, kidneys, and nervous system, as well as from abnormal hormone levels. Your endocrine system, organs, circulatory, and nervous systems can also be off kilter if you have undiagnosed, silent CD—again, without you having a clue. So which came first, the disease or the HBP? And in some cases, could gluten be the common denominator, a factor of HBP leading to so many diseases?

A 2002 study hypothesizes that blood pressure could be brought under better control in CD patients if the coexisting hyperhomocysteinaemia (high levels of homocysteine, a non-protein amino acid) were treated with essential nutrients. After adopting a GF lifestyle, supplemented by B6, folate, and iron as well as B12 shots, participants saw a return to normal blood pressure in 15 months.[19] I personally know of three individuals whose blood pressure dropped significantly after they adopted a gluten-free diet. In one of them it normalized.

The title of a 2007 study, *Successful treatment of portal hypertension and hypoparathyroidism with a gluten-free diet*, speaks volumes about the GF lifestyle by suggesting a causal link between IPH and some of the inflammatory, CD-associated disorders.[20] One particular type of HBP—idiopathic portal hypertension or IPH—is linked to anemia and splenomegaly (an enlarged spleen). A 2009 study in which the patient showed improvement in hypertension and other symptoms following a GFD suggests screening for CD. The patient had an unrecognized iron deficiency anemia.[21] Sometimes anemia may be the only sign of CD.

Low Pulse Rate

The story following suggests that a low pulse rate may also be linked to gluten.

Don't Ever Go Off that GFD, by Gale Pearce, PA-C

Some time ago my wife and I were on a trip where we visited a well-known smorgasbord restaurant. After eating a very small portion of Mongolian beef I began to feel very ill. By the time we got back to our hotel room, I was so weak I could hardly stand. I took my pulse and it was 28 (normal 60–100). It was time to visit the emergency room.

Once in the ER they verified my pulse rate and hooked me up to several monitors. The examining physician determined my heart was in a bigeminal rhythm. In other words, I had an actual heartbeat of 56, but only half those beats were being conducted into my body.

After being hooked up to the monitors for a while, I suddenly had severe cramping accompanied by diarrhea. The second the diarrhea was over I felt fine; I was ready to dance. When the physician asked what I'd eaten, I explained about the Mongolian beef. Her only comment was, "Whatever you do, don't you ever go off that GFD!" Later we went back to the restaurant and asked for a list of ingredients in the Mongolian beef. The only thing of concern was the soy sauce, which the label indicated contained wheat.

Stroke

Strokes are caused by a lack of blood flow to the brain. "Hyperhomocysteinaemia is considered to be a risk factor for cardiovascular disease (particularly stroke) and has been implicated in recurrent miscarriage and osteoporotic fracture, recognized manifestations of coeliac disease (CD)."[22] Moreover, "hyperhomocysteinemia or cerebral arterial vasculopathy ...and antiphospholipid syndrome . . ." are each considered to be part of the disease process of a stroke coexisting with CD.[23] Lowering high homocysteine levels may help prevent strokes,[24] and adhering to a GFD helps reduce homocysteine levels as well as increase folate levels.[25]

A 2010 study found dilated cardiomyopathy (a weakened, enlarged heart) and stroke in a young CD patient; as a result, researchers suggested that screening for CD should be considered in trying to identify the cause of stroke.[26] Autoimmune vasculitis of the central nervous system, along with vitamin deficiencies, may also play a part in stroke susceptibility. Thus patients who have suffered an ischemic stroke (one caused by blockage of a blood vessel to the brain), especially young patients, should be assessed for CD, even though they may not have gastrointestinal symptoms.[27]

People can have heart conditions at any age, but the older we get the more plentiful these disorders seem to become. A stable immune system and a good supply of nutrients are vital to keep the heart, vasculature, and blood healthy. If you're having heart, hypertension, or vascular issues you may want to consider testing to make certain CD is not at the *heart of the matter.*

There is a huge need for more studies connecting gluten to heart issues, but don't hold your breath that they'll be done anytime soon. And until more doctors hear about the few studies that have been done, you need to become your own health advocate. For more about heart-related issues, see Chapter 7 for *Finally, at Almost 40*, Lisa Vasile's story about her sister's heart palpitations. Also see Dick Stevens's atrial fibrillation story, *I Got My Life Back*, in Chapter 9, and read more about cardiomyopathy in Chapter 10.

Ocular Issues: The Eyes Have It!

I met Jack at a conference held by Dr. Kenneth Fine, and he was most eager to share his unusual, almost unbelievable story. After having problems focusing on fine print for years, Jack discovered Dr. Fine's stool testing (he'd already tested negative on blood tests for CD). The results changed his life dramatically.

A New Perspective, by Jack

I have five brothers and two sisters. As children, one brother and I had surgery for strabismus (abnormal alignment of eyes). The surgery straightened our eyes cosmetically, but as I struggled through school I was unable to concentrate and had difficulty focusing my eyes while reading. I got through my school years by listening to the teachers and participating in class rather than by reading the materials in depth.

I wet the bed until the age of 12 and didn't experience puberty until I was 15. In my 30s I developed chronic low back pain along with bursitis in my shoulder, and by the time I was 40 I was struggling with my vision once again. Then I started suffering from sinusitis and migraines. Since the doctors believed my sinuses were the cause of many of my symptoms, I decided to have sinus surgery, but it didn't help. In fact, for a time I actually got worse.

I was also plagued by restless leg syndrome and muscle twitches, and my brain was in a constant fog. My doctor referred me to a neurologist for the headaches and twitches and to an ophthalmologist who suggested he could surgically improve my eye infraction, which had worsened with age. The neurologist ordered an MRI that showed lesions in the white matter of my brain. He also thought I might have demylenation (damage to the myelin sheath around my nerves). He even considered MS, but at the end of the day I had no definite diagnosis. The doctor scheduled me for a follow-up MRI in a year.

At this point two of my brothers, who'd been diagnosed with celiac in 2002 and 2003, urged me to have a blood test for celiac disease. I agreed, but the results were negative. I decided to go on a gluten-free diet anyway.

Three months after starting the GFD I was feeling mentally sharper. At a pre-op appointment with my ophthalmologist, he said my eyes were much better and my corrective lenses were working just fine. In fact, the improvement was so significant he no longer recommended surgery. "What are you doing differently?" he asked. I told him it must be the GFD. He patted me on the shoulder, smiled, and said, "Don't tell anyone."

Obviously this doctor did not care to hear my answer and I quickly lost all respect for him. He was never going to consider gluten as playing a role in my condition or in that of his other patients. I was happy to avoid surgery, but I couldn't help feeling bad as I walked past all the moms and children in the waiting room who were preparing to go through what I'd endured as a child. By this time I was wondering if gluten had a role in preventing my brain from developing proper vision in the first place and if some of those children in the waiting room might benefit from a GFD as well.

I continued on the GFD and, month-by-month, I started feeling better. Later I eliminated all yeast from my diet, as recommended by a homeopathic doctor I started seeing. One year after going gluten- and yeast-free my sinusitis was gone, I had no more migraines, no more twitches or restless leg, no more chronic back pain, and no more visual deterioration. I started reading books for the first time in my life, completing some in a single weekend. This was a milestone for me, and I am determined to realize my newfound potential.

A year later, the follow-up MRI showed the lesions in the white matter of my brain had shrunk in size. No additional lesions were found on my spinal cord. Demyelination and MS were ruled out. The neurologist, who never acknowledged any connection between my gluten- and yeast-free diet and the elimination of my symptoms and reduced size of my lesions, said my symptoms and abnormal MRI were most likely "migrainous" in nature. I had to laugh when I heard his explanation; I walked out of his office with a new perspective on life.

Below are some significant points relating gluten to eye disorders from studies done between 2007 and 2011:

- Vitamin D "may protect against early AMD [age-related macular degeneration] in women younger than 75 years."[28] Does this mean that vitamin D deficiency may lead to macular degeneration? Again, more research is needed, but it's important to remember that those with CD may be very deficient in vitamin D.

- CD patients were found to have "a 1.7 fold increased risk of allergic conjunctivitis, allergic rhinitis, and eczema."[29]
- A "cataract as the presenting feature of celiac disease" may have evolved due to chronic diarrhea and hypocalcemia, characteristics of malabsorption caused by CD.[30]
- "Two cases of gluten sensitivity presenting as neuromyelitis optica" revealed no history of intestinal issues.[31]
- CD was diagnosed in a young girl with type 1 diabetes who had lost vision in one eye. On a GFD the uveitis (inflammation of the middle layer of the eye)[32] healed in two months and her meds were tapered off.[33]
- Keratoconus, a "cone-shaped protrusion of the cornea,"[34] was linked to a number of autoimmune diseases.[35] Most of these diseases are also linked to CD.
- A young child with "a hemorrhagic conjunctival lesion in the right eye" also showed signs of CD: abdominal extension, anorexia, difficulty digesting baby food and a short breast-feeding period. "The case was diagnosed with CD and the conjunctival tumor showed complete regression during gluten-free treatment." The diagnosis was conjunctival Kaposi sarcoma, a type of cancer.[36]
- Ophthalmoplegia or "paralysis of the muscles of the eye"[37] is a neurological issue associated with vitamin deficiencies,[38] and, as we know, vitamin deficiencies are often associated with CD.

In 1981, a study on the macular detachment of the retina linked it to a manifestation of various systemic diseases. Some are autoimmune diseases also linked to CD: rheumatoid arthritis, lupus, inflammatory bowel disease, and more.[39]

Another study found that ocular maladies appeared in 84 percent of patients with gluten ataxia.[40] Patients with irritable bowel disease (IBD), another malady often associated with CD, were also subject to eye-related issues (see Chapter 7). Researchers found that "ocular manifestations occur in about 10% of IBD patients," and that when the IBD is treated, the patients' eye problems improve.[41]

Glaucoma, "a neurodegenerative disease of the optic nerve," is "a leading cause of blindness in the world."[42] Diabetes, high blood pressure, and migraines can "affect blood flow to the optic nerve…" and are linked to the progression of glaucoma. Arthritis, hypothyroidism, leukemia, sleep apnea, and more may also play a role in the development of glaucoma, and type 2 diabetics should be tested often for glaucoma.[43] Two 2011 studies suggest that autoimmune mechanisms may play a part in the development of glaucoma;[44] another study found that autoimmune neuropathy may play a role in a specific type of glaucoma.[45]

Vitamins and minerals play an important roll in eye health. For example, cataracts are linked to deficiencies of vitamin A and calcium, and they may be prevented or their growth retarded if the patient adopts a GFD.[46] Corneal issues may also result from vitamin A deficiency.[47] Even chronically bloodshot eyes, night blindness, and/or unexplained blurred vision can improve on a GFD.[48] (For even more information about eye-related disorders, see the section on *Sjögren's Syndrome* in Chapter 10, as well as *Even the Dog* in Chapter 9, Melanie Krumrey's story about her son's fuzzy vision.) With so many eye-related issues potentially linked to CD, it seems only logical that those with eye problems might want to find out if they are malabsorbing.

Lung Problems

A study going back to 1981 found "a history of asthma or chronic cough" in a greater number of CD patients than in the control group, indicating a link between airway breathing issues and CD.[49] Instances of fibrosing lung disease with no known cause were also found in CD patients.[50] In another study, patients with hypothyroidism and other autoimmune diseases linked to various organs were found to have greater levels of lung dysfunction and inflammation than the controls, as measured by cough symptoms, shortness of breath, sputum, and wheezing.[51]

More and more research indicates that CD should be ruled out in the case of COPD, bronchial issues, and pulmonary hemosiderosis (bleeding in the lungs). If gluten sensitivity turns out to be contributing to your breathing problems, getting tested could lead to a new lifestyle where you can finally "breathe easy."

Bronchitis—Bronchitis is an inflammation in the main airways of the lungs. One study reported no clear cause for the chronic cough in 20 percent of the patients studied. All of the respiratory symptoms in one newly diagnosed CD patient improved significantly on a GFD, which suggested "a causal relationship between celiac disease, cough, and lymphocytic bronchoalveolitis [an inflammation that can lead to pneumonia]."[52] In another study, a patient with irreversible impairment to a portion of the bronchial tree showed improvement in symptoms once diagnosed with CD and on a GFD. Lung infections and intestinal complaints were frequent in his childhood, and a causal association between CD and breathing symptoms was implied.[53]

In my own case, I'd been prone to bronchial infections for years prior to going on a GFD in 2004. Since then I've had only one lung incident. I'd only been on the diet a few months and my gut hadn't quite healed when I came down with walking pneumonia after pushing through several late nights, early mornings, and a bout of air travel. I didn't listen to my body and I paid the price, but ever since I've been free of bronchial problems.

Chronic Obstructive Pulmonary Disease—Chronic obstructive pulmonary disease (COPD) has come to include asthma, bronchitis, and emphysema, where flow of air into the lungs is hampered. Chronic cough, shortness of breath, sputum, and wheezing are some of the symptoms. **Along with smoking, malnutrition and inflammation are recognized contributors to COPD.** A 2011 Swedish study concluded that "patients with CD seem to be at a moderately increased risk of COPD both before and after CD diagnosis."[54]

A 2010 study from the Netherlands found that patients taking vitamins A, C, D, and E, plus beta and alpha carotene, showed a turn for the better in the "symptoms, exacerbations and pulmonary function" of COPD.[55] An older study claimed that diet may have an effect on asthma and COPD and that intake levels of antioxidant vitamins, fish, fruit, magnesium, and sodium may influence the progression of these disorders.[56] Although studies are few, diet seems to be a significant component in the evolution of COPD.[57]

For those with untreated CD, however, malabsorption of vitamins is the name of the game, which means taking a handful of vitamins will do no good. If you or someone you love has COPD, it only makes sense to determine if gluten sensitivity may be making matters worse.

Sarcoidosis—I met Marion on a summer morning while we were both exploring local yard sales. It didn't take long to learn her story. Back in 2001 she'd been having some trouble breathing. When she went to her doctor she was told she had lung cancer and had three months to live. After seeing several more doctors she learned she didn't have lung cancer after all. In fact, the doctors didn't know *what* her problem was. Finally she was diagnosed with sarcoidosis (an inflammatory disease characterized by enlargement of lymph nodes in various parts of the body). Fortunately the disease had not yet affected her liver, kidneys, or eyes, but she still felt miserable. After having pneumonia three times in three years she went to a nurse practitioner who suggested she remove gluten from her diet. (Many alternative and more open-minded practitioners suggest adopting a gluten-free diet without testing to see how the patient responds. For information on testing options, see Chapters 16 and 17.)

She is now off all grains, dairy, and eggs, and doing just great. She no longer needs inhalers or several of her sinus medications, and the scar tissue in her lungs caused by the sarcoidosis no longer hurts when she breathes. Life is good.

As one study found, the increased chance of developing sarcoidosis among CD participants lends support to the idea that the two diseases are causally linked by one or more common elements.[58] The "immune characteristics of CD may be linked to an increased risk of sarcoidosis," reported another,[59] and an Irish study noted a genetic commonality between the two diseases, indicating that sarcoid patients should be screened for CD.[60] In fact, a study in 1999 revealed "a high frequency of gastric autoimmunity and gluten-associated immune reactivity in patients with sarcoidosis" in nearly 40 percent of the cases.[61]

The results of these and other studies point to the fact that genetic and immunological components seem to be contributors to both CD and sarcoidosis. In one case a 14-year-old girl with CD developed a condition doctors diagnosed as sarcoidosis affecting the skin. When the teenager followed a GFD, her condition improved; when she lapsed, it worsened. Other cases have been reported of CD patients with sarcoidosis affecting the lungs. In one of these patients, the sarcoid lung condition worsened whenever gluten was reintroduced.[62]

Idiopathic Pulmonary Hemosiderosis—Idiopathic pulmonary hemosiderosis (IPH) is marked by bleeding into the lungs and leaving behind deposits of hemosiderin, a form of iron. Anemia, clubbing (a thickening of the ends of toes and fingers, where the nails may curve downward), spitting up blood, and weakness are all signs of IPH.[63]

Patients with IPH, even if they have no gastrointestinal symptoms, should be screened for CD, particularly when acute anemia is present. Both maladies may profit from a GFD.[64] In fact, regularly screening of IPH patients for intolerance to gluten was recommended as far back as the early

1990s.[65] In a 1991 study, a patient with IPH linked to CD remained symptom-free on a GFD.[66] In another study, a patient with many symptoms of pulmonary hemosiderosis improved within two weeks on a GFD.[67]

There are far too many idiopathic, chronic conditions associated with nutrient deficiency and/or immune reactivity to ignore the potential link between them and gluten sensitivity, especially since in many of these studies, the condition improved when gluten was eliminated from the diet. For more on this topic, see the section on *Allergies and Asthma* in Chapter 8.

Chronic Cough, by Tom Graves

For many months, I was bothered by a hacking cough after meals and when turning over in bed at night. I don't remember where I learned that sensitivity to wheat can cause many problems, but I did suspect wheat might be involved. So, about a year ago I went off wheat entirely—no more gluten-containing scones, bagels, pasta, pizza, sandwiches, crackers, cereal, dinner rolls, etc. Within a week or less my coughing ended. I also felt better generally and I had more energy. Over the next four to six months I also lost 10 pounds without trying—a very positive and unexpected side effect.

Getting rid of gluten requires a whole new way of thinking about food. As I got into the GFD I realized almost all my between-meal snacking had been heavy carbohydrates. I hadn't appreciated how much carbohydrates affected me, but when it comes right down to it, except for replacing wheat flour in my diet with rice and other grains, I eat as I always have. The cough has not returned and the weight has stayed off.

You may have the best diet in the world, but if you are malabsorbing, many of the nutrients are going out the back door instead of keeping your cells happy and healthy.

Gall Bladder

Along with diabetes and obesity, CD can impact gallbladder health.[68] One study showed that patients with CD released lower levels of cholecystokinin or CCK (a gallbladder-regulating hormone) after a meal than those in the control group. Reduced CCK is linked to damaged villi, as well as to the invasion of intraepithelial lymphocytes (white blood cells found, among other places, in the lining of the gastrointestinal tract).[69] Seven years after being on a GFD I was shocked to find I was having gall bladder issues. I was in the best health I had been in for years and I had great energy. A trip to Greece, with a major indulgence in feta and yogurt as thick as soft butter, may have precipitated the problem. I'd been pretty much off dairy for a couple of years, but I'm half Greek and on this trip I pampered myself with up to five servings a day of these cultural favorites. By the time we started home I was feeling stiff, my usual complaint from indulging in dairy.

Three weeks later I had an attack that took me to the hospital. I'd been uncomfortable for a while, but one night when we were having dinner guests I experienced a heavy indigestive feeling up near my bra line, a bit to the right. I Googled *heart attack* smack in the middle of the *hors d'oeuvres, then said to my husband,* "Hon, I think you'd better take me to the hospital." Dinner was nearly ready, but the company had to fend for themselves. (On that occasion I made it back from the hospital with all my parts intact, but my gallbladder was eventually removed.)

My doctor mentioned that approximately 1 of every 100 patients has intestinal problems following gall bladder removal. About the same time I found a couple of references to post prandial issues, such as running to the john after a meal, being connected to gluten. Is it possible that the one percent has CD that was brought on by surgery?

In an article at celiac.com, Dr. Ron Hoggan says, "There just isn't much ambiguity there. If you've got celiac disease, you have gall bladder malfunction, of the sort that may well develop into atresia [blocked bile duct] and gallstones." Based on his research, Dr. Hoggan also asserts that gallstones in children are linked to CD.[70] Isn't it amazing how all of our organs are so intimately connected? No wonder various parts of the body can be affected by gluten without our knowledge until one part or another develops a major issue.

Spleen

Splenomegaly (enlarged spleen) is associated with numerous medical conditions, among them CD (see *A Celiac Disease Case History*, Seth Ames's story in Chapter 8). Research on the connection between CD and other spleen conditions has been going on for decades. As far back as the early 1980s, for example, a study of patients with CD found a significant number also had hyposplenism (reduced spleen function).[71] "**Splenic atrophy occurs frequently in patients with coeliac disease and is related to the severity of the disease and degree of [GF] dietary control.**"[72] In 1984 researchers determined that the severity of hyposplenism "increased with advancing age and prolongation of exposure to dietary gluten."[73] And a 1983 study found that three of six hyposplenic patients experienced *full* recovery on a GFD.[74] In other words, a GF lifestyle can positively affect how the spleen functions.

Kidneys

Is There Anything that Isn't Linked to Gluten? by Gale Pearce, PA-C

I'd been plagued with kidney stones since my early 20s, generally passing a stone each year. Since going on a GFD, however, I have yet to pass a single stone. Two years ago there were still 11 stones distributed between my kidneys. They were still there a year later, but this time they were ***significantly reduced in size*** and no new stones had formed. It would be interesting to learn if others with kidney stones experienced similar results after adopting a GFD. My informal impression from my own patients would suggest a relationship, of what pertinence I cannot ascertain.

A friend and one-time neighbor who suffered from both osteoporosis and anemia came close to needing dialysis. Her doctor explained that when her iron level is low, fluids build up to the extent that it affects her kidney function. He suggested she adopt a GFD *as much as possible*, but he did not suggest testing for gluten sensitivity, nor did he offer any formal coaching on how to live gluten free. Ever since she's been trying to be careful, and it's been more than a year since I've heard her mention the possibility of needing dialysis.

IgA nephropathy (kidney damage) is found in a large number of renal cases linked to CD, and several recent articles support the association of CD with kidney disease. One young patient with acute anemia and CD proceeded to develop nephrotic syndrome, a kidney disorder that causes protein to leak from the blood into the urine. Membranoproliferative glomerulonephritis (MPGN) is a particular type of nephrotic syndrome linked to gluten. After being on a GFD for six months MPGN was no longer an issue for the patient.[75] In another case, a 45-year-old patient with a number of worsening, 10-syllable conditions, saw the proteinuria (abnormally high level of protein in the urine) associated with his MPGN fully resolve once he was on a GFD.[76] Additional research sounds an even greater alarm: In one 2011 study, **patients with "biopsy-verified CD suffer[ed] increased risk of subsequent ESRD" or end-stage renal disease.**[77]

About a third of IgA nephropathy patients exhibit a "rectal mucosal sensitivity to gluten, but without signs of celiac disease..." This correlation prompted researchers to postulate that "subclinical inflammation to gluten" might be connected to the IgAN disease process.[78]

Macroamylasemia (MA), a normally symptom-free condition in and of itself, is characterized by high levels of an enzyme called amalyse in the blood. MA may also be an indicator of celiac disease. One study found **"a significant percentage of newly diagnosed patients with CD have macroamylasemia" and recommended that patients with MA or high amylase levels should be screened for CD.**[79] In one young CD patient who had MA as well as autoimmune thyroiditis, there was a decrease in the CD-linked "antibodies to amylase and to exocrine pancreas tissue" when the patient began following a GFD. This study reports that only a few cases of MA are found in the related literature and all of the children whose amylase levels were abnormal also exhibited "intestinal pain and trauma."[80]

Bladder

Before going gluten free in 2004 I had my fair share of urinary tract infections (UTIs). Since then I've had only two (both related to a failure to keep up with the hot tub chemicals). In one instance I was able to avoid antibiotics by drinking pure cranberry juice—no sugar—sometimes straight, sometimes mixed with water, and flooding myself with water well beyond the disappearance of any symptoms.

I've also noticed the need to cross my legs and squeeze when I sneeze exists no more; my bladder is much stronger than it was prior to adopting a GF lifestyle.

Interstitial Cystitis—For years Wendy Cohan suffered with interstitial cystitis—*cause unknown*, though some doctors believe this condition is an autoimmune disease. Wendy maintains two informative websites, www.glutenfreechoice.com and www.wellbladder.com, and her article at www.celiac.com, "Gluten Sensitivity and Bladder Disease," very convincingly associates interstitial cystitis with gluten. She has also written *The Better Bladder Book: A Holistic Approach to Healing Interstitial Cystitis and Chronic Pelvic Pain.*[81] She shares her story in the hope it may help others with similar problems. (Also see her allergy story, *Choices*, in Chapter 8.)

They Said, "No Cure!" by Wendy Cohan, RN

In sensitive individuals, gluten intolerance can affect all of the mucous membranes in the body (sinus, gut, mouth, and esophagus), including the lining of the bladder. In 1996 I was diagnosed with an incurable, progressive, painful disease called interstitial cystitis. The symptoms mimic those of a bad bladder infection, although most lab tests are negative for bacteria and antibiotics generally do not help. As a nurse, I knew how the bladder functioned and that it needed an intact lining to hold toxic wastes prior to elimination. So it made sense to me to try a dietary approach, and I had good luck immediately by eliminating such known bladder irritants as tomatoes, caffeine, chocolate, citrus, and alcohol, even though at the time most doctors gave diet little credit for a reduction in symptoms. In spite of my dietary changes, however, the disease continued to progress. Eventually I needed painkillers, antispasmodics, and other medications to enable me to function. Every urinalysis showed significant amounts of blood in my urine. I was one sick young woman, but no one ever tested me for food allergies or gluten intolerance or considered any contributive cause. No one suggested my symptoms were part of a systemic dysfunction in my body. The doctors acknowledged I had a painful disease, and they would prescribe as much pain medicine as needed, but they insisted there was "no cure."

I was no longer getting enough sleep to enable me to function well as a nurse, so I stopped working in order to rebuild my health. I was in constant pain. I began turning to alternative practitioners for help. I also started experimenting more with diet, as well as having food allergy and sensitivity testing done. Careful observation showed what did and did not affect my bladder. Eliminating gluten resolved a long-standing rash on my legs called dermatitis herpetiformis, so I kept on doing it [see more on this skin condition in Chapter 11]. After two years and a lot of alternative body work, my bladder began to significantly recover.

My urologist readily agrees that gluten negatively affects the bladder in some patients, and that, for these people, eliminating gluten leads to a reduction in symptoms. Still, there are almost no published journal articles linking gluten intolerance with bladder problems. Through my book and web sites, I am trying to get the word out: ***We do not have to live with constant pain, and what we eat can affect our health.***

If you've been told your ailment has no known cause, that it's incurable, or that it is genetic and there is *nothing you can do about it,* it's hard to keep on looking for answers. On the other hand, I have read over and over that certain disorders are incurable, yet when gluten is removed from the diet of those who suffer from them, marvelous transformations can happen. CD itself has a genetic component, and it is the only autoimmune disease with a *known cause.* If you've read this far, you know that gluten sensitivity can affect any part of the body in complex, interwoven ways that can have serious health consequences.

If your doctor has not suggested CD/GI testing for what is ailing you, it is most likely because research on the many gluten-associated maladies has not yet reached his ears, not because he doesn't have your best interests at heart. Help your doctor to help you by becoming a full partner in understanding how your body functions and how your health may be adversely affected by your diet. The tests outlined in Chapters 16 and 17 can help determine whether gluten is a contributor to your problems. If so, adopting a GFD may improve your health—and ultimately change your life—in ways you never could have imagined.

A Commodity of Oddities 15

No Symptoms

Doesn't it seem odd that one can have full-blown celiac disease (CD), including damaged villi, and have few or no obvious symptoms? That's one of the maddening aspects of this disorder: You may not know what's happening inside you until significant damage has been done. In fact, in one study, ***a third of the CD patients had no signs of CD.***[1]

Amazing Attitude, by Bonnie Zonghi

Our son, Brandon, was diagnosed with CD at age 13 [also see Brandon's sister's story, *Saving Bryanne,* in Chapter 7]. He'd tested negative years before and hadn't been exhibiting any symptoms, but given the fact that puberty was approaching, along with the potential genetic predisposition since his sister was already following a gluten-free lifestyle, I felt it was time to test him again. If he ***was*** gluten sensitive and passed puberty untreated, I knew it could affect his potential adult height as well as his general health.

As I write this it's been just over three months since Brandon started on a gluten-free diet [GFD]. His attitude continues to amaze us. We are so proud of how he has accepted his diagnosis and eats 100-percent gluten free. He hasn't noticed any difference in how he feels, but he has gained a welcome five pounds and grown an inch!

Pain

A woman I know had suffered for 10 years with a gnawing arthritic pain that migrated from her arms, neck, and back to her legs, knees, and shins. Five days on the gluten-free diet and the pain along with the reflux had disappeared.

The causes of pain are often difficult to pin down, but many people have experienced reduction or elimination of pain after adopting a GF lifestyle. Once the villi begin to heal, vitamins and minerals can go to work, refurbishing malnourished cells. Lower-back, shoulder, and pelvic pain may disappear. Bone and muscular pain, along with migraines and headaches, may also get better once the body has a chance to recover from the assault of gluten. Menstrual pain can subside. A dull, gnawing pain in your side, horrendous pain in your stomach, or the discomfort of reflux can evaporate on a GFD. Pain is nature's way of telling us something is wrong. Masking it with painkillers may make us more comfortable, but it does nothing to address the underlying cause. Abdominal pain, particularly, may be an indicator of serious problems.

In my own case, I have noticed the muscles in my buttocks and lower back, which tighten when I am accidentally hit with gluten, also seem to tighten and ache when I consume dairy. Even too much sugar seems to make me a bit sore.

Listen to your children when they complain of pain and are not feeling well. Bone and muscular pain in childhood may be the pangs of CD. Perhaps there is no such thing as "growing pains." As she explains below, Corinne experienced very unusual pain throughout her childhood; finally, as a young adult she traced it to gluten.

A Journey to Wellness, by Corinne Wilkens

My story begins early in life. Like most kids in America, each morning I would chow down a bowl of wheat-filled breakfast cereal before running to catch the school bus. And every morning at the bus stop I had sharp cramps.

I also had painful, aching feet from the time I was a small child. Whenever I went to a fair, the zoo, an amusement park, the aquarium, or on a class trip or other event that required me to stand or walk for more than 20 minutes, I was in constant pain.

And ever since I could remember I'd had gastrointestinal symptoms of every sort. I dreaded the mere suggestion of eating out, as my cramps would begin before the check even had time to arrive. Every night I would take an antacid or two before bed, and I often experienced what I liked to call "the feeling of having eaten a bowl of glass shards." When I sought help for these problems I received the "catch-all" diagnosis of irritable bowel syndrome.

Next there were the cluster headaches I began having in high school. I didn't know what they were, and back then they didn't have their own classification. After self-diagnosing the headaches in my early twenties, I thought *How lucky can you be?* Most cluster headache sufferers are male. They are also smokers and heavy drinkers; I am neither. One section of the headache book I read said cluster headaches could be caused by food allergies to things like wheat. *Sure*, I thought, chuckling. If only I had done more research at that point, I could have saved myself 15 years of suffering.

Three years ago I began hearing and reading more and more about the wheat thing. Then I read *Dangerous Grains;* it was amazing! I could have taken a red pen and just checked off the symptoms that applied to my situation. I knew right then and there that this was the answer to my problems; it explained so much.

I'm not particularly fond of doctors, needles, and invasive tests, and I don't really care about having an exact diagnosis of celiac disease, gluten intolerance, or wheat allergy. So against conventional wisdom and medical advice I just went on a GFD to see what would happen. I didn't notice a drastic change; in fact, it wasn't until a month went by and I attended a Renaissance faire that I had an astounding experience.

Due to my painful aching feet, I told the person who attended the faire with me that two hours was the maximum I could stay, and that when I said it was time to leave, we needed to leave! I knew my limits; on previous excursions I usually would have downed three painkillers by the half-hour mark. This time a half hour went by and I had no pain. An hour went by, then two, then four. We finally left after five hours, having seen and done everything we wanted to.

When I got back to our hotel I realized what a milestone this represented. In my whole life I had never done anything like this. I had grown up assuming everyone's feet hurt all the time, that it was just a fact of life. That day everything changed. What was different? I had worn the same expensive sneakers to the same faire the previous year, so it wasn't the shoes. I racked my brain for what seemed like hours. Finally it occurred to me: Could it be the GFD? This seemed impossible. How could something you *eat* cause such pain? But I could think of no other answer.

Now, three years later, I have no doubts. If I ingest even a crumb of something with gluten in it and then go shopping, my feet start to kill me within 20 minutes.

I stopped eating gluten in September 2003; I've never looked back. With all the wonderful gluten-free goodies on the market these days, I don't even miss the wheat. Well, to be totally honest, I do miss pizza; however, some great gluten-free pizzas are now becoming available.

I did eventually see an allergist and had a positive skin test for wheat allergy, although I believe my problems are more involved than just an allergy. From all indications I probably have an intolerance to gluten. Since I've never been tested I can't prove it but, truly, I know all I need to know. If I eat gluten I feel horrible; if I don't eat it I feel great!

Eating Disorders

Today it seems there's an article about eating disorders in almost every magazine. But are these eating disorders *always* caused by something purely psychological, or could they sometimes be connected with CD? Recently I heard of a young woman whose doctor thought she was starving herself; the tests he did showed she was anorexic. Fortunately, she was also tested for CD and—guess what?—the results were positive. Now on a GFD, the young woman feels like a million bucks. A person with CD may have a poor appetite. He or she may also be plagued with nausea and vomiting, hardly an incentive to chow down. Given the apparent explosion of eating disorders, potential links with CD beg for more research.

CD can prevail in conjunction with an eating disorder or it can be "masquerading as an eating disorder." **Eighty percent of patients in one recent study were able to "achieve or maintain remission from their celiac disease and their eating disorder."**[2]

CD can also *provoke* an eating disorder, even when treated, especially in adolescents. For example, one group of patients with CD experienced an increased rate of eating disorders, in particular bulimia nervosa.[3] A review from the United Kingdom found between 25 and 35 percent of children with CD also had anorexia.[4] CD may lead to "peculiar eating behaviors, restrictive eating, and/or vomiting accompanied by body dissatisfaction," found researchers in another study; they suggested CD screening for patients with bloating and nausea and noted that a GFD may alleviate such symptoms.[5] Another study concluded that "anorectic patients with severe anemia and malnutrition should be evaluated" for other conditions (such as CD).[6]

Oral Health Issues

Just like the rest of the body, our teeth and gums need vital nutrients to remain healthy, so it's not surprising that many dental and oral-health conditions are associated with CD. For example, since I've been on a GFD my gums no longer bleed when I brush, my bad breath is gone, and my fuzzy tongue has disappeared. In the past, I occasionally developed a canker sore, but no more. We hear a lot these days about the link between bad oral health and heart issues. But what is really causing these issues? Could gluten be playing a part in your oral health problems? If so, it's unlikely your dentist will raise the issue. I've asked several dentists and hygienists if they knew of the connection between CD and oral health. They did not and said no articles on the subject had been included in the professional journals they read. Once again, if gluten could be adversely affecting your health, it's unlikely you'll find out unless you raise the issue with your medical professionals.

Gray Teeth, by Mary

My daughter's symptoms were worse than mine. Beginning with the introduction of solid foods, she developed such severe stomach issues she was hospitalized twice before the age of two. She also stopped teething, though until that time she'd been teething at a normal pace. Her two front teeth started to discolor and her growth seemed to stop.

At this age she was given only the tTG, which came back negative. However, her symptoms got progressively worse. Fortunately my sister put me onto EnteroLab, and at about age three my daughter tested positive on Dr. Fine's stool testing. We started her on the GFD right away, and the results were amazing. It was like a new girl was born.

Dental-enamel defects in children are highly linked to CD that is not diagnosed and treated before the period of enamel formation. Screening for CD should be considered in those with enamel defects and aphthous ulcers (canker sores).[7] More cavities and a delay in tooth eruption and development of the lower jaw are CD features that put one at risk for malocclusion (askew or misaligned teeth).[8]

In some patients, **RAS or "recurrent aphthous stomatitis [mouth sores] may be the sole manifestation" of CD**. Those diagnosed with CD and following a GFD showed appreciable amelioration of symptoms.[9] RAS is found in nearly 23 percent of CD patients, and nearly 72 percent of CD/RAS patients in one study saw notable improvement on a GFD.[10] Outside of the laboratory, an alert and CD-educated dentist can suggest CD screening for his patients. Not only might such a suggestion prevent future oral health complications, for those who test positive and adopt a GFD, it could have a lifelong impact on their health overall.

Disappearing Symptoms: Sally's Story

An acquaintance of mine had just come from a dental cleaning. The hygienist couldn't believe how little plaque she had and what great shape her gums were in. Upon learning that Sally (not her real name) had been on a GFD for nine months the hygienist expressed, "Maybe your immune system is in much better shape."

Sally had suffered from stomachaches when she was a kid, and for most of her adult life she'd struggled with hemorrhoids and periodic bouts of diarrhea. Now that she's been on a GFD, the stomachaches and hemorrhoids are gone, but if she's hit with gluten, the diarrhea returns. She also broke her thumb some years ago, after which she suffered from arthritis in that hand, especially in damp weather. In addition to causing her pain, the arthritis was particularly troublesome because it meant she no longer had a full finger span on the piano. She also suffered from plantar fasciitis (a painful inflammation of tissue connecting the heel and ball of the foot).

After several months on a GFD, Sally's pain has all but disappeared and she's ceased being able to predict the weather. She can play the piano with ease, and she no longer needs stretching exercises for her feet before getting out of bed. In fact, other than supplements for osteopenia, she takes no meds at all, something her doctor finds remarkable considering Sally is 73 years old.

Auditory Problems

Is there a connection between hearing loss and gluten? Could it be that loss of nutrients needed to keep the fantastic inner ear machinery working is a contributing factor, or might an immune response be working its deviltry?

In one study, sensorineural hearing loss (SNHL) was found to be much more prevalent among the children with CD (40.6%) than among those in the control group. Could there be a link between the two? Much more research is needed but, in the meantime, hearing loss should be looked for among children with CD.[11] A study on mixed connective-tissue disorders (see Chapter 10 for more on autoimmune diseases linked to gluten) found that "autoantibodies, decreased levels of regulatory T cells, and overexpression of proinflammatory cytokines" may be involved in the development of inner-ear malfunction.[12] The link between CD and auditory deficit may be due to immune reactivity of autoantibodies and vasculitis.[13]

Recurrent otitis media, an inflammation of the middle ear, has been linked to food allergies. Although gluten/wheat wasn't mentioned in this particular study, eliminating the most common offenders—beans, citrus, eggs, milk, and tomato—led to a notable improvement. Reintroducing the allergen precipitated another ear infection.[14] It makes you wonder how many children have had tubes put in their ears when what was really needed was to take dairy and other allergens off their plates.

Lyme Disease

I wonder if the ability to fight off Lyme disease, a systemic nightmare for some people, might also be linked to CD or, at least, the road to recovery might not be so difficult if the patient had a strong immune system. Kathy suffered for 30 years with joint pain, migraines, allergies, and more before being diagnosed and treated for Lyme. Then she adopted a GFD. When I met her she looked and felt great. She was traveling with her mother who, after going gluten free herself, proclaimed, "Seventy is the new fifty!"

A Ticking Time Bomb, by Kathy

I was a successfully recovered Lyme patient following heavy-duty antibiotics, until an acute episode of food poisoning following a meal at a favorite restaurant left my recovery in jeopardy. I couldn't seem to get over it. I began to worry I was experiencing a Lyme relapse. I had migraines, peripheral neuropathy, fatigue, brain-fog, migratory joint pain, and deep, glandular sore throats that robbed me of energy. I was also plagued with constant nausea, IBS, and vomiting. I would feel better on the BRAT diet—bananas, rice, applesauce, and toast—as long as I stuck to the first three items. The minute I introduced toast, all heck would break loose and I would vomit uncontrollably. Something was definitely wrong!

Two decades earlier my allergist had run a celiac panel, but it was negative. At the time he was surprised; he thought it would confirm CD. My serum IgA had also been measured numerous times by my allergist/immunologists, so I knew it was low. [For more on IgA deficiency, see Chapter 16.]

This time, following a visit to the emergency room, I saw a gastroenterologist who again performed the standard tests for celiac, blood tests, including one to measure my IgA, and a biopsy. When the results came back, my IgA was still low, which led one doctor to comment that if the tests showed ***any*** antibodies it would be significant. (Now that I know IgA deficiency can skew test results, I believe this is what may have happened when I was tested for CD initially.)

While waiting for results from the blood tests and biopsy and continuing to feel miserable, a friend urged me to do the more sensitive testing at EnteroLab. Just as IGeneX is the best specialty lab for accurate Lyme testing, it made sense to me to use this specialty facility to test for gluten sensitivity. According to what I learned, the stool tests determine the presence of IgA antibodies where they are produced—in the small intestine. I was already out thousands for an ER visit and a gastroenterologist. A few hundred more for my own peace of mind was a drop in the bucket, especially compared to past medical bills.

The endoscopy showed I had patchy villous atrophy, but the cutting-edge testing from EnteroLab provided me with some real answers. Thanks to a strict gluten-free lifestyle I'm healthier than I ever imagined I could be, and I no longer worry about a Lyme relapse. Within several months of going gluten free, my long-standing anemia—with numbers that would *almost* break the low to normal range with B12 shots and iron—finally resolved itself. I began to feel better and better. In the past I'd always struggled with colds and the flu; now I recover quickly and I'm happy and energetic as opposed to depressed and fatigued.

In one way I'm lucky. Because I can't ingest any gluten without debilitating symptoms that will most likely land me in the ER, I'm not tempted. Still, I wonder. Was it really a sudden onset of CD that threatened my recovery and felt like a Lyme relapse, or was it a ticking time bomb that had been there all along and that may have left me vulnerable to chronic Lyme disease in the first place? I may never know for sure, but I've finally found lasting health. I've attended a few gluten-awareness conferences and am always amazed by how radiantly healthy the recovered patients are. I am grateful to be one of them.

Below are just a few of the many other ailments associated with gluten sensitivity. No doubt more will be linked to gluten in the future. It's very tempting to keep doing research to uncover more connections, but as my husband says, "Anne, you need to stop doing research and get this book out there!"

- Chilblains were the main manifestation in one case study of CD in a young girl. Researchers noted that chilblains "may accompany systemic illnesses including states of malnutrition and autoimmune diseases" and that, at least in this case, they got better once the patient was on a GFD.[15]

- The bottom line of another study was that children with Kawasaki disease (a blood-vessel inflammation disorder) have an increased prevalence of CD and thus should be screened for CD.[16]
- Numerous nail abnormalities may also be a sign of systemic disease. Search online for: "Nail Abnormalities: Clues to Systemic Disease" for a thorough chart on nail conditions and what they reflect.[17]
- Gluten-sensitive patients can be extremely sensitive to light. For example, I seem to be visually photosensitive; I can tell a light has been turned on even with hands covering my closed eyes. And it's not just humans that are affected. In one case, three Appaloosa mares developed a "severe photosensitivity dermatitis" triggered by gluten in the feed. When the feed was changed and the animals protected from the sun, the lesions healed.[18]
- In children with CD, pica—the craving for non-food substances such as clay or chalk—may be precipitated by micronutrient deficits such as iron deficiency.[19]
- In two separate cases, variable immunodeficiency (a compromised immune system due to a variety of causes) was linked to villous atrophy and improved when the patients adopted a GFD.[20]

There are an inordinate number of syndromes and autoimmune diseases that are idiosyncratic—in other words, they have no known cause. *CD is the only autoimmune disease with a known cause: gluten!* So no matter what your symptoms, disease or ailment—even if your doctor says it is *genetic* or *incurable*—take charge and do some research of your own. The information you find may help to transform your health! (Appendix A includes some helpful tips to help you get started.)

16 Gluten 102: Traditional Blood Testing

TESTING FOR CELIAC disease (CD) or non-celiac gluten intolerance (GI) is a tricky business. Research continues to identify more and more maladies that get better when gluten is removed from the diet, but old belief structures die hard. Many doctors still have a very limited awareness of the range of ailments associated with CD. Moreover, an understanding of gluten sensitivity beyond the classic, damaged-villi concept is practically non-existent in mainstream medicine (though it is more recognized by alternative practitioners).

Who Should Be Tested

As you know if you've read this far, it often takes years for CD to be diagnosed, years of impaired health, high medical bills, and lost opportunities that could often be avoided with a few simple tests. So who should be tested? Individuals at high risk for developing CD—**those with Down's syndrome, IgA deficiency, and/or type 1 diabetes, as well as first-degree relatives (parents, children, siblings) of CD patients—should be first in line.**[1] CD is also prevalent in children and adolescents with delayed puberty, dental-enamel defects, or Turner or Williams syndrome. Dermatitis herpetiformis, gastrointestinal symptoms, osteoporosis, persistent iron deficiency, and short stature, may plague children and adults who should be tested as well.[2] To my way of thinking, however, the testing scope should be even broader. *Anyone* with an autoimmune disease, cancer, gastrointestinal or skin issue, heart disease, infertility, or any other disorder or symptom mentioned in this book, especially anemia, fatigue, osteoporosis, and/or acid reflux, could benefit from being tested in order to determine if he/she is suffering from CD/GI.

Information on various testing options is included in both this chapter and the one that follows. Regardless of the approach you choose, however, it's important to remember the following:

- Blood test results will not be valid if you are already on a GFD. Therefore, you *must* keep consuming gluten until you have the tests.
- If you are taking heavy-duty drugs (immunosuppressants, steroids, and possibly others) and/or receiving treatments such as chemotherapy, your body may be unable to produce sufficient IgA antibodies for accurate test results.[3]
- CD has a genetic component. If you test positive, your parents, children, and siblings (and perhaps other relatives, especially if they are having symptoms) should be tested as well.

The Critical Four: Blood Tests Needed to Detect Celiac Disease

Traditional testing for celiac disease consists of blood tests followed (in most cases) by an endoscopic biopsy to confirm positive findings. However, many doctors are not up to speed on the full range of blood-test options. In this chapter we'll review four blood tests that, taken together, offer a comprehensive diagnostic tool for many people.

- Tissue Transglutaminase—tTG: IgA* (IgG if IgA deficient)
- Endomysial Antibody—EMA: IgA
- Antigliadin Antibody—AGA: IgA and IgG
- Total Serum IgA—IgA deficiency test

There are national support groups and celiac disease research centers that recommend slightly different blood-testing panels. Some don't mention the total serum IgA test, but if one is IgA deficient this test is critical. Most don't suggest the tTG: IgG, but this is important if one is IgA deficient. Others

* A new set of tests, the Deamidated Gliadin Peptide, or DGP: IgA and IgG, may be suggested in place of the tTG, though as of this writing not all labs offer this test. Two recent studies concluded that the tTG continues to be more effective than the DGP.[4] On the other hand, new studies are being done all the time, so it's important to watch for continuing information on this option.

don't recommend the antigliadin antibody (AGA) test, yet it's this test that may detect the newly recognized condition of non-celiac gluten intolerance (GI). And, as noted above, some groups recommend the DGP: IgA and IgG as more effective than the tTG. All this conflicting information, of course, is extremely confusing to the consumer. One would hope the future brings testing standardization to help both doctors and patients stay on the same page. *In the meantime, more-forward-thinking doctors and researchers believe the four tests highlighted above offer the best chance for an accurate diagnosis of CD.*

Traditionally, many doctors have ordered only one or two tests—usually the tTG or the tTG and EMA. These tests (as well as the DGP alternative) are limited to diagnosing CD in the blood. They will not identify non-celiac gluten intolerance. I've talked to far too many people who were told—when *the* test came back negative—that they didn't have CD but were still suffering from "something." This is why it's so critical to request all *four* blood tests *by name*, not just ask to be "tested for celiac disease." Hopefully, your doctor will order them without you having to make a special appointment, especially if you've had recent sick visits. In most cases, your insurance should cover them.

Once you've scaled this first hurdle, double-check the lab order *before* your blood is drawn to make sure the tests you are getting are the ones listed above. If your results are positive, even on only one test, your doctor may recommend an endoscopy to confirm damaged villi. However, ***even if you test negative on all four blood tests, or if you test positive but the endoscopy results are negative, you cannot assume you are not sensitive to gluten.*** Chapter 17 provides information on stool testing, an alternative method used to identify individuals who fall within a wide range of gluten sensitivity. These tests are 100 percent effective at recognizing CD and nearly 100 percent effective at detecting gluten sensitivity.[5]

What's It All About?—Antibodies

Antibodies (also known as immunoglobulins) are proteins created by the immune system to fight off antigens. Antigens—toxins such as chemicals, pollen, viruses, etc.—are seen by the immune system as foreign substances, and antibodies are the body's soldiers, designed to seek out and destroy these dangerous invaders.[6] If an individual is sensitive to gluten and/or to the casein in dairy products, his/her immune system treats these substances like any other invading foreign body; it fights to eliminate them, sometimes at a terrible cost.

In a real war, occasionally soldiers are killed by friendly fire. This same sort of thing can happen in the body. When antibodies can't distinguish between healthy tissue and an antigen, an immune response will attack and destroy healthy tissue. The result is known as an autoimmune disease.[7]

There are five types of antibodies: IgE, IgA, IgG, IgD, and IgM. IgE antibodies are used to test for allergies; IgA and IgG antibodies are used to test for intolerances. An *allergic response* to gluten might manifest itself through itching, hives, coughing, or runny-nose symptoms, or a more severe anaphylactic reaction that could result in death. An *intolerance* to gluten may have no symptoms, developing silently over months, years, or even decades before outward manifestations point to one or more signs and symptoms of CD/GI. Individuals with celiac disease (those whose villi are already damaged) may have IgA and/or IgG antibodies against endomysium, gliadin, or transglutaminase in their bloodstream. Some folks without damaged villi may have these same antibodies. For these individuals, researchers believe the antibodies are an indicator of things to come. If they continue to consume gluten, they may eventually develop the full-blown, damaged villi of CD.[8]

Tissue Transglutaminase Antibody (tTG)

A recent study noted that the amount of tTG (an intestinal enzyme) antibody in one's system correlates with the severity of the disease. In other words, CD does not emerge "fully formed"; instead, it develops on a *continuum* from its latent, potential, or silent form to end-stage celiac disease with severe symptoms.[9] Or, as another study puts it, the tTG antibody, when found in the blood, has been closely linked to "the acute phase of the disease."[10] **Early-stage CD damage can be detected with the tTG: IgA test,[11] but between 60 and 70 percent of patients with mild villi damage may not be identified if the only test they get is the tTG: IgA. And some who test positive on the tTG may have only borderline results.**[12]

In the past, borderline results have been largely ignored, but more recent research indicates they may be a valuable "early-warning system," allowing us to implement corrective measures before more damage is done. This is why using a panel of tests—especially the antigliadin antibody (AGA) test discussed later in this chapter—is so critical to a comprehensive diagnosis.[13]

Endomysial Antibody (EMA)

Most researchers agree that the EMA is a much better predictive tool than the tTG or, as one study reports, "***The EMA is virtually 100% specific for celiac disease.***"[14] On the one hand, this is good news; on the other, why wait until you have full-blown CD to discover you have a problem?

Even in patients without damaged villi, future damage can be *anticipated* when tTG and EMA antibodies show up in the blood.[15] One researcher in a 2009 Finnish study put it this way: "Endomysial antibody positivity without atrophy belongs to the spectrum of genetic gluten intolerance." This study also suggested that patients who exhibit endomysial antibodies would be aided by a GFD no matter how much intestinal damage they have.[16]

The EMA, like the tTG, is designed specifically to recognize damaged intestinal tissue, yet for a significant number of folks with active CD it can return a false negative. Relying on the EMA alone, in fact, has been shown to result in a rate of misdiagnosis approaching 20 percent.[17] Again, this is why the four-test panel is so important.

Antigliadin Antibody (AGA)

The antigliadin antibody (AGA: IgA) test appears to be more sensitive than either the tTG or the EMA in identifying milder intestinal damage. So as not to miss a large percentage of folks with CD, one study recommends "at least" combining the AGA with other screening tests.[18] When AGA tests were used in the past, however, they were thought to be almost *too* sensitive. About 10 percent of the "healthy" population test positive for gliadin antibodies,[19] and many with positive results do not show damaged villi on a follow-up endoscopy. Of course, that's exactly the point, but at a time when the only accepted definition for CD *was* damaged villi, the test results flew in the face of accepted medical wisdom. This is too bad, because a lot of people who were really quite gluten sensitive were sent home with a negative diagnosis and thus continued to suffer. These days AGA testing is barely on anyone's radar screen in the U.S. Only the most forward-thinking U.S. doctors recognize how beneficial this test is in diagnosing a sensitivity to gluten, regardless of whether one has full-blown celiac disease or non-celiac gluten intolerance.

I recently checked a number of national support groups and well-known CD clinic websites to see which ones suggested AGA: IgA and IgG tests. I was greatly disappointed. Some that do include AGA testing in their CD panel are the Massachusetts General Hospital Celiac Research Center, newly established by Dr. Alessio Fasano; the Celiac Disease Center at Columbia University Medical Center, directed by Dr. Peter Green; and Dr. Rodney Ford's clinic in New Zealand. At EnteroLab, a testing facility discussed in depth in Chapter 17, Dr. Kenneth Fine includes the AGA: IgA in his stool testing (IgG antibodies are not found in the stool).[20] On their website, www.gluten.net, the Gluten Intolerance Group also suggests including AGA: IgA and IgG testing along with the tTG and EMA.

In 1991 a study from the Netherlands found, after a gluten challenge with children, that AGA testing (both IgA and IgG) was 100 percent effective in detecting CD. Based in part on these results, the researchers suggested AGA testing could be used in place of the endoscopic biopsy.[21] (See more under *Testing Children* below.) Is there some reason this same logic wouldn't carry over to adults?

Other groups are also recognizing the value of AGA testing. One study states that since up to 85 percent of patients with CD have *no gastrointestinal symptoms*, it is essential to give the AGA test "in all cases of idiopathic ataxia" (lack of muscle coordination without a specific cause), especially since ataxia symptoms may fully resolve on a GFD.[22]

Gluten sensitivity, of course, can affect far more than muscles. Skin, nerves, blood, bones, tissue, and/or organs can also be adversely affected, and AGA antibody blood tests are often positive when there is *no* villous atrophy. This is why I feel so strongly that they should be included on every panel testing for CD/GI.

Recognizing the implications of test results can be another issue. As Phyllis Zermeno, clinical manager at EnteroLab, reports, "The IgG antibody is seen in the blood far more often than the IgA, but many practitioners do not put enough store in IgG test results to recommend their patients eliminate gluten." This is unfortunate, to say the least. The sooner gluten sensitivity can be identified, the sooner it can be treated with a GFD and the healthier the patient will be.

Total Serum IgA

A 2007 Italian study found that IgA-deficient patients (those who do not produce enough IgA antibodies) have "a 10– to 20–fold increased risk for celiac disease." It's easy to see why screening is essential for such individuals,[23] but the IgA portion of the tTG, EMA, and AGA tests discussed above may return a false negative in patients who are IgA deficient.[24] This discrepancy is why an ***"IgA deficiency in serum must always be excluded" when***

evaluating test results."[25] It is also why the IgG portion of the tests is so important. The tTG: IgG and EMA: IgG (though the latter is generally not given) are very effective in recognizing CD in patients with IgA deficiency.[26]

Deamidated Gliadin Peptides (DGP)

A 2010 Finnish study of the new DGP test found it to be better than the tTG and equal to the EMA in identifying CD in its initial phases (before villous atrophy).[27] An Italian study done about the same time defined combination of tTG, EMA, and AGA testing as the best approach, but their research also concluded that using the tTG: IgA and DGP-AGA: IgG together was a more effective diagnostic tool.[28] A third study found the DGP-AGA: IgG to be equal to the tTG: IgA.[29] In other words, the jury is still out. Like so many facets of this complex disorder, determining which tests are best to use, as well as whether one test or a combination thereof may someday replace a biopsy as the ultimate diagnostic tool, requires a great deal more research.

When someone is on a GFD, DGP antibodies disappear more quickly than tTG antibodies. One study suggested, therefore, that the DGP test could be helpful in overseeing GFD compliance in children. DGP antibodies may also surface before tTG antibodies in some children,[30] which could help doctors detect gluten sensitivity sooner.

Other Tests for CD

Researchers continue to seek more effective ways to diagnose celiac disease. Although none of the methods listed below—all developed since the year 2000—are in common use in the U.S. as of this writing, many suggest the need for further CD testing. Some may lead to future diagnostic breakthroughs.

- A new saliva test was introduced in Italy in 2011. Sensitive to the tTG antibody, this test is being used for CD screening in young children to promote early diagnosis.[31]
- A finger-prick blood test for recognizing CD and monitoring a GFD revealed a strong association with antibody and biopsy results.[32]
- Separate studies in Italy and Finland showed a strong relationship in CD patients between the degree of acute injury to intestinal tissue and the level of anti-actin antibodies. This correlation may offer a new tool for detecting severe villi damage.[33]

- Another study showed anti-ganglioside antibodies to be strongly associated with neurological diseases in CD patients. These antibodies may prove useful in detecting neurological issues in those with CD.[34]
- Other research found that "the inflammatory cytokines found in potential CD specimens strongly suggest that these inflammatory markers can be identified long before visible villous changes have occurred." Higher counts of intraepithelial lymphocytes have also been noted.[35]
- Researchers in a 2006 study determined that gliadin increases levels of zonulin (a protein in the intestine). High levels of zonulin amplify the chances of intestinal permeability,[36] and a breach in the intestinal barrier can lead to "both intestinal and extraintestinal autoimmune, inflammatory, and neoplastic [abnormal tissue growth that can turn cancerous] disorders."[37] The good news is that nearly half the participants in one study who followed a GFD for a mean of 9.7 years had normal intestinal permeability and biopsies, as well as normal antibody levels.[38]

Testing Children

In very young children with CD, tTG and EMA antibodies may not have developed,[39] but a 2009 Italian study concluded that for children less than two years old with no IgA deficiency, the AGA: IgG test was as effective as the tTG: IgA.[40] Another study recommended the use of both the DGP: IgA and IgG and the tTG: IgA and IgG to identify CD in children.[41]

Swedish researchers in 2008 suggested using the tTG: IgA and the EMA: IgA as a single marker for children over the age of 18 months. In children younger than 18 months, they concluded, a "combination of [the] AGA: IgA and tTG: IgA is optimal for identifying untreated CD."[42] I can't emphasize enough that the tTG and EMA tests are geared to recognize CD with damaged villi, while the AGA is more likely to detect a sensitivity to gluten in those with or without damaged villi, no matter the age of the patient. (Note: The antigliadin stool test, discussed in the following chapter, is even *more* sensitive than the antigliadin blood test and can be used to detect gluten sensitivity in very young children.)[43]

A friend just mentioned how so many more ailing folks are being diagnosed (I agree), but it is just the very tip of the iceberg of the more common symptoms and ailments, generally related to the gut. It will be decades before all the devastating and degenerative ailments affecting any/many parts of the body linked to gluten are recognized. The stories that follow illustrate just how little is understood on this subject by many of our health care professionals. This lack of knowledge not only keeps people sick, it has been my driving force in writing this book.

Susan's story is an excellent example of how people can have *negative* blood test results but *positive* stool test results. It also illustrates how important it is to have the total serum IgA test discussed above. Subsequently, although most everyone in Susan's family tested negative on the blood tests, they were identified through stool tests to be gluten sensitive. In fact, Susan is the woman who introduced me to Dr. Fine's stool testing, a connection that turned out to be a godsend.

CD and the Family Tree, by Susan G.

It all started with my son Andrew (the boys' names have been changed). Well, genetically, that's not true, but chronologically it was he who gave root to this particular aspect of our family tree. Andrew was a typical five-year-old, except that his height was that of a two-year-old. He had not grown in nearly three years and weighed a mere 26 pounds. Aside from his size he looked healthy, and he was smart, curious, and full of energy. What he wasn't full of was food! Even when offered high-calorie, kid-favorite foods like pizza, macaroni and cheese, and ice cream, Andrew just didn't like to eat. He would take a few bites and quickly be satisfied. He didn't complain but, nevertheless, we were worried. At first his doctor thought he was just a small kid, an assumption supported by the fact my husband and I are both relatively short. Then it was suggested we boost his calorie intake, giving him whatever he wanted to overcome a "picky-eater" syndrome. But picky eating wasn't the problem. Andrew didn't prefer one food over another. He didn't want *any* food.

Finally we were sent to Children's Hospital to consult with endocrinologists for what was suspected to be a hormone deficiency. It was there that a resident suggested, in addition to the hormone tests, Andrew be tested for celiac disease. I had read about celiac as a cause for short stature but hadn't really given it any credence. The resources I'd seen all cited severe gastrointestinal symptoms as the major manifestation of the disease. Andrew exhibited no signs of gastric distress, so imagine our surprise when three months later (evidently the physician in charge had been out of the country) we got a call: Andrew's blood work indicated he had celiac disease. He would need a biopsy to confirm the result.

From there things moved amazingly quickly. We were referred to a gastroenterologist who immediately scheduled Andrew for a small-intestine biopsy. Within two weeks we had the confirmation. The doctor told us we were lucky. "If you are going to have a disease, this is the one to have. It can be completely managed by diet." I remember feeling great relief but also great concern. What could I feed my child if he could no longer eat wheat, rye, oats, or barley?

Surprisingly, getting used to a gluten-free diet was not overwhelming. There were a lot of references available on the web, and we happened to meet an amazing couple right in our town whose daughter had celiac and who willingly shared their secrets with us. I'm not saying it was easy. We had to educate everyone, and we learned to pack our son's food wherever we went, but this was a small price to pay for Andrew's health.

The real difficulty came when we had to explain to family members that celiac is a genetic disease and, since we didn't know which side of the family carried the gene, it would be in their best interest to be screened. No one wanted to do this. After all, they all felt great ... had no symptoms ... wouldn't want to follow *that* diet. It was only after we gave them reference after reference about the various symptoms that could be associated with celiac and how even asymptomatic celiac disease can cause major health problems down the road that, one by one, they started getting tested.

For some the process was frustrating. Many of their physicians would not test for celiac. These doctors felt the tests were unnecessary, especially since most family members did not complain of the "typical" gastrointestinal symptoms associated with the disease. When the test results came back, everyone in my immediate family *tested negative*. Initially I was relieved, but then I started questioning. Right after Andrew was born I had developed arthritis symptoms. My doctor had said it sounded like an autoimmune issue, but he hadn't been able to uncover anything specific. Now I was learning that arthritis symptoms are common in those with celiac.

As I kept reading, I learned about a lab that did both a stool test for gluten sensitivity and a cheek-swab gene test. The lab was highly thought of in the celiac community, even though the testing methods were not "accepted" as standard methodology by most gastroenterologists. I decided to have the test. When the results were positive for gluten sensitivity I was not surprised. The tests also showed I had two copies of the predominant gene for celiac. Soon afterward I went gluten free and, guess what, my joint pain subsided. In addition, the hay fever allergies I'd been plagued with since childhood disappeared!

The more I studied the more I learned of other health problems associated with gluten. For example, my niece had many behavior issues, and since so many celiac references listed this as a symptom, my sister-in-law had stool tests done for my niece and for herself. Both tested positive for gluten sensitivity and both carried the dominant gene. After going gluten free my niece's behavior improved dramatically: no more outbursts, no more anger. And my sister-in-law discovered the "bloat" she had learned to live with disappeared and her energy soared!

After that, it was almost a domino effect. Another of my sisters decided to have her son and herself tested. She had been sick all during her childhood with bouts of strep throat and fatigue; as an adult she'd been diagnosed with chronic fatigue syndrome. My nephew was very small in size and didn't like to eat, much like Andrew. Their blood tests were negative but, again, they both tested positive on the stool test for active gluten sensitivity and the swab for the dominant celiac gene. My sister's physician, a well-known doctor specializing in celiac, suggested she try the diet. Within a couple of weeks of eliminating gluten, she started feeling healthier and my nephew started to eat. Today my once sickly sister, formerly sidelined with chronic fatigue, is a tri-athlete!

My older sister had had skin rashes for years (another sign of gluten sensitivity). In fact, her hands were so bad you could see bone through the dried, cracked skin. She'd gone to dermatologists and tried prescriptions galore, all to no avail. Based on the family experiences, she decided to go gluten free; she didn't even bother with the tests. The response was nothing short of miraculous. Her hands cleared up within weeks, and when she mistakenly consumed gluten, the horrible rash would appear again. The evidence of cause and effect was plain as day.

My youngest sister held out on getting tested until her daughter started to show symptoms. As an infant my niece had been hospitalized a number of times for uncontrollable vomiting. She also was small for her size and had skin rashes. After my sister was diagnosed with a thyroid disorder, an autoimmune disease closely associated with celiac, she decided to have the stool test and the gene test for her daughter and herself. Both tested positive—and nobody was surprised. Today both are on a GFD. My niece is a picture of health, and her mom doesn't get migraines anymore.

Our middle son, Sam, had a history of behavior issues and had been diagnosed with ADHD. He was also very small for his age and was being tested for hormone deficiencies. He'd tested negative on a number of blood tests for CD, so we decided to have stool and gene tests for him as well. I'm not sure why I waited so long to try the stool tests or why I simply didn't put him on the diet. Maybe I knew in my heart he would need *proof* before he'd agree to the diet changes. His tests were also positive and, like other family members, he has two copies of the predominant celiac gene.

Based on these results, we knew my husband would be gene-positive and that our oldest son, Brad, had to have the gene as well. The question was, did either of them have active gluten sensitivity? Both submitted to the stool test. My husband was shocked when he came back positive. Brad was thrilled when he came back negative!

Sam and my husband joined Andrew and me on a GFD without a problem. We were ecstatic when we saw a marked improvement in Sam's behavior and his attention span. It wasn't miraculous—he still has learning issues—but he's improved a great deal. Even more noticeable, after about six months he started to grow. His endocrinologist was surprised and quite pleased. "Keep at it!" he said. My husband hadn't thought he had any symptoms, but after a couple of months without gluten he no longer had a full, bloated feeling after he ate and an old acid-reflux issue had subsided.

Our oldest son continued to eat gluten. At his next physical, however, the doctor did another celiac blood test, this time adding in the total serum IgA. The results showed Brad was IgA deficient—previous test results could not be relied upon. Based on our family history, the doctor strongly suggested he go gluten free, but so far he's chosen not to do so.

As I write this we are an 11-member gluten-sensitive family. Some other family members tested negative, but none of them has had the all-important total serum IgA or stool tests. So far these folks are holding on to their negative results and have opted not to pursue the matter further, but at least they know the door is open.

Endoscopic Biopsy

According to traditional medicine, the gold standard for being diagnosed with CD is a positive endoscopic biopsy showing villous atrophy—damaged intestinal tissue. Those who test positive on the tTG or EMA—tests designed to identify this intestinal damage—are normally expected to have an endoscopic biopsy to confirm a CD diagnosis. Some newer research, however, suggests a biopsy may not be necessary if the results of certain tests are positive. And since biopsy results "may not detect patchy VA [villous atrophy] or milder enteropathy,"[44] they are not always definitive. If the microscope is not powerful enough to pick up mild damage, or not enough samples are taken, or the pathologist is inexperienced, results also may be compromised.[45]

One of the reasons the biopsy *gold* standard might one day become the *old* standard is a growing recognition that people without damaged villi can still be gluten intolerant. Not everyone who tests positive on the tTG and/

or the EMA has damaged villi—at least not yet. In fact, some researchers report that the extent of villous atrophy is in line with the strength of blood-test positivity.[46] In other words, the more damage to the villi, the higher the test score (unless one is IgA deficient, of course, in which case all bets are off). Even a low score, sometimes not recognized as indicative of celiac disease or even non-celiac gluten intolerance, is nothing to ignore. It could mean damage is beginning to happen.

Jane's story illustrates just this point, and it's a great example of why I'm writing this book. It makes no sense to give an endoscopy to someone who has not eaten gluten for any period of time. For the results to mean anything, the patient *must* keep consuming gluten until they've had the procedure. Moreover, standard protocol dictates that patients receive blood tests *first*, followed by an endoscopic biopsy to confirm CD if test results are positive. Despite Jane's weight loss and a compression fracture—significant tip-offs for CD—she was slipping through a veil of health care unawareness. And she is not alone.

A Misunderstood Subject, by Jane Landreth

When my doctor suspected I might have a gluten problem, he immediately ordered an endoscopy. The only thing I was told in preparation for this procedure was not to eat after midnight the night before. The doctor knew I hadn't been consuming gluten for three weeks prior to the test, but no mention was made of the fact that this might affect the results.

Knowing what I know now, I'm not surprised the results came back negative. Afterward, I had to talk the physician's assistant (PA) into doing a blood test. The results were also negative. Of course, the blood test should have been done *before* the endoscopy, but given the fact I was not eating gluten, the order of the tests was somewhat of a moot point. The "treatment" suggested for the cramping and gas I'd been having for three months, along with accompanying unintended weight loss, was to eat a regular diet and take peppermint-oil capsules for my discomfort. I declined.

My chiropractor gave me digestive enzymes to see if they would help my discomfort, but he also suspected gluten and suggested staying gluten free. More importantly, as it turns out, he X-rayed my back and discovered I had a compression fracture. It appeared the fracture was causing muscle spasms that literally were stopping my digestion, allowing partially digested matter to sit and ferment before moving on. I was relieved to find an answer for my problem, at least until both the chiropractor and a new family doctor pointed out that given my activity level and good eating habits, I shouldn't have had the fracture in the first place.

When I told the PA about the fracture and what the other doctors had said, her response was, "Oh my." I asked about further testing for gluten sensitivity, but she could see no need to do so since both the endoscopy and blood test had been negative. Since then I have continued to stick to the gluten-free diet and am feeling much better. My digestive issues and compression fracture resolved themselves within a month, and I've even gained some weight.

Jane was smart to listen to her body and her chiropractor in spite of her negative test results. I always urge people to get tested, but some don't have insurance, some don't like doctors, and some just want to "try" the diet. Seeing positive results in black and white is very helpful in maintaining a GF lifestyle.

The doctor wanted to challenge this mother's "failure-to-thrive" child—a child who had finally begun to grow—by giving her gluten so *another* endoscopy could be performed. Since the child was already responding favorably to a GFD, the common sense of this eludes me. Why make the child suffer needlessly?

180-Degree Turnaround, by Krissy Herrick

My four year-old daughter wasn't growing, and I'd been telling the pediatrician for three years that something was very wrong. She finally agreed to test her for CD, but both the blood tests and endoscopy were inconclusive. Based on research I'd done and my own battles with CD, however, I knew in my heart that my daughter was gluten sensitive. I decided to put her on a GFD diet. Within two days I noticed a difference. By the time of her annual checkup she'd made a 180-degree turnaround, gaining three pounds and growing three and a half inches. She'd also started to have regular bowel habits and to sleep much better—no more middle-of-the-night interruptions. Later the doctors wanted to do another endoscopy, but this would have required reintroducing gluten, something neither I nor my daughter wanted. She knew what made her tummy hurt and she'd become accustomed to checking with me before eating anything questionable. We decided against the test.

The obvious question, of course, is why would anyone want to wait until they have near-end-stage CD to find out they have a problem? Based on my own family's experience and the experience of so many whose stories are included in this book, I believe—to the tips of my toes—that the most sensitive tests currently available are the stool tests offered by Enterolab (covered in the next chapter). Since most of my family tested negative on the blood tests, yet all of us were positive on the stool tests and have found much greater health by following a GF lifestyle, I sometimes find it tempting to suggest people go directly to the stool tests. On the other hand, doctors need to learn more about this subject—from their patients, if need be—and the blood tests are more likely to be covered by insurance.

The route you take is up to you, but if you're "sick and tired of being sick and tired" a good first step is to learn more about how gluten sensitivity could be contributing to your particular health issues. When you're ready, have a conversation with your doctor about testing options. If you opt to have the blood tests, be certain—again, I can't emphasize this enough—to request the four tests listed at the beginning of this chapter. If the tests are negative and you're still feeling bad, I urge you to strongly consider the stool testing offered by EnteroLab. Dollar-for-dollar, it may be the best investment you've ever made.

CD has an identified genetic component, so if you receive a positive diagnosis of gluten sensitivity on either blood tests or the stool tests, it's critical that you encourage your relatives to be tested as well, especially parents, children, and siblings.

If you are gluten sensitive, the only way to rejuvenate your health and halt further degenerative damage is to adopt and follow a strict, gluten-free diet for life. Contrary to what many people believe, however, giving up gluten is not the kiss of death. Rather, for those affected by this ubiquitous protein, adopting a GFD may well offer the gift of a long and healthy life.

17 Gluten 103: Progressive Stool Testing

If you've been tested for CD in the past, you've most likely had blood tests—the tissue transglutaminase (tTG) and maybe the endomysial (EMA), though the EMA is costlier and more labor intensive. While useful diagnostic tools for many, the tTG and EMA are designed only to recognize CD with varying degrees of villous atrophy; they will not detect non-celiac gluten intolerance. The AGA: IgA and IgG tests are very good at detecting a sensitivity to gluten whether the villi are damaged or not. And the total serum IgA can measure whether someone is IgA deficient, in which case other IgA test results may not be valid. As discussed in the previous chapter, the tTG, EMA, AGA, and IgA total serum, given together, can help identify gluten sensitivity in many people.

Even under the best of circumstances, however, blood testing does not work for all, which is why I've devoted this entire chapter to stool testing, a cutting-edge option for identifying gluten sensitivity in a wide range of individuals, including some people with negative blood-test results. "**Stool testing for the antigliadin IgA antibodies is so much more sensitive than blood tests that the antibodies can still be detected in the intestine up to 1–2 years after beginning the GF diet** . . ."[1]

Chapter 16 reviewed the advantages and pitfalls of blood tests (and follow-up endoscopic biopsies) as diagnostic options. If, like many others, you are someone whose tests are negative, yet symptoms remain, you may be glad to learn more about the stool test option.

- Have you tested negative on blood tests designed to diagnose CD?
- Is your doctor resistant to your requests for specific tests and reluctant to review the information you provide?
- Is your doctor willing to order only one or two tests?
- Have you been through the mill trying to find out what ails you and you're still sick?
- Are you without health insurance or have a huge deductible and thus want to spend your money only once?

If any of these scenarios applies to you, it may be time for stool testing.

Stool Tests

Dr. Kenneth Fine, a board-certified gastroenterologist with years of experience in the field, is a progressive thinker among those espousing a broader view of gluten sensitivity. Because Dr. Fine is more interested in detecting a broad scope of gluten sensitivity rather than pinpointing CD specifically, he has developed specialized, patented stool tests for measuring an individual's sensitivity to gluten. EnteroLab, a "registered and fully accredited clinical laboratory specializing in the analysis of intestinal specimens for food sensitivities," offers stool tests that can detect antibodies produced in the intestine before they enter the bloodstream.[2] As a result, they can often identify gluten sensitivity where blood tests have failed.

If I seem biased toward stool testing, it is with good reason. Most of my family had negative results on the blood tests, even my daughter, who was fading away. Because doctors were so concerned about her health, they ordered an endoscopy anyway, but this, too, was negative. She tested positive, however, on the antigliadin IgA antibody *stool* test, and since adopting a gluten-free lifestyle her health has completely turned around. Had I not discovered EnteroLab, my health and that of my family could have continued its downward spiral. Many of those whose stories appear between these pages, along with thousands of others, I suspect, wish they had discovered stool testing long before they developed full-blown CD and its many accompanying ailments.

Because the "marker" for gluten sensitivity, the antigliadin (AGA) IgA antibody, is produced in the small intestine and thus can be picked up in the stool before it gets into the blood,[3] Dr. Fine asserts it will be produced long before tissue damage to the villi occurs. Recent research has found that early damage can also be revealed by tTG (transglutaminase): IgA, another antibody produced in the gut.[4] Given the source of antibody production in the small intestine, it only makes sense that stool tests could detect a wider range of gluten sensitivity than traditional blood tests.

Of course, stool tests are used for a variety of diagnostic purposes, but at EnteroLab they are employed specifically to detect antibodies such as AGA: IgA and/or tTG: IgA, among others. EnteroLab is currently the only facility offering a stand-alone AGA: IgA antibody stool test, as well as a three-part gluten-sensitivity stool panel that measures levels of antigliadin (AGA): IgA and tTG: IgA antibodies along with levels of fat malabsorption. However, more and more research is supporting this approach.

- A study done in Italy in 2011 noted that the presence of tTG: IgA antibodies, which are formed in the intestine, "seems predictive of future celiac disease." This study also found "a new form of genetic-dependent gluten intolerance ... in which none of the usual diagnostic markers is present." When genetically predisposed relatives of CD study participants adopted a gluten-free diet (GFD), their symptoms resolved and their tTG antibodies vanished.[5]
- Another 2011 Italian study found that "fecal assays for ECP [eosinophil cationic protein] could be used to identify FH [food hypersensitivity—to milk protein and gluten] in patients with IBS [irritable bowel syndrome]."[6]
- According to Finnish gastroenterologist Dr. Katri Kaukinen, when antibodies are found "in vivo [live cells] in small-intestinal mucosa ... it is possible to find even more reliably patients having celiac disease in its early stages." In 2008 Dr. Kaukinen and his colleagues went on to suggest that once the diagnostic panorama has been widened to include non-celiac gluten intolerance, damaged villi "will no longer be the gold standard in the diagnosis of celiac disease."[7]
- A 2005 Finnish study concluded that CD can exist even when villi are normal and thus "mucosal transglutaminase 2-specific IgA deposits can be utilized in detecting such patients with genetic gluten intolerance."[8] Transglutaminase (tTG) deposits are also found in the small intestine and can be excreted in the stool; hence the importance of Dr. Fine's fecal testing for early detection and prevention.

- In a 2004 German study one CD patient had normal blood screening, but was high in stool AGA and tTG testing. Study conclusions stressed how important fecal antibody testing is for patients who are serum negative but have signs of CD.[9]
- A 2002 study from Italy found that endomysial antibodies [EMA] were revealed in the blood, culture media, and stool samples of all untreated CD patients. Finding EMA in fecal samples is verification that this antibody, like the AGA and the tTG, is *also* created in intestinal mucosa. EMA stool testing could be used to further clarify ambiguous biopsy results.[10]

EnteroLab uses the same FDA-approved kit for stool testing that other labs use for blood tests. Some of the tests offered are described below. More information can be found on the EnteroLab website: www.enterolab.com.

A Range of Options

Gluten Sensitivity Stool Panel—This valuable, three-part series includes the antigliadin (AGA) and tTG: IgA antibody tests as well as a microscopic fat malabsorption test. (If your body is not absorbing fats, it can be an indication of damaged villi.) Many people who are sensitive to gluten are also sensitive to the casein protein in dairy products and/or to eggs, soy, etc. If you suspect you may be one of them, you can add on tests to measure these intolerances.

Antigliadin Antibody Stool Test—If your budget is really tight, the AGA: IgA (antigliadin antibody) test will tell you whether or not you are gluten sensitive. If the results are positive, you could then order other antibody tests such as the tTG or food intolerance tests within a couple weeks.

Genetic Mouth-Swab Test—If it turns out you *are* sensitive to gluten, you may want to consider ordering the genetic mouth-swab test. Knowing your genetic predisposition can be helpful, especially if you have first-degree relatives (children, siblings, or living parents). Second-degree relatives (aunts, uncles, cousins) with health issues may benefit from testing as well. If you are IgA deficient you could order the gene test to see what your hereditary predisposition is for celiac disease and/or non-celiac gluten intolerance.

Other Sensitivity Tests—EnteroLab offers tests for other food sensitivities: milk, soy, egg, and dietary yeast, as well as a new food panel that measures sensitivity to corn, oats, rice, beef, chicken, pork, tuna, almonds, walnuts, cashews, and white potatoes. For some people, one or more of these food sensitivities can also wreak havoc on your body.

Dr. Fine answers many questions about gluten sensitivity, colitis, and more on his website, www.FinerHealth.com. Also, be sure to read "Who should be screened for gluten sensitivity?" at the bottom of the section on "Frequently Asked Questions About Gluten Sensitivity." You may be amazed at what you discover.

The cost of stool testing at EnteroLab is out-of-pocket, but the test may be retroactively covered by your insurance, and the lab provides a coded invoice for your convenience. Once I began to understand the genetic nature of gluten sensitivity, I ordered a series of tests for my entire family that included the AGA: IgA and tTG: IgA antibody stool tests plus tests for malabsorption, genetic markers, and dairy intolerance. The results were educational to say the least! For one thing, I learned from the fat malabsorption test that I was not absorbing fat and important nutrients properly—and I didn't have to have an endoscopic biopsy to find out! Stool testing uncovered the gluten sensitivity that was causing most of the fatigue, allergies, and ill health in my family. It was the best money we ever spent.

Disclaimer*: I have no affiliation, financial, or otherwise, with Dr. Fine or EnteroLab; I am simply a strong believer in the work they do.*

Testing Children

According to Dr. Fine, "Stool testing for IgA antibodies can be done as early as 12 months in a symptomatic child and 18 months in an asymptomatic child. This is not true for serum (blood) testing, as serum testing is often falsely negative at any age."[11] Since gluten in the mother's diet, as well as any IgA antibodies she may be producing in reaction to gluten, can pass through breast milk to the child, the lab does not recommend testing children who are being breastfed until at least six months after they've been weaned. Otherwise, it would be unclear from the test results as to whether antibodies came from the mom, the child, or both. It also would be important to test the mom, since she might be reacting to gluten as well.[12]

A Must-Read

In a lecture by Dr. Fine titled "Early Diagnosis of Gluten Sensitivity: Before the Villi Are Gone," he explains in a common-sense way why stool testing is superior to blood testing. The points below are taken from this essay:[13]

1. "We can diagnose the problem before the end stage tissue damage has occurred, that is 'before the villi are gone,' with the idea of preventing all the nutritional and immune consequences that go with it."
2. By the time you have a "biopsy showing villous atrophy…associated bone, brain, growth, and/or gland problems are all but guaranteed."
3. In "people with intestinal symptoms, but normal blood tests and biopsies, the antigliadin antibodies were only inside the intestine (where they belong if you consider that the immune stimulating gluten also is inside the intestine), not in the blood."
4. "Gluten sensitive individuals who do not have villous atrophy (the mass of the iceberg), will only have evidence of their immunologic reaction to gluten by a test that assesses for antigliadin IgA antibodies where that foodstuff is located, inside the intestinal tract, not [in] the blood."

You can find a transcript of this lecture at www.FinerHealth.com or www.EnteroLab.com. After you've had a chance to review it, you may want to share it with your doctors. The EnteroLab site also has a slide show with additional information about gluten sensitivity.

Stool testing is sensitive, non-invasive, and reasonably priced. If you are experiencing *any* of the symptoms or maladies mentioned in this book—especially if you've tested negative on blood tests designed to diagnose CD—I urge you to investigate this alternative. Why wait until antibodies show up in your blood or until your villi are severely compromised? You might even want to make stool testing your first choice, especially if you don't have health insurance.

The choice is simple. If you are "sick and tired of being sick and tired," especially if you've gotten nowhere with diagnostic blood tests, seeking out stool tests may be one of the best decisions you ever make. But remember, no matter where you fall on the continuum of gluten sensitivity, ***if you test positive for an intolerance you need to follow a strict, gluten-free diet (GFD) for life.***

Progressive Blood Tests

Cyrex Laboratory offers progressive antibody blood testing for a number of autoimmune disorders/conditions. If you tested negative on the traditional blood tests and the progressive stool tests and are still ill you may want to consider using Cyrex Labs. Check at http://www.cyrexlabs.com.

A Lousy Inheritance 18

THE GENETIC PICTURE of celiac disease (CD) and non-celiac gluten intolerance (GI) is complex and ever evolving. Two particular genes have been linked to CD, the HLA-DQ2 and the HLA-DQ8. Human leukocyte antigens (HLA) are present in most tissues and are strongly linked to autoimmune diseases.[1] About 95 percent of CD patients have the DQ2 gene. Most of the remaining 5 percent have the DQ8.[2] The DQ2 and DQ8 gene tests can be used to exclude CD, so if your results are negative for both consider yourself lucky; it's likely you'll never develop the disease.[3] Conversely, although 30 to 40 percent of the general population has at least one of these genes, only one to two percent of the population actually develops CD.[4]

Still other genes have been associated with CD. For example, research done between 2008 and 2010 has:

- "Identified 39 nonHLA risk genes.... Most of the coeliac disease-associated regions are shared with other immune-related diseases, as well as with metabolic, haematological or neurological traits, or cancer."[5]
- Found four new genes linked to CD and rheumatoid arthritis, in addition to confirming two previously discovered gene locations.[6]
- Revealed "more than a dozen new susceptibility loci for celiac disease."[7]

The more research that's done, the more we know about the overlap between celiac disease, non-celiac gluten intolerance, and a myriad of disorders and symptoms. This is why genetic testing is so important if you or any of your family members have chronic ailments.

What ailments have manifested themselves among members of your family? As illustrated by Cecile's story below, fatigue, depression, moodiness, anemia, pain, weight gain/loss, gut issues, allergies, miscarriages, arthritis, osteopenia or osteoporosis, and skin issues are just some of the many maladies linked to gluten sensitivity.

A Typical American Family, by Cecile

This is a story about a typical American family (all names have been changed)—Bart, the father; Cecile, the mother; and Marie and Oliver, the children. The family heritage is a mixture of Scottish, English, French and German, with bits of Dutch, Irish, and Spanish mixed in. There was never a mention of celiac disease or other food related problems on either side.

I was born healthy, if a little underweight. When I was five years old I had walking pneumonia. At seven I had double pneumonia, which is when iron deficiency anemia was discovered and treated. As I grew up the only health problems I had were bad cramps each month and, in my 20s, problems with my knees. At times they would swell, pop, and grind; then they began collapsing with no warning. It felt like they were out-of-joint. When my husband and I decided to have children I had two miscarriages before my daughter Marie, was born and another miscarriage before giving birth to my son, Oliver. Both children were born healthy and the doctors offered no reason for the three miscarriages.

A combination of depression and anxiety, accompanied by urgent intestinal issues I refer to as "Mississippi Mud," led me to Dr. Peter Green's book, *Celiac Disease: a Hidden Epidemic* and from there to seek CD testing, although my symptoms never prompted my doctor to suggest any tests. A well-known clinic recommended the endomysial antibody (EMA) blood test. The results were negative but I wasn't convinced. Something was definitely wrong and I knew I had to keep looking for answers. Finally, through EnteroLab stool testing I discovered I was highly intolerant to gluten, casein, and soy; I also have two gluten-sensitive genes. Eighteen months after eliminating the offending items from my diet I have more energy and am able to better control my weight. After 20 years my intestinal issues are finally "normal," but my reaction to these intolerances, if accidentally ingested, is swift, from diarrhea and immediate rectal itching to a paranoiac depression and fatigue with arthritis pain.

I was recently diagnosed with osteopenia, as well as stage II osteoarthritis in my knees. In the past when my knees were bothering me, I used to wear patches for the pain and go down steps sideways or backwards. Since being gluten free I no longer have knee pain. In fact, walking, dancing—even aerobic exercise—is no problem unless I go off the diet; then the aches, pains, and stiffness return. And I take no medication except vitamin D3 and calcium citrate.

I was nearly 60 years of age by the time stool tests revealed my intolerance. Looking back, I realize I've probably been sensitive to gluten since childhood.

My daughter, Marie, had a few ear infections about the age of nine months but was otherwise healthy until the fourth grade, when she came down with a bad case of chicken pox. The following summer she developed asthma. After allergy tests showed she was allergic to mold and dust mites, she was successfully treated with allergy drops, but she continued to be troubled by asthma for nearly 30 years. She had pain in her joints, particularly in her knees. At times it was so bad she thought she might need a knee replacement. She's also suffered from depression, dry skin rash, trigeminal neuralgia, and carpal tunnel syndrome. [In one study about 20 percent of CD patients had carpal tunnel.[8] Could this disorder, a form of neuropathy, also be linked to gluten?]

Marie had the gold standard of testing for celiac disease—blood tests and an endoscopic biopsy. All were negative. Then she, too, submitted stool samples to EnteroLab and discovered she was intolerant to both gluten and casein and that she has one gluten-sensitive gene and one celiac gene. As I write this Marie has been gluten free for seven months. She's seen some improvement in her asthma during this time, but the most remarkable change is that her knee pain is gone!

My son, Oliver, developed chronic ear infections when he was just a month old. By the time he was two and a half he had tubes in his ears. He had problems as a child with milk and intestinal gas, and he would frequently burp while talking. He caught chicken pox at the same time as his sister, and the following summer developed petit mal epilepsy. When we did allergy testing on him, he had positive results for tree and grass pollen. The day he started on the allergy drops, his epilepsy was gone. He also had dry skin and as an adult developed itchy blisters on his feet [possibly undiagnosed dermatitis herpetiformis].

Oliver was the first to read about gluten problems and went gluten free without being tested. The blisters went away. Recently, he gave himself a gluten challenge, and the blisters returned almost immediately. His new wife wisely chose to adhere to a gluten-free diet through her pregnancy and remains on the diet since she is nursing the baby. When the child is old enough, they'll have her genes tested, too. Thank heavens for my son's investigations. If he hadn't come across information about gluten sensitivity, we might all still be suffering.

For many years my husband, Bart, was relatively healthy. His only problem was scoliosis and a mold allergy that brought on bad moods. Then he contracted Lyme disease, which led to fibromyalgia. A few years later he developed intestinal issues and underwent the traditional EMA blood tests for CD. The results were negative. Through stool testing however, he, too, was diagnosed with gluten sensitivity, along with an intolerance to casein and soy. After going gluten free his fibromyalgia pain and intestinal issues are gone, and he has much more stamina.

Gene tests revealed Bart has one gluten-sensitive gene and one celiac gene, which might go a long way toward explaining a family history of wasting disease on his Scottish father's side.

Kay, a recently retired professor from Simmons College, is a dear friend who induced me to getting back on a bike after decades of not riding. She's a few years older than me and has had a hip replacement, but she and her husband were planning to do a bike/barge trip from Paris to Bruges and urged me to join in (my husband had already signed on). With a bit of nudging I thought, "If Kay can do this, I should be able to, too!" I only had a week and a half of training around our hilly town before we set off, but I was able to keep up with the "Chain Gang" on half-day excursions in France and Belgium. What a time we had, riding with our spouses and good friends. And since three of us on the barge were gluten free, the chef mostly cooked gluten free for everyone. On pasta night, he even made up special, gluten-free pasta.

Kay's story is a good example of the many detrimental threads of gluten sensitivity and what a variation of "colorful" symptoms these threads can weave within a single family.

A Family Saga, by Kay, EdD

I am writing this from my perspective as a granddaughter, daughter, mother, and grandmother. One of my early memories is hearing my grandmother in the bathroom in the middle of the night, and again at dawn, releasing noisy gas followed by diarrhea. From the age of six I spent my summers on Cape Cod with my grandparents. I often slept with my grandmother because my grandfather snored so much he slept in the guest room. I never knew why my grandmother had so many gastric problems, but her nocturnal emissions woke me every night.

When I was in my early 20s my father, then in his early 50s, developed the same symptoms. At first he was diagnosed with being sensitive to corn, which he dutifully eliminated from his diet. Twenty years later, in his early 70s, he was diagnosed with celiac disease and cut out all gluten products.

When my husband and I retired from teaching we celebrated our first fall without a teaching schedule with a trip to Prince Edward Island just after Labor Day. Fresh corn was at its height, and we had corn fritters with breakfast, corn chowder for lunch, and corn in some form as a vegetable at night. By the end of the trip I had such a case of diarrhea that it took two years, many doctor visits, and a variety of medications to clear it up. A colonoscopy showed I had collagenous colitis. My gastroenterologist didn't know why I'd developed this disease, though he agreed corn might be a likely suspect. After that I eliminated all corn from my diet and became an expert at reading labels to find the myriad of ways corn products are used in everything from ketchup to soy sauce to ice cream. When my bowels finally returned to normal, I breathed a sigh of relief.

Several years later I suddenly developed strong nasal allergies. I would sometimes sneeze 20 times in 5 minutes, and my nose ran continuously. When I visited an allergist, however, the skin tests showed nothing. "You don't have any food allergies," this doctor reported, "and certainly not to corn." He scoffed at the idea of food sensitivities. [Some doctors believe enzyme-linked immunosorbent assay testing (ELISA) may be more definitive in revealing food sensitivities.]

My nasal allergies continued. When I caught a cold they were even worse. After having three colds that turned to bronchitis and then to pneumonia, I was sent to a lung specialist. He said that he didn't care what caused my runny nose and sinus infections; his job was to *treat* them. He tried a variety of ways to dry me up, including antibiotics. Finally he found a treatment that worked: one pill that lasted for 12 hours during the day, another than lasted for four hours at night. After about two years my runny nose and postnasal drip cleared up, as long as I kept taking these medications.

I then had about a year of good health before my bowels began to act up again. About this time—by now I was 68 years old—I met Anne Sarkisian. She told me about some of her family's experiences, shared information about the genetic nature of gluten intolerance (up until then I'd never considered my problems might be hereditary in nature), and told me about Dr. Kenneth Fine and the stool- and gene-testing procedures offered by EnteroLab. These tests seemed much less invasive than others I'd read about, so in the fall of 2007 I carefully followed the testing directions. The results came back positive. Not only was I sensitive to gluten, I also have two genes that correlate with gluten sensitivity—one from each parent.

At the same time—again, at Anne's suggestion—I was reading *Dangerous Grains*. The authors related that according to the Centers for Disease Control

(CDC), there is a strong correlation between gluten sensitivity and non-Hodgkin's lymphoma. I was shocked, because my mother had died from this form of cancer in 1963. The book also noted the link between type 1 diabetes and gluten sensitivity. My first husband had had type 1 diabetes. Realizing my son may have inherited a gene from both his father and me, I immediately called my son, Jon. Fortunately, Jon did not have diabetes like his father, but for years he'd had problems with digestion, and he was having more and more bouts of unexplained nasal allergies.

Jon and his wife, Laura, have two children. Their daughter had no symptoms, but their son has had problems with digestion. Explaining the genetic nature of gluten sensitivity, I offered to pay the lab fees if Jon would agree to tests for himself and his children.

All three tested positive for gluten sensitivity. Each had two genes, one inherited from each parent. Jon's wife has not been tested, but she also may have a gene linked with gluten sensitivity. She also has rheumatoid arthritis, another autoimmune disease associated with gluten sensitivity. It's difficult to believe that all of these associations are mere coincidence.

"The proof is in the pudding," my mother always said. Last fall, three generations of our family joined my father (the fourth generation) in a gluten-free lifestyle. Are we feeling better? My nasal allergies have improved greatly, and I've been off medication for this condition for several months; my bowels also improved rapidly. Last winter I had two colds but no bronchitis or pneumonia.

My daughter-in-law has seen a lessening in her arthritis pain. Since she's not been formally tested for gluten sensitivity, from time to time, she'll challenge her system and eat food containing gluten, like the special garlic bread she had on a recent visit to a local restaurant. The next day she felt fine, she reported, but for five days thereafter her joints felt like they were on fire each time she moved. She is now more determined than ever to stay gluten free.

Jon's digestive and nasal-allergy issues have improved as well. To me, however, the most dramatic proof of his sensitivity to gluten came within hours after he'd eaten some tabouli. He'd forgotten that bulgur comes from cracked wheat and ate almost a whole helping last summer before his hostess reminded him. He was up all night sneezing and blowing his nose.

Neither of my grandchildren has shown such dramatic changes, but my grandson says his tummy does feel better when he avoids gluten.

In our quest for good health, four generations of our family (my father recently turned 100) continue to work at being gluten free and to avoid the pitfalls of hidden gluten. We are lucky to live near bakeries and markets that carry gluten-free baked goods, and Laura is developing tasty recipes for brownies, chocolate chip

> cookies, and pie crust. Jon is working on a show-stopping pizza crust, and I'm on a hunt for a bread and hamburger roll recipe that everyone might like.
>
> Feeling better gives us the motivation to remain gluten free. The hardest part is explaining our new diet to our friends and helping them to understand there is still a lot we can eat. It is certainly much easier to be gluten free now than when my father was diagnosed with CD 40 years ago.

In my case *everyone* in my immediate family—my husband, three children, and four grandchildren—was affected. If both parents have two genes, the child would inherit two gluten-related genes, one from each parent. If a parent has one gluten-sensitive gene, the child would have a 50/50 chance of inheriting it. And so this very common and unhealthy demon continues from one generation to the next.

19 The Gluten-Free Lifestyle: Say It with a Smile

The Gluten-Free Diet–You Don't Just Try It

The gluten-free diet (GFD) is actually misnamed. It's not a diet; it's a lifestyle. If intolerant to gluten, your health depends on making an absolute, lifetime commitment to living without it. This is one reason it's important to get tested. Seeing positive results in black and white will help you stick to the diet when you're tempted to be careless. Some alternative health care professionals may suggest you not consume gluten for somewhere between two to three weeks and a few months, and then see how you feel when it is reintroduced. The idea is this: If you begin to feel really good without gluten and not so good with it, you have an answer to your problem. This is one approach, but getting a real handle on a gluten-free (GF) lifestyle may take several months. If you are, indeed, gluten sensitive but inadvertently ingest even small bits of the stuff during your "test" period, your problems may keep happening, which could in turn lead you to conclude that your issues aren't gluten related after all. Removing gluten from your diet can also interfere with blood-test results, so should you wish to be tested later, you'll have to start consuming gluten again. And if living gluten free has already made you feel better, reintroducing this protein (called a gluten challenge) might be very unpleasant. It could even be hazardous. (For one young woman's experience with a gluten challenge, see www.GlutenSensitivity.net, click on Personal Experiences and choose "Su's story.")

Fortunately, antibodies persist in the stool after they're no longer discernable in the blood,[1] so if you've had little or no gluten for a while and decide to get tested, you might consider stool testing.

Nigel's story is an example of someone who listened to his body, found information about gluten online, went on a GFD without testing, and found greater health. Although this route worked for him, his recommendation is that anyone with health issues strongly consider being tested.

Diet in a Fast-food Nation, by Nigel Wolovick

Good diet is the key to good health. As a child my diet was probably typical of most kids in the U.S. I consumed an abundance of pizza, pasta, and bologna and cheese sandwiches. I remember wondering why I had such a hard time swallowing these foods, but kids don't know how to fix this kind of problem. They can give feedback to their parents and ask for different foods, but many parents perceive such complaints as "Oh, my child is whining again." Children love to moan and whine, it's true, but they also complain when something really doesn't seem right to them.

By the time I reached adulthood there was always new information circulating among my friends about some disease or other. In fact, I think it was a friend who tipped me off to an online article on celiac disease. I'd been looking at other diseases, including some genetic ones that make you feel ***dead*** all the time. Was celiac like that?

I had a good friend who had celiac disease, and one day she explained the symptoms to me. Our talk brought back a flood of memories, one of which was the kicker: One day, after eating ice cream in a waffle cone at a miniature golf course, I felt sick to my stomach. Rushing to the bathroom, I felt a burning in my anus. I also noticed some blood in this area. At the time I didn't know what to make of it. Now I realize it was the beginning of hemorrhoids, a side effect of pushing hard for long periods of time to go to the bathroom. I also thought how I'd often had to sit on the toilet for an hour, trying to have a bowel movement, and sometimes still be unsuccessful. I consulted three different doctors but none seemed the least bit concerned about an 18-year-old guy with hemorrhoids and no energy.

I'd had other problems of gradually increasing severity since childhood. For instance, I had frequent back pain and I never had dreams, but my digestive problems were the worst. In addition to difficulty with my bowels, my abdomen was often painful. It would feel as though I'd eaten contaminated food that had somehow stopped all digestive activity. I soon learned to rub my tummy and to have empathy for others who lived in pain. And the treatment doctors prescribed for my hemorrhoid flare-ups—a synthetic fiber—was no cure.

By the time I finished my first year of college I felt bloated and run down all the time. Finally, after talking with my friend, everything made sense; I diagnosed myself with celiac disease. Very quickly I experimented with eliminating all wheat from my diet. It took several weeks to notice any sort of change. Days would pass when I was gluten free, but then I'd lust after something with wheat and give in. Every time I did my energy dropped and my gut felt like it was being attacked. So I'd swear off gluten again until my mind would second-guess me and I'd "fall off the wagon." At that time in my life I believed I could fix any problem simply by wishing it away, so it took me a long time to come to terms with my condition. Eventually I consoled myself over the loss of my favorite gluten-laden treats and adopted the GF lifestyle wholeheartedly.

The positive results of my decision were so obvious I never felt the need to check up on my status with tests. On the other hand, if I'd had formal test results to confirm my self-diagnosis, perhaps my transition to a GF lifestyle might have been less rocky. So please, if you have the opportunity, get tested! I realize that for many people this is scary advice. Even if they suspect gluten may be their problem, they don't want to know for sure. They fear the lifestyle changes they'll have to make if they test positive, and they don't want to give up their favorite foods. These are legitimate concerns, but think about it. Would you rather eat pizza than be energetic, alive, and healthy?

My aim is to inspire someone who suspects he or she may be gluten sensitive to test it out. Try going a week or two without any gluten at all, then reintroduce it. If you notice a difference, you'll know it's time to get tested and you'll have a pretty good idea of the changes you may need to make.

It's been four years since I learned about the effects of gluten on my body and started changing my life. Since then I've lost 15 to 20 pounds from switching to a good green diet. I eat mostly certified-organic, living foods that slightly invigorate me as soon as they hit my palate. I eat foods that make me feel light and joyful with energy, not weighed down and stuffed. I can wake up to any time I set my alarm. I can excrete normally. I am alive. I no longer feel like an eternal victim of fatigue. I am still healing, but I feel so much better than before I started on a GFD. I no longer spend an hour on the toilet and I only get a cold once a year or so. (Back in high school, I had a cold nearly every other month.) I've also inspired members of my family and friends to eat less wheat.

Here in California, gluten-free options are everywhere. I look forward to the day when this is the case across the country. I also look forward to a time when adequate testing for gluten sensitivity is available for anyone who seeks it.

Just as doctors need to be educated about adequate testing protocols and the numerous symptoms and maladies associated with gluten, dietitians and nutritionists need to be taught to help their clients implement a gluten-free diet. There is a *huge* gap between being diagnosed with gluten sensitivity and getting a handle on a GFD, and too many people are left to figure it out for themselves. I've heard from folks who were handed a couple pages of written information with no verbal explanation whatsoever. Neither my daughter nor I received even that much. I've also heard—many times over—of instances in which a patient was referred to a dietician or nutritionist and the patient knew more than the professional.

Many doctors paint a bleak picture about the feasibility of following the diet, and this type of negativity needs to be turned around. In fact, health care professionals should stress the importance of *100 percent compliance* (99 percent isn't good enough to avoid further complications). Otherwise the illness will continue and can lead to a continuum of degenerative and life-compromising ailments. Yes, less gluten is better than more, but the *tiniest bit* can keep damaging your villi and causing havoc in other parts of your body.

For most people, learning to cope with the diet on their own may be challenging. This is why education is so important. In terms of comprehensive health care, expecting people to handle the GFD alone is unacceptable, yet many people have been left in exactly that position. To make certain you are not one of them, be sure to check out the information in the following chapter. As you will learn, there are many ways to get help as you scale the GFD learning curve.

Living Well Without Gluten and Dairy, by Bridget Skjordahl

Most people want to know what it's like to live *gluten free*. All I can say is, once I began to see positive results (in my case, within a few weeks) I was hooked. Sure, there are inconveniences, but the benefits far outweigh them. My diet "evolved" over time as I moved through a series of peaks, experimented with different brands, felt fantastic, got bored, had a pizza, suffered prolonged consequences resulting in what seemed like a loss of two weeks of my life, expanded my knowledge, committed to wellness, and eventually felt wonderful.

I've had several incidents of "inadvertent" exposure, generally when eating in a restaurant or at a social function, but I get better at handling these situations all the time. In fact, my journey has been as much spiritual as physical. It has forced me to question and deal with all sorts of issues regarding self-esteem, shame, and deservedness. I had to question my definition of *polite*. I had to overcome my conditioning to not create a *fuss* in order to be able to ask for exactly what I need when ordering food in a restaurant. I had to get comfortable with calling attention to something I originally considered a weakness. I had to develop new strengths and learn to accept that which I could not change. In short, I had to master the art of treating myself with compassion.

I am still learning what my body will accept and what it will not, discovering what foods, brands of foods, etc., are GF and which are not. I continue to refine my practice of a gluten-free, dairy-free lifestyle, but at the same time I'm expanding my food choices by experimenting with new foods, new recipes, and new cooking techniques.

As I experiment I'm delighted to find I actually *prefer* many of the gluten-free and dairy-free alternatives such as rice noodles, GF waffles, almond, rice and coconut milks, olive and coconut oils, and buckwheat instead of oatmeal.

As my strength and stamina increase I'm more able to expend the effort to refine my diet even further. In turn, my health continues to improve. I never feel deprived, and I am blessed to have a number of allergen-free options available in my community and online. On occasion, I do get a little bored with the choices I've already discovered. That's when I know it's time to learn something new. I rely heavily on all the resources available to me, including brainstorming with my nutritionally savvy and celiac-aware doctor, seeking out new foods and ideas at my local natural food store, and searching the Internet.

Experimenting helps me stay on track, but now that I've experienced such profound improvements in the way I feel, I never lack the motivation to be 100 percent GF. There is no food temptation worthy of the hell I go through when something inadvertently slips by.

It has long been my belief that illness tends to serve two purposes—either a vehicle of transition to the hereafter and/or a teacher and catalyst for change, an initiation into the next level of awareness.

For me living gluten-free/dairy-free has been just such a catalyst, providing innumerable opportunities to heal old wounds and to support and serve a higher vision of myself. Intolerances may seem an odd place to look for answers to these sorts of problems, yet sometimes they offer a simple and most elegant solution. Eliminating a food or group of foods or substances from one's life requires no expensive prescription drugs, no ongoing monitoring by a doctor, no formal therapy sessions, no surgery, and no side effects—unless you consider wellness a side effect! In fact, taking this course of action is completely within your control—a self-managed solution to what ails you.

These days I feel like a different person, better than I have in more than 15 years. I hope that by sharing my story, someone else also may be guided in a direction that brings them relief. (See Bridget's main story in Chapters 6 and 9.)

Benefits Far Outweigh the GFD Effort

Remembering the severe illnesses caused by gluten for so many members of my family makes it easy for me to stick to this lifestyle. I wouldn't consider eating a crumb of the stuff—not even if a friend baked something special for me. On one occasion I completely forgot to ask our friends what they were planning for dinner. As the hostess pulled a casserole from the oven I asked in a panic what was in it. Unfortunately, the mushroom soup she'd used contained gluten. I was completely apologetic, but I *could not and would not* have any. I would have been happy with just the salad, but her husband ran to the freezer for a steak and broccoli and wouldn't hear of doing otherwise. I felt terrible, but I wouldn't indulge. Gluten is poison for me, for my family, and for millions of others who don't have a clue.

Yes, there is a learning curve in adopting a GF lifestyle, but when you consider the alternative of a downward-spiraling path to poor health, it's frankly not that tough. A little effort on your part can reap huge rewards if you put your best foot forward, and every day you're successful you'll be practicing preventive medicine.

GF foods are very plentiful, and the competition to improve their flavor and texture is *huge*. The following chapter contains many tips on successfully adopting and maintaining a GFD, and there are many informative websites to help you work through some of the challenges (see Appendix B). Gluten-free cookbooks can be found in bookstores or ordered online, and a wealth of recipes can be found on the web. Even eating out is becoming less of a challenge as more and more restaurants and chains offer gluten-free options.

Just as Tasty, by Gale Pearce, PA-C

Based on my experience, the changes associated with a GF lifestyle are not nearly as onerous as many people imagine, especially when the benefits are taken into account. When we're at home, my wife and I eat as well as we did prior to making the change, and our food is every bit as tasty. Friends and family have been extremely cooperative, and with a little care a nice meal in a restaurant is very possible without violating any gluten issues. We also are seeing more and more food manufacturers alter product content in order to claim gluten-free status in their advertising.

Eating Better from Scratch, by Melanie Krumrey

At first it was very challenging to come up with tasty, gluten-free foods, but when your child's health is in jeopardy you don't look back. I joined a support group in my town, collected recipes, read books, found cookbooks with gluten-free recipes, and forged ahead. Honestly, we eat better now—fruits, vegetables, fish, chicken, beef, eggs, nuts, rice, and potatoes. Things highly processed like cookies, prepared foods, and breadstuffs are usually off-limits because they contain wheat. Anything with a long list of ingredients is off-limits as well: canned soups, salad dressings, sauces, etc. And I've made us free from corn syrup, MSG, and food dye. I spend a lot of time in the kitchen, but I'm often thankful that some foods are no longer an option at our house. For baked goods I use alternative flours—mostly rice, tapioca, potato, bean, and nut. Almost everything we eat is made from scratch, but we do indulge in ready-made frozen waffles, pancakes, brown rice wraps, sandwich bread, and pizza crusts available from health-conscious chains such as Trader Joe's and Whole Foods.

A Minor Distraction, by Tom Graves

Initially, adopting a gluten-free diet was both stressful and extremely inconvenient. Two things helped. First, my wife is an excellent cook, with a great curiosity about food. Second, various segments of the food industry are responding to a growing public demand for gluten-free options. We've found cookbooks and flourmills, as well as packaged pastas and other commercially available foods that provide tasty and nutritious alternatives to foods once made exclusively from wheat. What started out as a major ordeal has become little more than a minor distraction.

So just how much gluten is *too* much? The proposed FDA guidelines (under review the last seven years) that a product can be labeled *gluten free* if it contains less than 20 ppm (parts per million) has just been accepted in August 2013. Twenty ppm is so small as to be practically nothing—in other words, another indication that you should *never* consume gluten. ***Even crumbs can send some people to bed or the hospital for weeks***. For others, the internal damage is so minimal they won't even know it's going on, but make no mistake, over time damage is still being done. In one case study, for example, intestinal healing was hampered in a patient who consumed "just a milligram of gluten every day for 2 years…"[2]

Gluten sensitivity is a most insidious malady, so it's important to remain ever diligent in following the diet. This is especially true for children, whose stature can be affected in their growing years. Some people may experience an intestinal backlash from "even microscopic amounts of gluten." For those who are strict about following a GF lifestyle, however, the damage will heal.[3]

Delia (not her real name) told me of her gut-wrenching experiences when she inadvertently ingested gluten. Unknowingly she had grabbed a regular loaf of bread at the health food store, threw it in the freezer, and didn't reach for a piece until a month later. After one slice of toast she was beset by diarrhea and vomiting; she thought she had food poisoning. A month or so later she had two pieces of bread and, again, was violently ill with vomiting and diarrhea, followed by great fatigue. She probably should have gone to the hospital, but she was careful to keep hydrated and after a few weeks she recovered. Then her wheels began to spin and she tracked down her problems to the frozen bread she had grabbed by mistake. Even crumbs make many folks ill.

My husband, Vahan, and I discovered and fell in love with Stephen Kishel's abstract metal sculpture (www.stephenkishel.com) when we attended a wedding near Hilton Head. Stephen, and now his wife, Gloria, understand the benefits of an *absolute* GF lifestyle, and it was awesome to have him so openly interested in my website. Not only that, as a computer guru he was full of ideas to get my message out there.

Path to Better Health, by Stephen Kishel

Dear Anne: Until I met you I really felt as if I was one of a very small minority with gluten intolerance; no one really understood my dietary restrictions. The truth is, while I had a pretty good idea what I could and could not eat, I was still making mistakes that were slowly eroding my health.

In speaking with you I learned things that have helped me significantly. Number one is that many people with gluten intolerance may also have issues with dairy products and don't know it. When I eat gluten I get stomach cramps and diarrhea within less than an hour. Although I had no such obvious symptoms from eating dairy, when you suggested I try going dairy-free for a week or two I felt it was worth a try.

I knew I needed to try ***something*** different. In the previous year I'd put on about 20 pounds and outgrown all my size 36 pants. Since I'm six foot six inches tall, the extra weight didn't worry me too much by itself. On the other hand,

I know weight gain is one of the warning signs of diabetes. Eye problems are another, and I'd had my share over the previous three or four years, everything from needing reading glasses to undergoing surgery for two separate instances of detached retina.

Another precursor of diabetes is frequent urination, also common in men my age experiencing prostate problems. I was getting up once or twice a night to use the bathroom and also craving sweet drinks, like orange juice, in the middle of the night. Needless to say I was beginning to worry about my health. Perhaps this is why I was so receptive to your suggestion. As they say, "When the student is ready, the teacher will appear."

My wife decided to join me in the experiment. After just a week she had less pain in her back and arms and more energy. She started doing stuff around the house she'd previously left to me, like washing the car, mowing the lawn, and sweeping the decks. She even began to get up in the morning and make coffee for me.

I was seeing some changes as well. Within a few days I was sleeping all night without the usual trip to the bathroom. My wife said I wasn't snoring as much, either. After three weeks we both noticed we were losing weight. Clothes that had been tight were now comfortable. Encouraged, we kept up the diet. After a time, even our skin became softer and smoother and, in my case, some of the skin tags and red spots on my body started to fade and shrink.

These days our snoring is gone, we sleep better, and we can wear our old clothes. In fact, my wife has abandoned her size 14 jeans in favor of her daughter's size 8. Not only is she feeling great, she's looking great, too. (Now I'm sometimes up at night for another reason!)

As I write this it has only been eight months since the two-week test that got us started on a path to better health, but what a difference it has made. Thank you for your encouragement and suggestions. Please keep up the good work and finish your book soon, for the benefit of those who are gluten sensitive and for the hundreds of thousands of others, not yet diagnosed, who don't even know they need it.

Sincerely, Stephen

Accidental Gluten Challenge, by Gale Pearce, PA-C

I'd been on a GFD for some time when I needed to be hospitalized for back surgery. During my hospital stay I had to fight continuously with the dietary department, since they had no standardized GFD alternative to a regular diet. Even the hospital dietician was of no assistance in maintaining my GFD status. This lack of support for hospital patients needs to be addressed both locally and as part of the national certification process for dieticians and nutritionists. Fortunately, I got out of the hospital without ingesting gluten, but it wasn't easy.

In two other instances I wasn't so lucky. One episode was the result of a restaurant meal made with soy sauce containing wheat. In that case, my CD demonstrated a cardiac element I hadn't been aware of previously (see the story of Gale's cardiac episode, *Don't Ever Go Off that GFD,* in Chapter 14).

The second episode added an unpleasant postscript to my back surgery. Upon discharge from the hospital (still gluten free) I was given an oral pain medication. Nine tablets and four days later I was deep in the throes of gluten ataxia. The package insert revealed that the medication contained pre-gelatinized starch. After switching to a generic-equivalent made with cornstarch, everything returned to normal within 48 hours.

Compliance

As early as 1989 researchers found that for those with CD, a normal, everyday diet containing gluten, or even a reduced-gluten diet (one where all gluten has not been eliminated), carried an increased risk for certain cancers, including those of the mouth, esophagus, and pharynx, as well as lymphomas. Conversely, a GF lifestyle played a role in *reducing* the chances of developing malignancies linked to CD. CD patients, therefore, are advised to pay strict attention to maintaining a GFD for the rest of their life. This same study reported that participants who followed a "GFD for five years" had a cancer risk similar to the general population.[4]

"Both benign and malignant complications of coeliac disease can be avoided by early diagnosis and a strict compliance with a gluten free diet."[5] The problem, of course, is that significant numbers of folks in the general population remain *undiagnosed* and thus are not following a GFD. What about their level of risk? Might they be the ones developing much of the cancer among the public?

Not sticking to a GFD 100 percent of the time is the main reason some CD patients either fail to respond as well as they might or, even worse, develop a resistant refractory sprue (see Chapter 13). To help people avoid noncompliance, it's essential they receive comprehensive counseling on how to implement and maintain their diet, along with continued monitoring and support.[6] Children diagnosed when young have the best record of compliance; adolescents and those who are mass screened experience the greatest number of lapses.[7]

Patients on a GFD may be screened by blood or stool testing to see how well they are adhering to the diet. However, one study found that the tTG: IgA antibodies, often used to check compliance in adults with CD, "are poor predictors of dietary transgressions. Their negativity is a falsely secure marker of strict diet compliance."[8] The title of one 2011 study—*Mean platelet volume could be a promising biomarker to monitor dietary compliance in celiac disease*—points to ongoing efforts to help those on a GFD lead a healthier life.[9]

Unfortunately, while an absolute GF lifestyle is essential to keep things from getting worse, it's not always a guarantee they will get better. One study involving children found that even though the kids on a GFD showed significant growth and greatly improved intestinal tissue, their villi did "not normalize even after [being on the diet for] 2–3 years."[10] Another study revealed that only 21 percent of participants had normal villi, whereas 69 percent had partial villous atrophy (VA) and 10 percent had total VA, even though all seemed to respond well to the diet.[11] Such reports, as sobering as they may be, also provide a strong incentive for early testing to nip gluten sensitivity in the bud—if possible before villi are damaged.

Regardless of where you are on the continuum of gluten sensitivity, following the tips in the next chapter will go a long way toward helping you embrace and maintain a gluten-free lifestyle.

Regardless of where you are on the continuum of gluten sensitivity, following the tips in the next chapter will go a long way toward helping you embrace and maintain a gluten-free lifestyle.

One Bite at a Time 20

Begin at the Beginning

If you are gluten sensitive, choosing to go gluten free could be one of the most important decisions you ever make. Adopting a gluten-free diet (GFD) is not easy, however, and achieving 100 percent compliance isn't something you master in a few days or even a few weeks. Here's how to begin.

1. Cut out the major toxic staples: regular bread, pasta, cookies, crackers, and so forth; then experiment with some of the tasty gluten-free (GF) substitutes.
2. Minimize junk food. Just because something is gluten free doesn't mean it's nutritious. Give your villi a chance to heal by eating a healthy diet. Fresh fruits and vegetables are better than cake and cookies—even gluten-free cake and cookies—every time.
3. Read through the hints and tips in this chapter and start to implement them one step at a time. Like anything worth mastering, going gluten free comes with a learning curve, but the slope is never too steep and, if you look around, you'll find many helping hands along the way.

I've been on this diet for nine years now, and I still goof up every now and then. When I do, it's a chance for me to learn something new and pass it on to my kids and grandkids. For example, the other day I was out to eat and forgot to ask how the scrambled eggs were prepared until after I'd eaten them. Oops! They were cooked on a flat grill also used for pancakes, which means my eggs more than likely came with a gluten "chaser." (Read on to learn more about cross contamination.)

Gluten-Proof Your Kitchen

Gluten is very sticky stuff, which makes contamination a huge issue. The littlest bit can keep the degenerative process going in your gut, even if you don't feel it. Fortunately, contamination can be avoided by taking a few simple precautions, all of which soon become second-nature. Hints for avoiding contamination in restaurants are included later in the chapter. Here's what to do in your own home:

1. Invest in new cutting boards, colander, strainer, rolling pin, wooden spoons, and toaster. A toaster oven may come in handy, and you can buy reusable toaster bags to use when traveling.
2. If folks in your household double-dip—spreading mustard, mayo, etc., on bread and then sticking the knife back in for more—gluten crumbs adhering to the knife can contaminate an entire container. So either keep your own jars of staples like peanut butter, jam, and mayo or adopt the one-dip rule: Always use a clean knife, no double-dipping. Label your own jars.
3. Be very careful with outdoor grills, flat grills, and pans. I maintain a gluten-free grill and don't let any strangely marinated foods on it. If you're toasting regular buns for company, do so in the oven or wrap in foil to heat on the grill.
4. When making cupcakes use paper liners or dedicated pans.
5. If your kitchen contains foods with and without gluten, think about how you store things like crackers, cereal, and cookies so gluten crumbs don't accidentally fall into GF foods. One way to keep gluten-free foods separate is to place them on a higher shelf, in a separate cabinet, and/or in plastic containers.
6. Keep your mixer ultra clean or use two. Flour dust in the air may take a few hours to settle and can land on anything; it also can be inhaled.
7. Some people have a dedicated bread machine. Since making gluten-free bread takes fewer steps, however, others find it just as easy to use a mixer and bake it in the oven.

It took me an entire year to clean out my pantry shelves, but I didn't use anything if I wasn't sure it was GF. If you maintain a dual GF/non-GF kitchen, stickers on the outside of food containers help everyone—especially kids—quickly identify products that are gluten free. To avoid the hassle, some entire families go gluten free when they're eating at home. It's just easier.

Watch for Other Sources of Contamination

When looking for sources of contamination, think outside the box. Pay attention to lipstick, toothpaste or lotions (hands touch food)...in other words, anything that goes in or on the mouth. Even kissing someone who's just had a bite of pizza or who is wearing lipstick containing gluten is a cross-contamination issue. Pharmaceuticals—over-the-counter or prescription—can also be a problem. Some are labeled GF but others contain gluten and, at least for now, manufacturers are not required to label drugs with allergen information. A list of drugs without gluten can be found at www.glutenfreedrugs.com. When in doubt, check with your pharmacist; if needed, some medications can be especially prepared for you.

Art Supplies—Art supplies can be a source of contamination for anyone who is gluten sensitive, but especially for children since little fingers often go into mouths. For a list of gluten-free art supplies, check www.adventuresofaglutenfreemom.com

Know the Enemy: What's Allowed and What's Not?

There's no getting around it: On a gluten-free diet there's a lot of stuff you can't eat. There's also a lot of stuff you can. So before getting started on specific do's and don'ts, let me emphasize how many gluten-free substitutes are now on the market. With focus and creativity you can enjoy a varied, delicious diet without compromising your health. In other words, you can have your cake (albeit, gluten-free cake) and eat it too, but you "gotta follow the rules."

To begin with the obvious: You *cannot* consume wheat, barley, rye, or oats (a toxic quartet sometimes referred to as WBRO). You also can't eat bulgur, durum, einkorn, farro, kamut, semolina, spelt, or triticale. And yes, in their natural form oats are gluten free, but in the U.S. almost all are contaminated with wheat unless they come from a specially grown, GF source. Many shopkeepers also may tell you spelt is okay—I've run into this more than once—but it is not.

You *can* use a wide variety of other flours: amaranth, bean flour, buckwheat, flax, millet, montina (Indian rice grass), potato, quinoa, rice, sorghum, tapioca, and teff. However, even then it's important to buy only certified-gluten-free grains and flours. Those that don't contain gluten naturally can be contaminated from a nearby wheat field while growing or a nearby source in your grocery. Avoid buying anything from bins. Contamination from other scoops or dust from flour in the bin next to that gluten-free rice you're putting in a bag may travel home with you as an unwanted guest.

The Labels—Always read labels! If a product contains wheat, new rules from the FDA (Food and Drug Administration) require that it says so on the list of ingredients. "Contains wheat" lets you know right away this product is not for you. For items without this cautionary statement, you still must scrutinize the ingredients list for rye, barley (malt), spelt, kamut, and/or other ingredients not allowed on a GFD.

Companies are constantly changing ingredients, so for items not marked gluten free you must read the label every time you buy a food product. If you run across an ingredient you aren't sure about, call the company. You might even suggest they try to find a replacement for a gluten-containing ingredient. For an extensive list of safe (and unsafe) ingredients, see www.celiac.com. Additional resources are listed in Appendix B.

The Temptations—If you're looking at a box of cereal, cake mix, brownie mix, etc., or you're in the bakery staring at rows of fresh-baked goodies, it's a pretty sure bet they all contain gluten. So be certain not to eat *anything* from the following list unless it's clearly labeled gluten free.

- Breading, coating, and crumb mixtures.
- Cakes, cookies, crackers, bread, muffins, bagels, scones, biscuits, etc.
- Communion wafers (an acceptable version may be available).
- Croutons.
- Gravy and sauces.
- Pasta and noodles.
- Stuffing.
- Thickeners.

The Intruders—In a world where almost every packaged food contains a long list of ingredients, many of which are hard enough to pronounce let alone identify, it shouldn't be a surprise to find gluten lurking far and wide. When buying one of the products listed below, be sure to check the label before plopping the box or can into your shopping cart.

- Baking powder.
- Broth, bouillon, canned or boxed soups, and soup bases.
- Cereals: rice and corn cereals—yes, they may be "wheat-free" but they often contain barley malt. (To be on the safe side, always buy cereals labeled gluten free.)
- Cold-cuts and prepackaged, processed meats (hot dogs, sausage, patties, veggie burgers).
- Imitation bacon and imitation seafood.
- Marinades, salad dressings, soy sauce, and other such sauces.
- Miso, seitan, and tofu.
- Nut mixes, rice mixes, or anything with a seasoning or flavoring packet.
- Self-basting poultry, marinated meats, or meat injected with broth (poultry and pork). And make sure hamburger is *pure* meat. Extenders often contain gluten, not to mention other controversial additives you might well want to do without.
- Soba noodles (made primarily from buckwheat but can contain wheat flour).

The Stealth Candidates—Until I had to think about it, it never occurred to me that gluten might be in some of these products, but these days I question, question, question. To make sure gluten isn't creeping into your diet, read labels, ask questions, even check with the manufacturer if need be. But ***when in doubt, leave it out!***

Unless "gluten free" is printed on the label, here are some of the items I've learned to watch out for.

- Artificial colors and flavors and natural colors and flavors, when manufactured in the U.S. or Canada, are generally safe; if made elsewhere they may contain gluten.
- Some brands of brown rice syrup, used as a sweetener, are made from barley. (The Lundgren brand is gluten free.)
- Buckwheat is naturally GF, but products made with it may have added flour.
- Caramel color is GF if made in the U.S. but can contain barley if imported.

- Hard cheese is GF. Some processed cheeses and non-cheese foods are not.
- Sour cream, spreads, and dips may or may not contain gluten.
- Dextrin, an ingredient in many packaged foods and in some dietary supplements and medications, is usually made from corn, but it can be made from wheat. Check labels carefully.
- Frozen French fries and instant potatoes may have added flour or seasonings. And anything frozen with a sauce is likely to contain gluten in one form or another.
- Pure, unadulterated herbs and spices are fine; seasoning mixtures may contain gluten. If individual ingredients aren't listed for a particular spice combo, consider buying tins or jars of your favorite individual spices and creating your own seasoning blends.
- Hydrolyzed vegetable protein, despite its name, may not actually be "vegetable" at all (unless you think of wheat as a vegetable). The source should be listed on the package. If it's not, beware.
- Maltodextrin, another common additive, is usually made from corn, but never assume anything without reading the label.
- Malt or malt flavoring is normally derived from barley, in which case the product containing it is not gluten free. If the flavoring is derived from corn, it's okay.
- Modified food starch is also made from corn in most cases, but again, be sure to verify.
- MSG (monosodium glutamate) made in the U.S. is gluten free; if it's made elsewhere it may contain gluten.
- Most soy sauce or soy sauce solids contain wheat. Two delicious, gluten-free alternatives are San-J Organic Wheat Free Tamari Soy Sauce and Bragg Liquid Aminos.
- Rice crackers are usually GF, though some can contain other flours or soy sauce.
- Malt vinegar is not gluten free; distilled vinegars are—the gluten protein does not survive the distillation process, though some very sensitive folks may still have an issue with distilled vinegars if made from a gluten source.

- In the U.S. and Canada wheat starch is not considered gluten free. The celiac community in Europe is less stringent and permits it; personally, I wouldn't use it.

Drink Me?—A few generations ago beverage choices were pretty simple: coffee, tea, milk, water, juices, and substances containing alcohol. Today grocery shelves and vending machines are filled with an incredible array of ways to quench one's thirst, all for a price, of course. To make certain you pay only at the cash register and not for days or weeks thereafter, it's important to pay attention to the following:

- Flavored anything may contain gluten. Keep an eye out for malt or barley.
- Plain, pasteurized milk from cows (whole, 2% or skim) is gluten free; flavored milk may contain gluten. Some soy, nut, and rice milks may contain barley.
- "Real" beer is definitely off limits, but there are a number of very good gluten-free beers on the market.
- Wine is fine, but wine coolers, flavored spirits, iced teas, and some sodas may contain gluten. Distilled alcohol (bourbon, Scotch, rum, etc.) without additives or flavorings, is supposed to be fine, but some very sensitive people have a problem.
- Pure juice is fine. Check the label of any juice drinks (though in most cases they're loaded with sugar rather than gluten).

Meat and Wheat—Plain meat—beef, chicken, pork, etc., is gluten free. Meat or cold cuts labeled as having "added broth" or "natural flavors" may well contain gluten. The only way to know for sure is to call the company that makes them. The USDA (United States Department of Agriculture), which governs the sale of meat products, has different rules than the FDA. Under FDA regulations, manufacturers must list whether a food contains one of the top eight allergens (the ingredients most likely to trigger food allergies). These include: eggs, fish and shellfish, milk, peanuts, tree nuts (almonds, cashews, walnuts, etc.), soy, and wheat. The USDA does not have this requirement. If a meat product contains "added broth" or "spices," there's no way to tell from the label what's in the broth or spice mixture.

Many cold cuts are naturally gluten free. To avoid cross contamination with those that are not, call the store the night before to place your order. Make it clear that you are gluten sensitive and ask that the meat department cut your order first thing the following morning on a clean blade. Many people ask to have the first two slices of their order discarded, with the thought that any gluten left on the blade will stick to the first slices cut. If your market is not familiar with the requirements of a GFD, look upon this as a chance to educate them. And, of course, always be sure to give them a big thank-you.

So What Can I Eat?

If by now your head is spinning from the "do-nots," try not to worry. To begin with, foods containing gluten are not a large part of a healthy diet for *anyone*. Fresh fruits and vegetables, meat (with the caveats listed above), eggs, and dairy products offer rich and varied sources of culinary delight. For foods that do contain gluten—breads, pasta, cakes and cookies, pizza crust, and more—there are literally thousands of gluten-free substitutes, with more popping up all the time. Gluten sensitivity is not going away. As more people are diagnosed and more companies adapt to capture this share of the market, the taste and texture of GF foods will only improve.

Dining Out

Okay, let's face it, your days of popping into any fast-food place, grabbing a burger and fries, and paying zero attention to what might be in them are gone forever. Bow your head in mourning. Take 30 seconds to feel sorry for yourself. Now hear the good news: With a little forethought you can enjoy delicious restaurant meals without compromising the GFD.

Most restaurants are willing to bend over backwards to accommodate their clientele; they want you to show up in the first place and they want you to come back. Before trying out a new restaurant, call early in the day when the chef or manager is apt to be less busy and ask if he or she is familiar with the requirements of a gluten-free diet. Does the restaurant have a GF menu? Is the wait staff familiar with gluten-free substitutions and the diet in general? Regardless of the answers you receive, always be pleasant and offer a big thank you.

Some restaurants publish a list of ingredients for all their dishes. Especially in establishments without a gluten-free menu, this information can be invaluable in making wise choices. (And when the list is posted on the web, you can even check it out before you go.)

If you haven't determined before arrival whether or not the restaurant has a gluten-free menu, ask about one even before you're seated. Even in restaurants that don't, the wait staff is almost always accommodating and willing to learn, but you need to mention—on every visit—that you are sensitive or intolerant to gluten. A busy waiter cannot remember everyone's food issues, and you are dependent on him or her to clearly notify the chef of your preferences. In appreciation for this extra consideration, don't forget to leave a nice tip at the end of the meal.

I used to think when a member of the wait staff asked, "How sensitive are you?" it meant he or she didn't understand the issue. Recently, I got a different slant. In talking with the manager of one particular restaurant that takes food allergies very seriously, I learned that when the wait staff asks "How sensitive are you?" they are seriously looking out for your health. The reason: a very large percent of folks who claim to be gluten sensitive are not that careful. Such patrons often wind up nibbling on bread or tasting someone's gluten-laden dessert, which sends mixed messages to restaurant personnel.

The bottom line, of course, is that someone who is gluten sensitive should have *no* gluten—it's not a matter of degree. If some restaurant workers don't know this, it's not surprising, since many gluten-sensitive *patients* don't know this. Even if they refrain from nibbling on the rolls, these folks indulge in French fries cooked in the same oil as all the breaded and battered stuff without a clue that their fries may be coated with a gluten "breading."

Occasionally the wait staff goes too far in the other direction, assuming that corn, potato, and/or rice also are off-limits. However, unless you are specifically sensitive to these foods, they're fine as long as they aren't cooked or flavored with gluten.

The following tips are designed to make your dining-out experiences both pleasurable and positive.

Alert: Make sure the restaurant has a method in place to alert the chef to a GF order.

Appetizers and the universal breadbasket: Before the waiter brings the pre-meal breadbasket I love to ask, "Do you have any gluten-free bread?" I know full well most restaurants don't, but if they hear the question enough, perhaps one day they will. Sometimes a fine restaurant will serve crudités and dip in lieu of bread, a very nice touch and always very much appreciated. You might ask your favorite restaurant if they'd consider it. If you order an appetizer, the universal rules of contamination still apply. In other words, eating the top but leaving the cracker doesn't cut it.

Bagels and toast: If you do run across a restaurant that serves gluten-free breads but doesn't have a dedicated toaster, you need to request that your bread be toasted in an oven, preferably on a clean pan or a sheet of foil.

Breakfast: If eggs are scrambled on a grill there is a huge chance of contamination. The same goes for bacon, hash browns, and even GF pancakes. Ask nicely for your order to be pan-cooked. Also make sure your scrambled eggs are just eggs. Some restaurants add pancake batter. Who would have thought!

Chicken wings: This ubiquitous snack food presents two potential problems: the coating added for flavor and method in which the wings are cooked. Even when the coating is gluten free, if the fryer used for wings is also used for everything else in the restaurant, you'll need to pass.

Corn chips: Many Mexican restaurants serve corn chips that are deep fried with everything else. If you're visiting a restaurant for the first time and you're not sure, take your own corn chips so you won't have to do without. (Assuming the salsa is gluten free, make sure you put some on your plate or in a separate dish—no sharing a common bowl with dining companions who are dipping corn chips with gluten.) If you enjoy your meal and would recommend the spot to others, you might suggest to the manager that the restaurant offer GF corn chips in the future since it would be good for business.

French fries: Fries present similar problems. If they are prepared in the same friolater as breaded or battered food there will be contamination. To be gluten free, fries must be potatoes only—no spice- or flour-mixture coating unless it's a GF coating—and they must be cooked in a dedicated fryer used only for foods that are gluten free.

Gravy: Gravy thickened with corn flour is okay; gravy thickened with wheat flour is not. (And scraping the gravy off is unacceptable.) A reduction sauce is usually fine, but double check to make sure it has no flour. As odd as it sounds, even au jus sometimes has added flour.

Meatballs and coatings: Meatballs usually contain breadcrumbs. Make sure the ones you order are safe before adding them, or the sauce they were cooked in, to your gluten-free pasta. The meat in recipes such as chicken marsala may be drenched in flour before it's sautéed. Experienced chefs can sauté without wheat flour, perhaps using cornmeal or a gluten-free flour mixture to create the same tasty dish.

Salads: Sometimes croutons are not mentioned on the menu as a salad ingredient, and occasionally I forget to specifically request no croutons. When that happens I have no qualms about asking for another salad (not just one with the croutons picked off), especially if I've previously alerted the waitress to the fact that I'm gluten sensitive. The way I look at it, it's a learning experience for both of us.

Sandwiches: As tempting as it may be, it does you no good to eat the insides of a sandwich and leave the bread.

Soups: Many soups are made from a base containing gluten. Fine restaurants, which often make their broth from scratch, are more apt to be up on the GFD. I never order soup unless I'm in a very fine restaurant and even then I always ask about the ingredients.

Vegetables: Vegetables should be safe, but I've heard of restaurants that actually warm their vegetables in pasta water. Again, it pays to ask.

The tips above will help most of the time, but despite the best intentions of all involved there will be times when you are inadvertently "glutened." This has happened to me several times. On one occasion I downed nearly an entire dinner of supposedly-gluten-free eggplant parmesan before the chef came running out and apologized profusely; he had served the wrong meal. The following day I was tired and my legs felt heavy. By day four the muscles in my legs, pelvis, and lower back had seized up to the point I was walking in a bent-over position. The discomfort lasted three to four days and gluten was the only explanation for what had happened. Nothing had changed except my diet.

Another time I ordered a gluten-free pizza. Wow! The first bite was delicious, the second bite was fabulous, and the third bite was just too good to be true. Sure enough, another mix-up in the kitchen.

The Gluten Intolerance Group (GIG) has developed a Gluten-Free Food Service Training & Management Certification (GFFS) to help meet strict gluten-free standards for participating food service establishments to "provide a high level of consumer confidence."[1] If you'd like to help your favorite eateries and food services to get up to speed on the GFD, you can find out more about GFFS at www.gluten.net.

When invited to a friend's house or a party, always offer to bring a gluten-free dish. Really good friends will want to accommodate you, so feel comfortable in quizzing them about "What's for dinner?" and educating them a bit on the realities of gluten-free ingredients and food preparation. When your children are invited to a party or play-date, always provide snacks and goodies so they don't feel left out. Also offer the hostess a new, small cutting board she can keep gluten free for cutting fruit, cheese, etc., on this and future play dates. If the hostess seems interested, you also might lend her a copy of this book so she can become familiar with the GFD and how very important it is to keep your child safe from gluten.

When traveling, make sure neither you nor gluten-sensitive family members are caught short. I almost always bring nuts, dried or fresh fruit and/or gluten-free crackers or cereal with me. I can live without bread.

Traveling?

Search online for “gluten-free restaurant cards” for the phrases you need—in a variety of languages—to keep you safe from foods containing gluten. Check with the airlines to see if they have an option for gluten-free meals. And be sure to check out Bob and Ruth’s Gluten-free Dining and Travel Club at http://www.bobandruths.com/.

It’s All Relative

In a perfect world we could eat anything we wanted, any time we wanted, as much as we wanted. In a perfect world we wouldn’t have cancer or earthquakes or homelessness, either. So, yes, there are times when you may feel deprived, resentful, sad, or a hundred other emotions because you can’t eat gluten. On the other hand, unlike many medical conditions, “what ails you” can get better just by changing what you eat. Remembering this fact—especially when smells emanating from the bakeshop in the grocery are driving you nuts—can go a long way toward achieving a sense of perspective.

The most important thing you can do is to take it one step at a time. Believe me, I didn’t do this overnight, but if I can do it, anyone can do it. As time goes on and you learn about the products, processes, and intricacies of cooking at home and dining out, the pieces will start to fit together. Eventually, living gluten free will become second nature.

Here is a list of resources that can help:

1. **National, state, and local support group**s (see the list in Appendix B). A good place to begin is to join a local support group. You’ll meet people already familiar with the diet who are eager to help you; in time you may want to help others.
2. **Periodicals** such as *Gluten-Free Living* (www.glutenfreeliving.com) and *Living Without* (www.livingwithout.com), both of which are excellent.

3. ***The Gluten-Free Bible*** by Jax Peters Lowell and ***The G-Free Diet*** by Elizabeth Hasselbeck. Both are excellent resources for those following a GFD. Many other books on gluten are listed in Appendix B.

4. ***The CSA Gluten-Free Product Listing***, published by the Celiac Sprue Association. This publication lists numerous GF food products along with safe and unsafe additives, 800 numbers for many companies, and more. You can order it at celiacs@csaceliacs.org or by calling 1-877-CSA-4-CSA. I highly recommend it.

5. ***The Essential Gluten-Free Grocery Guide***, published by Triumph Dining. Now in its fifth edition, this book is a huge asset when you're first getting started. It's even available in downloadable format for those who prefer electronic readers.

6. **Health-conscious grocery stores.** Trader Joe's and Whole Foods publish lists of their gluten-free products. Local co-ops may have similar lists; some even have an in-store nutritionist familiar with GFD requirements who can familiarize you with GF products in the store and offer tips for food preparation at home. What does your local market provide? If you ask for a list of GF products and they don't yet have one, you may be just the catalyst they need to accommodate this growing slice of the market.

7. **Recipes.** Recipes for delicious gluten-free dishes can be found on an avalanche of websites. Numerous gluten-free cookbooks also provide instruction and inspiration. If your local library doesn't have several from which to choose, request that they buy some.

8. **Handheld devices/smartphones**. For many people, smartphones have become like a fifth appendage. Now there are apps designed specifically to make gluten-free grocery shopping and dining out even easier.

9. **The Internet**. The web is invaluable for finding information on almost any topic, but there is also plenty of misinformation out there. To be certain the facts you gather about gluten sensitivity come from reputable sources, stick with the sites of national support groups and university research centers, as well as reputable celiac-related sites such as www.theglutenfile.com, www.celiac.com, www.glutensensitivity.net, www.toxicstaple.com, and www.x-gluten.com.

10. **Travel**. Glutenfreepassport.com is full of ideas to remain GF while traveling or dining out. It also has translations you can print regarding your gluten intolerance.

Twenty years ago there was almost no support by the food industry for a GF lifestyle. Even as late as 2000 there were few gluten-free products on the market, and a good many of them tasted pretty bad. "Cardboard" comes to mind. Today things are much different. When companies like King Arthur, General Mills, and Anheuser-Busch are introducing gluten-free alternatives, you know it's an idea whose time has come.

The fact that most of us have difficulty dealing with change was provocatively illustrated in Spencer Johnson's 1998 bestseller, *Who Moved My Cheese? An Amazing Way to Deal with Change in Your Work and in Your Life*. As you learn to deal with your own version of this question—"Who re-moved my gluten?"—consider yourself fortunate that you know both the cause of and the cure for your problem. Honor the past by bidding gluten a proper farewell over a last meal of wheat pasta; then turn, face forward, and take the first step on your new path toward wellness.

21 Dairy, Dairy, Quite Contrary

After becoming gluten-free (GF) I felt a heck of a lot better, but after two to three years I realized something else was also attacking my body. When I rode or sat for more than an hour it hurt to unbend to get moving again, and on occasion I had mild lower-back discomfort. I was beginning to understand why some people waddled from side to side when they walked. I had read that dairy could act just like gluten, so I decided to try eliminating dairy from my diet as well. Voila! My stiffness and discomfort disappeared, along with a bothersome postnasal drip, stuffiness, and the need to constantly clear my throat and breathe through my mouth at night. I've felt much better ever since, but I do miss cheese. It had been a huge part of my life for years.

Arthritis Pain 98 Percent Gone, by Angela T., APRN, CRNA

After finding a gluten-free, casein-free bread and reading the story of the woman who created it, I was inspired to remove dairy from my diet. She mentioned that eliminating dairy and gluten not only helped her gastrointestinal tract, it reduced her "arthritic" pain. I'd been having terrible pain in my lower back and pelvis, but after I eliminated dairy for just over a week the pain almost disappeared. I have been dairy-free for eight months now and my joint pain is 98 percent gone. [Angela also follows a gluten-free diet (GFD). Read her autism story in Chapter 9.]

Diana and I met at a gluten-related conference. I was traveling alone and she and her mate were very friendly to me. Diana is intolerant to many proteins, but her life is good unless she accidentally ingests one of them.

Psoriasis, by Diana Sheridan

During a three-hour initial appointment, my new physician said he was sure I was gluten intolerant. I had already had a blood test for wheat intolerance with negative results. Unconvinced, this doctor recommended Dr. Fine's stool test and connected me with EnteroLab (www.EnteroLab.com).

From the age of 20 I'd also suffered with psoriasis. A couple of years ago I learned that dairy was a major contributor to psoriasis, and as soon as I stopped eating it, my psoriasis disappeared.

In addition to gluten and dairy, I'm intolerant to soy and eggs. Just give me fresh fruits and vegetables, rice, quinoa, legumes, and animal proteins, along with nuts and seeds, and I'm fine.

Coleen confided that she was very intolerant to dairy. If she consumes any accidentally, she suffers from both intestinal problems and myalgia. She also follows a GF lifestyle, though not always 100 percent.

Twenty Minutes to Misery, by Coleen

About 12 years ago I started working at a health food store, in charge of the produce and prepared food department. As part of our job we had to participate in at least one cleanse class given by a nutritionist.

I had never done such a thing and decided to get a head start. I began three weeks beforehand and by the time the "real" class came along I was able to pass with flying colors. However, I'd lost way too much weight so I slowly began to introduce some of my favorite foods. This is when I found out that wheat, dairy, and sugar were no longer my friends. I would get bloated, constipated, and irritable—all within 20 minutes after eating. Looking back, I realize I'd had these intolerances all along but had never paid attention to the signals my body was giving me.

Working at the health food store and having a passion for whole foods helped me adopt a different way of cooking and a new lifestyle. I'm not a fanatic but I have a total awareness and am constantly learning more. Sometimes even wheat-free/gluten-free products irritate me. I think it's the whole processed-food thing.

Many people who know they are lactose intolerant have no idea they may be gluten intolerant as well. Conversely, because the lactase enzyme is produced in the tips of the villi, a high number of those whose villi are damaged from gluten may also be sensitive to dairy. In a study done in 1986, beta-lactoglobulin (whey protein), casein, and ovalbumin (egg-white protein) antibodies were found in 36 to 48 percent of CD patients.[1] To be on the safe side, some health care professionals suggest newly diagnosed CD patients eliminate dairy for six months to a year to give the gut time to heal.

Casein, a dairy protein, can mimic gluten in its detrimental effects, so it's not surprising dairy intolerance affects many of the storytellers in this book. Arthritis/rheumatism issues, skin problems, pain, mucus, and intestinal symptoms can clear up when dairy products are removed from the diet.

If you are having health issues that persist after adopting an absolute GF lifestyle, you might consider being tested for dairy and/or other intolerances (egg, soy, yeast, and more). Also check the section on *Refractory Celiac Disease* in Chapter 13. Some folks who have been diagnosed as *allergic* to dairy (or wheat, eggs, etc.) may actually have an *intolerance.* The testing they had just didn't go far enough to find out. And some folks use the word allergic when they mean intolerance. Tests for intolerances measure IgG and/or IgA antibody levels. Tests for allergies typically measure IgE antibody levels. To learn more about antibodies, antigliadin antibodies, and allergies, you may want to peruse Internet sites such as MedlinePlus (www.nlm.nih.gov/medlineplus/healthtopics.html) from the National Institutes of Health.

Almost three decades ago a study from London reported that proteins found in chicken, cow's milk, fish, rice, and soya—in addition to gluten—could "induce gastrointestinal symptoms and/or small intestinal mucosal damage." This same study reported the case of "a child with unequivocal gluten and cow's milk protein-induced enteropathy."[2]

"In the complete absence of symptoms cow's milk protein can … continue to cause damage to the small intestinal mucosa… ."[3] In other words, ***dairy can act much like gluten, causing villous atrophy.***

Here's a summary of some significant studies from 2007 to 2010 on the hazards of consuming dairy:

- A 2010 Italian study suggested that doctors might be suspicious of a cow's milk allergy in children who exhibit some of the following sudden symptoms: acute asthma with severe respiratory distress, acute urticaria/angioedema (hives/edema), anaphylaxis, dry cough, laryngeal edema, rhinitis, vomiting, and wheezing. Delayed reactions may include atopical dermatitis, blood in the stool, colic, constipation, chronic diarrhea, enterocolitis syndrome, gastroesophageal reflux disease, iron deficiency anemia, poor growth (food refusal), protein-losing enteropathy (inability of the body to absorb protein) with hypoalbuminemia (low levels of albumin in blood serum), and chronic vomiting.[4] Many of these symptoms sound like clones for symptoms of gluten sensitivity.

- A 2010 Swedish study revealed that nearly half the study participants with IgA nephropathy, a kidney disease, revealed a "rectal mucosal sensitivity to soy or CM [cow's milk]" and concluded that an immune reaction to these antigens may be linked to the development of IgA nephropathy in some patients.[5]
- Restricting gliadin and cow's milk antigens, reported a 2009 study from Serbia, may prevent "celiac disease and some premalignant conditions, like monoclonal gammopathy of undetermined significance (MGUS)," which disappeared when gluten and casein were removed from the diet.[6] MGUS, although a benign condition for most people, can sometimes develop into multiple myeloma, a type of cancer that attacks the body's plasma cells.
- Another study hypothesized that some youngsters with chronic constipation react positively when dairy is eliminated from their diet.[7]
- In addition to the gastrointestinal symptoms of CD, a large percentage of patients with primary Sjögren's syndrome have a sensitivity to cow's milk exhibited by irritable-bowel-syndrome-like symptoms.[8]
- Nearly half the CD patients in one study showed a "mucosal inflammatory response similar to that elicited by gluten." The casein protein appeared to be the culprit.[9]
- A young boy with eosinophilic esophagitis (brought on by an intolerance to cow's milk) and CD also suffered from asthma, eczema, and type 1 diabetes. Shortly after following a six-food elimination diet excluding gluten and milk protein along with eggs, peanuts, seafood, and soy, his stomach pain subsided, he no longer needed the puffers for reactive airway, and his eczema healed. He gained weight, his need for insulin decreased, and eventually his esophagus returned to normal.[10]

As far back as 1975, a study of infants with atopic eczema, diarrhea, failure to thrive, recurrent respiratory infections, and vomiting "concluded that the malabsorption syndrome with cow's milk intolerance is a clear-cut clinical entity" and is very similar to other malabsorption syndromes.[11] One study from 1989, as the title suggests, found an *association of serum IgA antibodies to milk antigens with severe atherosclerosis.*[12] Another reported that between 30 and 60 percent of newly identified CD patients exhibit lactose intolerance.[13]

Much more research is needed to identify the effects of dairy and other proteins on immunological reactions, damaged villi, and the resulting malabsorption of vital nutrients. In the meantime, you can read more in Chapter 7 about the connections between the dairy protein and various intestinal problems, as well as under *Allergies and Asthma* in Chapter 8 and *Lung Problems* in Chapter 14. And remember, just like gluten, if you are intolerant to dairy you should avoid the offending protein.

22 Motivation Breeds Creation

ANNA HAD BEEN dealing with a special diet for years, but once she was diagnosed with dermatitis herpetiformis and a biopsy confirmed celiac disease, her life took on a new direction. The creator of Breads from Anna® (www.breadsfromanna.com), she produces baking mixes that are gluten, soy, nut, and rice free. Several are free from corn, dairy, and yeast as well. All mixes from this company have been developed to be as nutritious as possible, as well as GMO free. Anna also travels widely teaching cooking classes.

Meeting the Challenge, by Anna Sobaski

For many years I suffered from stifling fatigue, among numerous other feelings of discomfort, but it wasn't until a rash appeared on my elbows that my dermatologist diagnosed me with dermatitis herpetiformis (DH) and exclaimed, "No more gluten." Almost the next thing out of his mouth was a prediction that I wouldn't be able to stick to a gluten-free diet. Having lived with type 1 diabetes, and the culinary discipline this entails, for the previous 26 years, his lack of confidence did not sit well with me. *Don't tell me I can't do this diet!* I thought.

I accepted the challenge, but it didn't take long to realize I was facing a very big loss. Food, eating out, and feeding my family and friends was a much bigger part of my life than I had realized. After trying to make the best of it, which included stripping my kitchen of all foods containing gluten, eating out rarely, and watching invitations to eat with family and friends dwindle, I decided the situation required an all-out change.

So I signed up for cooking school, a very special school with a very special philosophy: Food and health are connected, and a special diet does not mean deprivation. This decision put me on the path to a new career: creating an array of delicious, gluten-free foods traditionally made with wheat flour. I am currently working on a cookbook, and my goal is to develop delectable, gluten-free mixes so others who are gluten sensitive can prepare a wide range of delicious baked goods with minimum effort.

I met Lee in 2006 at the 12th International Celiac Disease Symposium in New York City. A man of creative genius with non-gluten flours, he readily agreed to share his story. Anyone diagnosed with gluten sensitivity is ecstatic to discover his mouthwatering, gluten-free products at Whole Foods markets around the country.

Gluten-Free Lee: Lee Tobin's Story as told by his wife, Agnieszka Stachura

Serendipity: (1) an aptitude for making advantageous discoveries accidentally; (2) being in the right place at the right time.

It started with a rash. In the spring of 1996 I developed a painful, blistering, itchy rash on my elbows and knees. Maybe it was poison ivy. Maybe, as my girlfriend suggested, I'd gotten it from scrubbing the bathroom floor too vigorously. Whatever the cause, it wouldn't clear up on its own and it was too maddening to ignore. After weeks of discomfort, my family doctor referred me to a dermatologist. I was lucky. One good hunch and a small skin biopsy later and her initial diagnosis was confirmed.

"Dermatitis herpetiformis!" my future mother-in-law gasped when we called her; "This is a form of celiac disease, a reaction to the presence of gluten in digestive tract." (Okay, she's a doctor who trained in Eastern Europe, so it made sense that she knew what it was. I'd never heard of it.) Her prescription was simple: "You cannot eat wheat." More specifically, she explained, I could no longer eat wheat, rye, barley or, given the likelihood of cross contamination, oats.

The path forward seemed simple enough. After all, I was a cook. I worked for Whole Foods Market, champion of fresh, minimally processed foods. Healthy eating has always been important to me, so I had no junk-food habit to break. How difficult could it be to live without four basic grains?

The optimism lasted about a week. Conscious efforts to convince myself that this new diet would not be a hardship could not silence the misgivings. I was at work when, surrounded by the familiar fragrance of warm cake and loaves of rising bread, the enormity of my loss finally struck. *No more cereal. No more bread. No morning oatmeal. No Thanksgiving stuffing. No birthday cake.* I stumbled to my manager's office and I cried.

One month and 12 bags of rice cakes later, I began experimenting with recipes and offering the imperfect results to local celiac support group members. Their encouragement and support convinced me to ask Whole Foods for permission to begin a small, in-store gluten-free baking program. Soon (after thorough scrub-downs), the Chapel Hill Whole Foods Bakery was gluten free one afternoon a week.

My product list quickly grew from five to twenty-seven items. We started fielding requests for mail order and out-of-state shipping. Could we ship to Alaska, to Denver, to Mobile? What about zucchini bread? Wedding cake? Donuts? The gluten-free baking program was outgrowing the store. What we needed was a bakehouse, a centralized, dedicated space in which gluten-free products could be prepared, baked, and frozen, then shipped to Whole Foods stores around the country.

Once again, serendipity kicked in. I presented a business plan; it was accepted. The Whole Foods Market Gluten-Free Bakehouse was dedicated in Morrisville, North Carolina, on October 4, 2004, and my gluten-free products now ship to Whole Foods stores as far away as Vancouver.

When I started my gluten-free life, the choices for fresh baked goods were limited. My first gluten-free experiments were simply an attempt to feed myself. Today, dedicated bakehouses, storefront bakeries, and a growing number of celiac-aware restaurants make life with celiac easier every day. A few weeks ago I propped my rash-free elbows on the kitchen table and started in on a bowl of certified-gluten-free hot oatmeal, sprinkled liberally with dried cranberries and brown sugar. Never mind that it was 90 degrees outside. It was my first bowl in 11 years, and I wouldn't have it any other way.

Many people diagnosed with celiac disease or gluten intolerance have found a new career in the support of tasty, gluten-free food. And since only a small percentage of those with gluten sensitivity have been diagnosed, new opportunities to serve this expanding market will exist for years to come. Some people will prepare and sell specialized foods and/or help restaurants offer GF options. Some will open stores or bakeries or totally gluten-free eating establishments. Some will go on educational speaking tours or create websites and/or Facebook pages. And some, like me, will write books!

Health Care Despair 23

AFTER FINALLY TRACKING down the cause of her family's health problems, Cara has become a champion to the gluten-sensitive community. Her website, www.theglutenfile.com and FaceBook page under The Gluten File, provide a wealth of information and support.

Health Care Systems, by Cara

What is wrong with our health care system when a patient with serious health problems can find answers on the Internet that have somehow eluded their flesh-and-blood physicians, doctor after doctor, year after year? Is the problem that unless a remedy involves a prescription drug or surgery, our doctors aren't in tune with it?

In my experience, doctors seem to believe nutritional deficiency is uncommon. It's not! In fact, when you consider all the disease states that result from food sensitivity and nutritional deficits alone, it's mind-boggling. Nutrition is one of nature's building blocks; without it our bodies cannot function properly. So why do so many doctors ignore nutrition completely? If a total nutritional assessment was included in every well-health checkup, how many health problems could be prevented down the road?

Rising health care costs? When I think of the alphabet of tests and procedures my family has been through—blood tests, CT scans, echocardiograms, endoscopies, EEG, EKG, EMG, Holter monitor, MRI, tonsillectomy, tympanostomy tube surgery—not to mention courses and courses of antibiotics and other prescription drugs, I can only wonder. Had doctors identified our gluten sensitivity in the beginning, how many of these tests, procedures, and medications might never have been needed?

At one point I was suffering from symptoms of B12 deficiency, but I saw eight different specialists over three years before one finally thought to check my B12 levels. Thank goodness this doctor was a neurologist who realized that B12 deficiency could persist in someone within the low-normal limits of the range. Along the way I encountered an alphabet soup of specialties: cardiology, gastroenterology, gynecology, neurology, ophthalmology, psychiatry, and urology. However, each specialist looked only at his or her piece, missing completely that something systemic was going on. It was evident to ***me*** that all these symptoms must be somehow related, but when I tried to relay this concept to each new specialist by reviewing symptoms outside his or her area of expertise, my efforts served only to advance notions of hypochondria or somatic illness.

Once my B12 deficiency was finally diagnosed I stumbled upon the neurology forums at BrainTalk (www.braintalkcommunities.org). There I learned how often a B12 deficiency is missed and how most doctors don't know how to properly test for it even when it occurs to them. Symptoms of B12 deficiency can overlap with symptoms of MS, celiac disease, gluten ataxia, Alzheimer's disease, Lyme disease, lupus, and more, so testing should be considered for patients with all of these disorders. Had I stumbled upon the BrainTalk forums when my symptoms first began, I might have been diagnosed within weeks rather than years.

Why are so many neurologists not looking for these things, particularly in a child with a family history of autoimmune disease and nutritional deficiency? A child plagued with unexplained rashes and hives? Dental-enamel defects? Stomachaches?

Why did it take two years of daily diarrhea before my youngest daughter was referred to a gastroenterologist? My pediatrician had indicated my daughter's problems were not uncommon…nothing to worry about. Thank goodness for the new pediatrician who entered the group and pronounced, "That's not right!"

I offer my family's experience as an example of how important it is to take an active role in your health care. Do research; network with others having similar symptoms. The right doctor can make all the difference in the world, so work until you find a doctor you trust who is willing to partner with you in your quest for good health. If you don't find the right one the first time, don't be afraid to change. Request copies of all lab tests and procedures, learn what they mean, and keep a home file. Above all, trust your instincts.

Higher Level of Suspicion, by Gale Pearce, PA-C

The biggest flaws in the current treatment of CD and gluten intolerance are: (1) the low level of suspicion among medical professionals; (2) their lack of knowledge about proper testing procedures; and (3) their hesitation to prescribe a gluten-free diet (GFD), mostly because they are convinced it is impossible to follow. To combat these issues we need a battery of highly motivated, knowledgeable lecturers in our medical schools and in the medical community at large to provide accurate, up-to-date information on the many forms of this disease. I'm convinced that if such a plan were implemented, not only would many more gluten-sensitive folks receive a proper diagnosis, we also would see significant reductions in many diseases not even thought of as related to gluten.

Further research into the gluten connection may reveal it to be the stimulus for a cascade of health issues we currently lump under the heading autoimmune disease: type I diabetes, juvenile rheumatoid arthritis, Crohn's disease, multiple sclerosis, migraines, ADD, ADHD, autism, and more than a hundred other conditions that plague mankind. I am happy to add my story to the many in this book in hopes it may help foster a wider recognition of the many symptoms that can be gluten related. (See Gale's ataxia story in Chapter 9.)

Much of our health care paradigm is shaped by pharmaceutical companies and by major governmental bodies such as the National Institutes of Heath (NIH), the Centers for Disease Control and Prevention (CDC) and the American Medical Association (AMA). If research on the hazards of gluten is not pursued and disseminated by these groups, the majority of individual doctors and other health care professionals, no matter how dedicated, will remain in the dark, and far too many patients will be given one prescription after another to treat something that, in many cases, can be managed by diet alone.

For those who are intolerant, gluten is a toxic staple, affecting their quality of life and destroying their health. If you suspect you or someone you love may be one of them, make a commitment today to find out by pursuing one of the test options outlined in Chapters 16 and 17. If you determine that gluten sensitivity is your problem and subsequently adopt a gluten-free diet, the return on investment may net years of improved health for you and your family.

24 Brevity or Longevity?

AT AGE 86 John is a strong ski and bike enthusiast. He talks with a smile on his face, as well he should; he could have been six feet under in his sixties instead of climbing mountains two and a half decades later.

Reaching the Peak, by John Pepper

Before being diagnosed with celiac disease (CD) at age 60, I had no energy. I could bike 30 to 40 minutes but then I needed to lie down; the fatigue was tremendous. When the doctor mentioned that I would need to give up gluten I kiddingly said, "I never liked the stuff anyway," not knowing what it was. There were few gluten-free (GF) products then, and those that existed I had to order from Seattle. Now that the diversity and quality of GF products has increased significantly, sticking to the diet is so much easier. Besides, my wife has become a pro at adapting recipes to the GF lifestyle.

In the good weather I now bike 30 to 40 miles a day, sometimes more. In the winter I ski 10 runs at Wildcat and after lunch go out for some cross-country skiing. I climb Tuckerman's [slope on Mt. Washington in New Hampshire] annually, but I must confess it takes a bit longer each year.

A lean, lovely, and alert woman, Terry had celebrated her 90th birthday when we met at an exercise class. One day we were chatting about the effects of gluten and Terry, being very interested in her health and wanting to feel more energetic and perhaps a little less stiff and tired, decided to get tested for gluten sensitivity by having the four blood tests outlined in Chapter 16. Terry's story is the perfect example of doctors not recognizing that weak-positive tTG results may suggest some villi damage. Even negative results on all four blood tests cannot definitively rule out gluten sensitivity, as it may be detected by the more sensitive stool tests.

Going Strong: Terry's Story

The results from three of Terry's blood tests were negative. The fourth, the tTG, showed a weak positive, but her doctor, like much of the medical community, did not consider this to be indicative of a problem with gluten. His diagnosis: Terry was "not gluten intolerant."

Based on her tTG result, however, Terry decided to submit a stool sample to EnteroLab. The results were positive. Not only is she sensitive to gluten and dairy, the tests showed she was malabsorbing and had two gluten-sensitive genes.

At 90 years of age it was hard to learn a whole new way of dealing with food, but Terry attributes her continued longevity to enthusiastically trying to follow a GFD, eating very healthily for decades, supplementing her diet with vitamins prescribed by her naturopath, and having a strong faith. She gets help with shopping, cooking, and daily life activities, but otherwise functions very independently, and her memory is far superior to mine. With her great attitude and commitment to living life to the fullest, now at 94, she is truly a treasure.

Having read an article and seen a picture of this energetic 90-year-old, I needed to track her down. Barbara, who is lucky to have survived childhood, was ill for nearly half a century before being diagnosed with celiac disease and told to adopt a GFD. Her story is a testament to how effective the GF lifestyle can be in dramatically turning around one's health.

Thriving at Ninety-two, by Barbara Wasson

I was about five years old in 1923 when I began suffering from constipation and diarrhea, a lot of bloating, and sometimes pain, nausea, and vomiting. I was told then I had celiac disease, but back then no one knew what to do about it; many children with similar symptoms died. I was lucky to have survived, but I was very anemic and also developed rickets. My doctor put me on a diet of bananas and rare liver! The liver helped the anemia and the bananas didn't upset my stomach. No one said anything about not eating grains, however, so in addition to my "staples" of bananas and liver, I ate shredded wheat for breakfast every morning.

Until I was a junior in high school I was the smallest person in my class. Finally, my eye doctor discovered I wasn't growing because of a parathyroid problem.

He prescribed some medicine for this condition and I started to grow—I even grew an inch after I got to college. Now I'm about five-and-a-half feet tall.

My intestinal issues continued through high school and, to a lesser degree, through college and beyond. When I was 48, I went with my family to Aspen, Colorado, on a two-week vacation. Aspen is a lovely town, and at that particular time it was quite crowded. Service was slow, but every restaurant offered specialty breads, which we ate to keep us happy until the food arrived. We also took recipes away with us to make interesting breads at home.

Is it any surprise my gastrointestinal symptoms returned with a vengeance? Our doctor was also our next-door neighbor, so I went over to see him. "This is acting like the celiac disease I had as a child," I said.

"Celiac, what's that?" he replied.

At the time my cousin was head of the Indiana Medical Center. When my father told him about my failing situation he insisted I come to the Center to be checked out. I checked in and was immediately placed in the terminal section with leukemia and cancer patients and others too sick to be helped by their doctors—not an encouraging beginning. The tests, including an endoscopic biopsy, went on for 10 days. At the end the doctors said, "You have a classic case of celiac disease. Go home and don't eat wheat, oats, rye, or barley products for the rest of your life."

It took awhile to get used to reading the labels on everything, but I gradually got better and started exercising, something I'd been too exhausted to do before. These days, though I recently turned 92, I still teach piano about 30 hours a week and continue to drive myself wherever I want to go (though I no longer drive much at night).

I've been on a gluten-free diet for over 40 years, which probably makes me one of the oldest celiac survivors. My villi have long since healed, and I'm not quite as sensitive as my granddaughter, Tiffany Shaw-Diaz (see her story in Chapter 8), but I still pay very close attention to everything I eat.

What continues to baffle me is how friends, family, and acquaintances who have serious, degenerative, and/or life-threatening issues won't at least *try* to enhance their health by screening for gluten sensitivity. It's only blood and stool testing; it's not snake oil. Some people just can't imagine that any medical information could be valid unless it comes directly from their doctors. And then, of course, there are folks who are stuck on the fact that they could "never give up bread" or that they "love pasta." I love pasta too—gluten-free pasta—and there's not much I've given up in order to get my health back.

Frankly, even if I could never eat *any* kind of pasta again, it would seem a small price to pay for the possibility of adding years of health to my life.

As a family we were extremely fortunate to have uncovered the negative role gluten was playing in our lives and to see dramatic improvements in our health after embracing a gluten-free lifestyle. I just entered the eighth decade of my life, but I feel far better than I did when I was 40. "We are what we eat," the old adage goes. So if you are eating gluten, could it be eating you? You'll never know unless you get tested, but if the answer turns out to be yes, the solution is simple: Delete the wheat and discover just how enchanting life can be.

A Empowerment

INCREDIBLE RESEARCH HAS been done on the devastating effects of gluten—more research than you can imagine. Once you begin to dig a little you may be amazed at what's available. In fact, you might feel inundated, since more and more studies are coming out that link gluten to a variety of diseases. It's easy to use the Internet to tap into research around the world, so even if your health issues are genetically linked, very rare, or deemed incurable, I strongly encourage you to do some searching. You also may find it helpful to peruse the databases at your local hospital or college library to explore a specific topic in greater depth.

Even if you don't find any information on your particular malady or chronic condition today, this doesn't mean that a link may not be discovered in the future. Therefore, if you're "sick and tired of being sick and tired" or have any chronic issues, I urge you to consider being tested for gluten sensitivity (specifics on available test options are outlined in Chapters 16 and 17).

Here are some tips on how to make your time at the computer as effective as possible:

- Surround the topic you are searching for with quotation marks if it is more than one word (for example, "peripheral neuropathy" or "atrial fibrillation").
- Add the word *gluten* or the term *"celiac disease"* to your search.
- Add the word *pubmed*. PubMed is a service of the U.S. National Library of Medicine that will direct you to reliable research from around the world. (If you leave *pubmed* out, you may find additional research, blogs, websites, etc., so try it both ways.)

- Use the word *and* or *not* between subjects to narrow your search.
- To find the most recent articles or research results, narrow your search to a year or even three to six months by using Google's Advanced Search feature.

Below are some examples of effective search entries:

- "atrial fibrillation" and "celiac disease" and pubmed
- lupus and gluten and pubmed
- dementia and "antigliadin antibodies" and pubmed

When you find information that's helpful, don't forget to print out copies for yourself and your doctors.

B Helpful Resources

You may find the resources listed below of particular help as you begin to learn more about gluten and its effects on the human body. The Bibliography contains a more comprehensive list. As you begin your own research you will find that information about celiac disease and non-celiac gluten intolerance (CD/GI) is a never-ending, constantly changing river that grows and evolves as additional research brings new information to light.

Books about Gluten Sensitivity

Breaking the Vicious Cycle™, by Elaine Gottscall (2004) a book about The Specific Carbohydrate Diet™ that may benefit those suffering from intestinal issues who are not able to digest carbohydrates well.

Celiac Disease: A Hidden Epidemic, by Dr. Peter H. Green and Rory Jones (2006; revised edition 2010) gives a thorough overview of celiac disease and explains how intimately the gut is connected to other organs and to major illness. An excellent read.

Cereal Killers: Celiac Disease and Gluten-Free A to Z, by Ron Hoggan, EdD, and Scott Adams (2010). (Adams is the founder of http://www.celiac.com and the publishing company Watersideworks.) This collection of essays leaves no topic of gluten sensitivity untouched. The authors advocate for Dr. Kenneth Fine's stool testing (http://www.EnteroLab.com) and recognize the expanded view of gluten sensitivity beyond celiac disease.

Dangerous Grains: Why Gluten Cereal Grains May Be Hazardous to Your Health, by James Braly, MD, and Ron Hoggan, EdD (2002). This is an eye-opening book. Check out the appendix for a list of over 200 symptoms and maladies connected to gluten. Hoggan is dedicated to spreading the word about the nasty and degenerative effects of gluten.

Get the Iron Edge, by Ron Hoggan, EdD, Watersideworks (2008) explains iron deficiency: how it affects learning, memory, and health; the tests necessary to detect it; and how to correct it naturally.

The Gluten Connection: How Gluten Sensitivity May Be Sabotaging Your Health, by Shari Lieberman, PhD, CNS, FACN (2007) explains the negatives associated with traditional blood testing for CD. The author gives great credence to the stool testing at EnteroLab and speaks of Dr. Aristo Vojdani's extensive research. More great information.

The Gluten-Free Bible, by Jax Peters Lowell (2005) is an indispensable book for those embarking on a gluten-free diet (GFD). It covers many aspects of living a gluten-free (GF) lifestyle.

The Gluten Syndrome, by Dr. Rodney Ford (2007) asserts that gluten may cause numerous disorders involving 10 different organs, not just the gut. Many of Dr. Ford's patients test negative for gluten in the intestine but positive for gluten antibodies. Check out his website, http://www.doctorgluten.com, for more great information and easy-to-read books.

Recognizing Celiac Disease, by Cleo Libonati (2007) is a comprehensive, well-documented work listing more than 300 signs, symptoms, and associated disorders linked to gluten. This book should be on the desk of health care professionals in every discipline of medicine. It is an easy-to-use tool for anyone who has health issues or is interested in disease prevention.

Wheat Belly, by William Davis, MD (2011) documents the history of wheat from the time of early man. Dr. Davis reveals the drastic changes that have taken place over the last 50 years in genetically modifying wheat so it contains more gluten. He also explains the effect wheat has on our metabolism and its role in the development of numerous degenerative diseases.

Wheat Free, Worry Free, by Danna Korn (2001) is filled with information. The author, a driven mom who has become an authority on gluten sensitivity, has also written Kids with Celiac Disease (2001) and Living Gluten Free for Dummies (2006).

Books about a Gluten-free Diet

The G-Free Diet: A Gluten-Free Survival Guide, by Elisabeth Hasselbeck (2009) contains everything you need to know to lead a gluten-free lifestyle.

Gluten-Free Diet: A Comprehensive Resource Guide-Expanded and Revised Edition, by Shelley Case (2010)

Gluten-Free Nutrition Guide, by Tricia Thompson (2008)

Periodicals

Gluten Free Living—http://www.glutenfreeliving.com

Living Without—http://www.livingwithout.com

Simply Gluten Free —http://simplygluten-free.com

Websites about Gluten Sensitivity/Research

Celiac.com—http://www.celiac.com, created by Scott Adams, provides a wealth of information written by open-minded doctors and advocates, including substantial information on every aspect of celiac disease and non-celiac gluten intolerance.

Doctors—The following forward-thinking doctors support antigliadin antibody (AGA) testing that may detect a sensitivity to gluten beyond CD:

Kenneth Fine, MD: http://www.EnteroLab.com and http://www.FinerHealth.com. Early Diagnosis of Gluten Sensitivity: Before the Villi are Gone is a must-read essay on the superiority of stool testing. (See http://www.finerhealth.com/Essay/.)

Rodney Ford, MD: http://www.drrodneyford.com/extra/doctor-gluten.html

Marios Hadjivassiliou, MD: You will find most of his research at https://sites.google.com/site/jccglutenfree/halloffame.

Scot Lewey, MD:

- ezinearticles.com/?Diagnosing-Celiac-Disease-and-Gluten-Sensitivity&id=239028
- http://www.celiac.com/articles/1101/1/Gluten-Sensitivity-A-Gastroenterologists-Personal-Journey-Down-the-Gluten-Rabbit-Hole-by-Dr-Scot-Lewey/Page1.html

Thomas O'Bryan, DC: http://www.youtube.com/watch?v=BhHwq8eErxs

Aristo Vojdani, PhD: "NeuroImmunology: From Leaky Gut to Leaky Brain" at www.publichealthalert.org/Articles/scottforsgren/neuroimmunology.htm

The Gluten File—http://www.theglutenfile.com, by storyteller Cara, provides significant updated research and an expanded list of more forward-thinking doctors. Excellent site.

The Gluten Syndrome—http://www.theglutensyndrome.net, offers valuable information. The site is authored by Olive Kaiser, a dedicated advocate who works tirelessly to educate doctors and the public about the dangers of gluten. Another must-read.

X-Gluten.com—http://www.x-gluten.com was created by Anne Sarkisian to highlight important information about testing for celiac disease and non-celiac gluten intolerance.

Websites about a Gluten-free Diet

Beth Israel Deaconess Medical Center—http://www.bidmc.org/celiaccenter offers useful information for gluten-sensitive individuals under "Basics of the Gluten Free Diet."

Canadian Celiac Association—http://www.celiac.ca/pdfs/gfdiet.pdf offers an excellent explanation of grains and other food products as well as lists of safe and unsafe foods, GF substitutions, and more.

Celiac.com—http://www.celiac.com has safe and unsafe lists, alternative flour information, cooking tips, recipes, informative articles, and much more.

Celiac Sprue Association—http://www.CSAceliacs.org is the place to order the CSA Gluten-Free Product Listing, which is updated annually. This book includes lists of thousands of GF products, safe and unsafe foods, GF companies, alternative flours, 800 numbers for many food companies, and more.

Gluten Intolerance Group (GIG)—http://www.gluten.net/learn/gluten-free-diet.aspx offers "The Gluten-Free Diet Nutrition Guide," by Cynthia Kupper, Executive Director of GIG, free for downloading. GIG sponsors a gluten-free food service awareness program at http://www.glutenfreerestaurants.org/. Here you can find out which restaurants around the country have gone through the training.

Healthy Villi—http://www.healthyvilli.org is an advocate for the celiac community of New England. This site contains a helpful list of New England restaurants catering to those on a GFD.

Other Websites of Note (*a few of many*)

American Celiac Disease Alliance—http://www.americanceliac.org/about-us/ (Spanish available)

Autism Network for Dietary Intervention (ANDI)—http://www.autismndi.com/

Celiac Disease Foundation (CDF)—http://www.cdfresourcedirectory.com offers a directory of gluten-free resources.

Food Allergy and Anaphylaxis Network—http://www.foodallergy.org/

GFCF [Gluten Free/Casein Free] Diet Intervention—Autism Diet—http://gfcfdiet.com/

Gluten-Free Drugs—http://www.glutenfreedrugs.com/ (scroll down)

It's Not Mental—http://itsnotmental.blogspot.com/

My Brain Health—http://www.mybrainhealth.org/files/Gluten-induced_neurological_disease_Feb_8_2011.pdf is a power point presentation on how gluten can affect the brain in numerous ways, ranging from inattention to seizures.

Recognizing Celiac Disease—http://www.recognizingceliacdisease.com/21.html "contains over 300 Signs, Symptoms, Associated Disorders and Complications directly or indirectly resulting from celiac disease."

DVD

Unlocking the Mystery of Wheat and Gluten Intolerance, by Dr. Thomas O'Bryan and Sueson Vess substantiates the devastating effects of gluten with some great research—a must-see DVD.

National Support Groups

CCA: Canadian Celiac Association—http://www.celiac.ca

CDF: Celiac Disease Foundation—http://www.celiac.org

CSA: Celiac Sprue Association—http://www.csaceliacs.org

GIG: Gluten Intolerance Group of North America—http://www.gluten.net

NFCA: National Foundation for Celiac Awareness—http://www.celiaccentral.org

Many countries have national support groups.

Education and Research Centers

Celiac Center at Beth Israel Deaconess Medical Center
http://bidmc.org/CentersandDepartments/Departments/DigestiveDiseaseCenter/CeliacCenter.aspx

Celiac Disease Center at Columbia University
http://www.celiacdiseasecenter.org

Celiac Disease Clinic at Mayo Clinic
http://www.mayoclinic.org/celiac-disease/

Massachusetts General Hospital Celiac Research Center
http://www.celiaccenter.org/

University of Chicago Celiac Disease Program
http://www.cureceliacdisease.org

Support Forums

- http://www.Braintalkcommunities.org
- http://www.Neurotalk.psychcentral.com

C Acronyms and Definitions

FOLLOWING IS A partial list of *acronyms* used within the book. The first time a term is used in each chapter it is spelled out, followed by the acronym in parentheses.

AGA—*antigliadin antibody*—a test that detects sensitivity to gliadin, a part of the gluten protein

AID—*autoimmune disorder*—a condition in which the body mistakenly attacks its own tissue

BMD—*bone mineral density*

BMI—*body mass index*

CD—*celiac disease*—an immune response to gluten that damages the villi in the small intestine

CF—*casein free*

DGP: AGA—*deamidated gliadin peptide/antigliadin antibody*—another test used to detect CD

DH—*dermatitis herpetiformis*—a chronic skin condition producing an itchy, blistery rash on elbows, knees, etc., that is often a manifestation of celiac disease

EMA—*endomysial antibody*—an important test in the detection of celiac disease

EPI—*exocrine pancreatic insufficiency*—a condition in which the pancreas does not produce enough enzymes to digest food

GF—*gluten free*

GFD—*gluten-free diet*

GI—*non-celiac gluten intolerance*—a condition in which the patient does not have villous atrophy but may have major health issues linked to gluten

IDA—*iron deficiency anemia*

IgA, IgG, and IgE—immunoglobulins that attack antigens (see definition of these terms under *Antibody* below)

tTG—*tissue transglutaminase*—an enzyme linked to celiac disease; often the only test given to detect celiac disease is the tTG: IgA

SIBO—*small intestinal bacterial overgrowth*, a condition that may need to be ruled out in cases which do not respond well to a strict gluten-free diet

Definitions used throughout the book are based on information from *Black's Medical Dictionary*, 42nd ed., as well as the online sites MedlinePlus, Merriam-Webster, MedicineNet, and Free Dictionary. Where U.S. and British/Canadian spellings of a medical term differ—for example, celiac (coeliac), anemia (aenemia), pediatric (paediatric)—the U.S. convention is used in almost all cases unless the term is part of a direct quote.

Antibody—one of the five classes of immunoglobulins: IgA, IgD, IgE, IgG, and IgM. The immonoglobulins IgA and IgG, which reveal intolerance, and IgE, which reveals allergy, go on the defensive to help protect the body when they detect a foreign invader such as gluten, a virus, or bacteria.

Antigen—a foreign invader such as gluten, dairy, a virus, etc., that the body sees as dangerous.

Autoantibody—an antibody that destroys one's own tissues, resulting in an autoimmune disease.

Autoimmunity—a condition in which one's own tissues are destroyed by the immune system, leading to autoimmune disease.

Celiac sprue—another name for celiac disease.

Differential diagnosis—one or more diagnoses from which the correct diagnosis will be revealed after further investigation. Much of the research throughout this book suggests that celiac disease should be added as a differential diagnosis in trying to determine the cause of numerous ailments.

Enteropathy—a disease of the intestine.

Extraintestinal—occurring outside the intestinal track.

Gluten enteropathy—another name for celiac disease.

Histological—a term pertaining to cell or tissue structure.

Idiopathic—refers to a symptom or condition whose cause is unknown.

Inflammatory cytokines—proteins such as interlukin or interferon that help regulate the immune system and cause inflammation when they get out of control.

Mucosal—an adjective describing the mucous membrane that lines the gastrointestinal tract and other parts of the body.

Myopathy—a muscle disorder.

Refractory—a condition that is difficult to treat or cure.

Subclinical—a description of symptoms that may be either mild or not yet apparent but are nonetheless indicative of an underlying disorder.

Endnotes

Introduction

1. *University of Chicago*, "Celiac Disease Facts."
2. Ford, *The Gluten Syndrome*, 48.
3. *University of Maryland School*, "Researchers Identify Key."
4. Fine, "About EnteroLab."
5. *University of Maryland*, "Celiac Disease Is More Prevalent."
6. Libonati, *Recognizing Celiac Disease*.

Chapter 1 – Crazed

1. *National Foundation of Celiac Awareness*, "Defining, Diagnosing."
2. Fine, "Early Diagnosis of Gluten Sensitivity."

Chapter 2 – Angry Gram: Family Saga

1. Fine, "Early Diagnosis."
2. Fine, "Can I Be Tested?"
3. Korn, *Wheat-Free, Worry-Free*.
4. Elfström, "Risk of Primary Adrenal Insufficiency."
5. Fine: Explanation of lab results from EnteroLab.

Chapter 3 – A Whirlwind of Illnesses

1. Green et al., "Characteristics of Adult Celiac," quoted in Talley et al., "Epidemiology of Celiac Sprue."
2. Braly and Hoggan, *Dangerous Grains*, 186–202.
3. Libonati, *Recognizing Celiac Disease*.
4. Green and Jones, *"Celiac Disease,"* 3.
5. *University of Maryland School*, "Researchers Identify Key."
6. Fine, "About Enterolab."
7. Green et al., "Characteristics of Adult."
8. Fasano et al., "Prevalence of Celiac Disease."
9. Caja et al., "Antibodies in Celiac Disease," quoted in Lohi et al., "Increasing Prevalence of Coeliac," Mäki et al., "Prevalence of Celiac Disease," and Vilppula et al., "Increasing Prevalence and High," respectively.
10. Freeman, "Risk Factors in Familial Forms."

11. Zwolińska-Wcisło, "Frequency of Celiac Disease."
12. *Mayo Clinic*, "Mayo Clinic Study Finds."
13. Fasano, "Clinical Presentation of Celiac."
14. Green and Jabri, "Coeliac Disease."
15. Murray, "The Widening Spectrum."
16. Hamilton, "Gut Check: Belatedly."
17. Green et al., "Characteristics of Adult."

Chapter 4 – Gluten 101

1. Hoggan, "Gluten Intolerant, Gluten Sensitive."
2. Hadjivassiliou et al., "Gluten Sensitivity: From Gut."
3. Catassi and Fasano, "Celiac Disease Diagnosis."
4. *University of Maryland Medical*, "Researchers Find Increased Zonulin."
5. Lee and Green, "Celiac Sprue."
6. McGowan, Castiglione, and Butzner, "The Changing Face."
7. Schreiber et al., "Atypical Celiac Disease."
8. Vilppula et al., "Increasing Prevalence."
9. Braly and Hoggan, *Dangerous Grains*, 186–202.
10. Libonati, "*Recognizing Celiac Disease.*"
11. Brandimarte, Tursi, and Giorgetti, "Changing Trends in Clinical."
12. Bardella et al., "Silent Celiac Disease."
13. Green, "The Many Faces of Celiac."
14. Ludvigsson, Brandt, and Montgomery, "Symptoms and Signs."
15. Gasbarrini et al., "Celiac Disease: What's New."
16. Wahnschaffe et al., "Celiac Disease-like Abnormalities."
17. Biagi et al., "Intraepithelial Lymphocytes."
18. Järvinen et al., "Villous Tip Intraepithelial Lymphocytes."
19. Kaukinen, Collin, and Mäki, "Latent Coeliac Disease," quoted in Kuitunen, Savilahti, and Verkasalo, "Late Mucosal," and Hogberg et al., "Anti-endomysium."
20. *University of Maryland School*, "Researchers Identify Key."
21. Troncone and Jabri, "Coeliac Disease and Gluten."
22. *University of Maryland*, "Researchers Identify Key."
23. Beck, "Clues to Gluten Sensitivity."

Chapter 5 – Misdiagnosed from Coast to Coast

1. *National Digestive Diseases Information Clearinghouse*, "How is Celiac Disease?"
2. Catassi et al., "Detection of Celiac Disease."
3. Kostopoulou, Devereaux-Walsh, and Delaney, "Missing Celiac Disease."
4. Fine, "Early Diagnosis."

Chapter 6 – Systemically Intrusive, Ever Elusive

1. Halfdanarson, Litzow, and Murray, "Hematologic Manifestations."
2. *Recognizing Celiac Disease*, "Celiac Disease Symptoms."
3. Phyllis Zermeño, Clinical Manager at EnteroLab, e-mail message to author, December 8, 2011.
4. Vojdani, "The Role of Mucosal Immunity," slide 66.
5. Duggan, "The Great Imitator."

Chapter 7 – More Than a "Gut Feeling"

1. Hungin et al., "Irritable Bowel Syndrome," quoted in Talley, "Irritable Bowel."
2. Murray et al., "Effect of a Gluten-free Diet."
3. Murray et al., "Bowel Habits."
4. Usai et al., "Co-morbidity of Irritable Bowel."
5. Korkut et al., "The Prevalence of Celiac Disease."
6. Verdu et al., "Clinical Onset of Celiac Disease."

7. Verdu, Armstrong, and Murray, "Between Celiac Disease."
8. Leeds et al., "Is There an Association?"
9. Mayberry, Smart, and Toghill, "Familial Association."
10. Green et al., "An Association between Microscopic."
11. Glas et al., "Novel Genetic Risk Markers."
12. Matteoni et al., "Celiac Disease is Highly."
13. McCashland et al., "Collagenous Enterocolitis."
14. Wolber, Owen, and Freeman, "Colonic Lymphocytosis."
15. Heap and van Heel, "The Genetics of Chronic."
16. Tursi et al., "High Prevalence of Celiac," quoted in Cottone et al., "Familial Occurrence."
17. Schedel et al., "Association of Crohn's Disease."
18. Di Tola et al., "Anti-tissue Transglutaminase Antibodies."
19. Jankowiak and Ludwig, "Frequent Causes of Diarrhea."
20. Lomer, Parkes, and Sanderson, "Review Article: Lactose Intolerance."
21. Ojetti et al., "High Prevalence of Celiac Disease."
22. Vernia, Di Camillo, and Marinaro, "Lactose Malabsorption."
23. Drut and Drut, "Lymphocytic Gastritis in Pediatric."
24. Stancu et al., "Collagenous Gastritis."
25. Vogelsang, Oberhuber, and Wyatt, "Lymphocytic Gastritis and Gastric."
26. Martinez, Israel, and White, "Celiac Disease Presenting."
27. Al Furaikh and Al Zaben, "Recurrent Small Bowel Intussusceptions."
28. Mushtaq et al., "Small Bowel Intussusception."
29. Marconi et al., "Transient Small-bowel Intussusceptions."
30. Suares and Ford, "Prevalence of, and Risk Factors."
31. Kiefte-de Jong et al., "Infant Nutritional Factors."

Chapter 8 – Typically "Atypical" Symptoms

1. Aszalós, "Neurological and Psychiatric Aspects."
2. Jones, D'Souza, and Haboubi, "Patterns of Clinical Presentation."
3. Halfdanarson, Litzow, and Murray, "Hematologic Manifestations."
4. Suárez et al., "Iron, Folic Acid."
5. Annibale et al., "Efficacy of Gluten-free Diet."
6. Grey-Davies, Hows, and Marsh, "Aplastic Anaemia in Association."
7. Acquaviva et al., "Celiac Disease in a Patient."
8. He and Wang, "The Impact of Anemia."
9. Khemiri et al., "Screening for Celiac Disease."
10. Ivanovski et al., "Erythrocytic Transglutaminase."
11. Cuoco et al., "Link between Helicobacter Pylori."
12. Lazzari et al., "Sideropenic Anemia."
13. Patwari et al., "Clinical and Nutritional Profile."
14. Lukowski et al., "Iron Deficiency in Infancy."
15. Fayed et al., "Prevalence of Celiac Disease."
16. Mody, Brown, and Wechsler, "Refractory Iron Deficiency Anemia."
17. Kapur et al., "Iron Supplementation in Children."
18. Souroujon et al., "Serum Ferritin Levels."
19. Patwari et al., "Clinical and Nutritional."
20. *Merriam-Webster,* s.v. "Myeloproliferative," http://www.merriam-webster.com/medical/myeloproliferative (accessed August, 15, 2012).
21. *TheFreeDictionary,* s.v. "Neoplastic," http://www.thefreedictionary.com/neoplastic (accessed March 27, 2012).
22. Carroccio et al., "Extreme Thrombocytosis."
23. Dupond et al., "Thrombocytosis of Celiac Disease."
24. Nelson et al., "Thrombocytosis in Patients."
25. Halfdanarson, Litzow, and Murray, "Hematologic Manifestations."
26. Bianchi and Bardella, "Bone in Celiac Disease."
27. Capriles, Martini, and Arêas, "Metabolic Osteopathy."

28. Science Daily, "Gluten-free Diet Alone;" Zanchi et al., "Bone Metabolism."
29. Mora et al., "Reversal of Low Bone Density."
30. Byrne et al., "Disabling Osteomalacic Myopathy."
31. Zofková, "Celiac Disease and Its Relation."
32. Jones, D'Souza, and Haboubi, "Patterns of Clinical."
33. Stazi and Trinti, "Risk of Osteoporosis."
34. Stenson et al., "Increased Prevalence of Celiac."
35. Ludvigsson et al., "Risk of Fractures."
36. Leslie et al., "Celiac Disease and Eosinophilic."
37. Sinha et al., "Cervical Esophageal."
38. Nachman et al., "Gastroesophageal Reflux Symptoms."
39. Usai et al., "Preventing Recurrence of Gastroesophageal."
40. Maieron et al., "Celiac Disease and Intestinal."
41. Sinha et al., "Cervical Esophageal."
42. Wright, "The Major Complications."
43. Stein and Siewert, "Barrett's Esophagus."
44. Black's Medical Dictionary, s.v. "Metaplasia," 428.
45. Jordá and López Vivancos, "Fatigue as a Determinant."
46. Zipser et al., "Presentations of Adult Celiac Disease."
47. Westerberg et al., "New Strategies for Diagnosis."
48. Sanders, Evans, and Hadjivassiliou, "Fatigue in Primary Care."
49. MedlinePlus, "Food Allergy," http://www.nlm.nih.gov/medlineplus/ency/article/000817.htm (accessed September 14, 2011).
50. Palosuo, "Update on Wheat Hypersensitivity."
51. Tronconi, Parma, and Barera, "Celiac Disease."
52. Berni Canani et al., "The Diagnosis of Food."
53. Palosuo et al., "A Novel Wheat Gliadin."
54. Bittner et al., "Identification of Wheat Gliadins."
55. Mark, "Pediatric Asthma."
56. Kero et al., "Could TH1 and TH2 Diseases."
57. Ludvigsson et al., "Celiac Disease Confers."
58. National Heart Lung and Blood Institute, "National Asthma Guidelines."
59. Fasano and Counts, "Editorial: Commentary on."
60. Farkas et al., "Association of Celiac Disease."
61. Medical News Today, "What Is Edema?"
62. Djuric et al., "Celiac Disease Manifested."
63. Cheng et al., "Body Mass Index."
64. Harvard Medical School, "The Benefits and Risks," 1, 3.
65. Libonati, Recognizing Celiac Disease.
66. Hadithi et al., "Effect of B Vitamin."
67. Durand et al., "Psychiatric Manifestations."
68. Khazai, Judd, and Tangpricha, "Calcium and Vitamin D."
69. Werder, "Cobalamin Deficiency."
70. Hoţoleanu, "Hyperhomocysteinemia."
71. Neffati et al., "Hypocholesterolemia and Celiac."
72. Libonati, "Hypoglycemia," 104.
73. Atikou et al., "Celiac Crisis with Quadriplegia."
74. MedlinePlus, s.v. "Hypokalemia," http://www.nlm.nih.gov/medlineplus/ency/article/000479.htm; s.v. "Rhabdomyolsis," http://vsearch.nlm.nih.gov/vivisimo/cgi-bin/query-meta?v%3Aproject=medlineplus&query=rhabdomyolysis++&x=11&y=15 (accessed March 27, 2012).
75. Merriam-Webster, s.v. "Tetany," http://www.merriam-webster.com/medical/tetany (accessed March 27, 2012).
76. Peña Porta et al., "Hypokalemic Rhabdomyolysis."
77. Zerem et al., "Atypical Manifestations."
78. Kuloğlu et al., "Celiac Disease: Presentation."
79. Oregon State University, "Micronutrient Information Center."

80. Djuric, Zivic, and Katic, "Celiac Disease with Diffuse."
81. Cameron et al., "Celiac Disease Presenting."

Chapter 9 – Neurological Dilemmas: The Mind-blowing Hazards of Gluten

1. Libonati, "Recognizing Celiac Disease," 89–94.
2. Hadjivassiliou and Grünewald, "The Neurology of Gluten."
3. Hadjivassiliou et al., "Gluten Sensitivity: From Gut."
4. Hadjivassiliou and Grünewald, "The Neurology of Gluten."
5. Zelnik et al., "Range of Neurologic Disorders."
6. Dietrich and Erbguth, "Neurological Complications of Inflammatory."
7. Hagen et al., "Neurological Diseases."
8. Kozłowska, "Evaluation of Mental Status."
9. *National Institutes of Health*, "Vitamin B12."
10. Kieslich et al., "Brain White-Matter Lesions."
11. Ghezzi and Ghezzi, "Neurological Manifestations of Gastrointestinal."
12. TheFreeDictionary, s.v. "Homocysteine," http://medical-dictionary.thefreedictionary.com/homocysteine (accessed January 27, 2012).
13. Werder, "Cobalamin Deficiency."
14. Poloni et al., "Gluten Encephalopathy."
15. Obeid, McCaddon, and Herrmann, "The Role of Hyperhomocysteinemia."
16. Wilhelmus et al., "Transglutaminases and Transglutaminase-catalyzed."
17. Mayo Clinic, "Mayo Clinic Discovers Potential."
18. Usai et al., "Frontal Cortical Perfusion."
19. Pitner and Bachman, "A Synopsis of the Practice."
20. Mayo Clinic, "Mayo Clinic Discovers Potential."
21. Fine, "About EnteroLab."
22. MedicineNet, "Asperger's Syndrome?" http://www.medicinenet.com/asperger_syndrome/article.htm (accessed April 1, 2012).
23. Wasilewska, Jarocka-Cyrta, and Kaczmarski, "Gastrointestinal Abnormalities in Children."
24. Horvath and Perman, "Autistic Disorder and Gastrointestinal."
25. Il Messaggero.it, "The False Discovery."
26. Cade et al., "Autism and Schizophrenia."
27. Millward et al., "Gluten- and Casein-free."
28. Atladóttir et al., "Association of Family History."
29. Merriam-Webster, s.v. "Purkinge Cell," http://www.merriam-webster.com/medical/purkinje%20cell (accessed April 1, 2012).
30. Vojdani et al., "Immune Response to Dietary."
31. Morris and Agin, "Syndrome of Allergy, Apraxia"; Science Daily, "Scientists Characterize New Syndrome."
32. Genuis and Bouchard, "Celiac Disease Presenting."
33. Elder, "The Gluten-free, Casein-free."
34. Niederhofer and Pittschieler, "A Preliminary Investigation."
35. Sinn, "Nutritional and Dietary Influences."
36. Mousain-Bosc et al., "Improvement of Neurobehavioral Disorders."
37. Konofal et al., "Iron Deficiency in Children."
38. Braly and Hoggan, Dangerous Grains, 149 quoted in Kozlowska, "Evaluation of Mental Status," and Paul et al. 1985, paraphrased by Reichelt in "The Effect of Gluten."
39. Merriam-Webster, s.v. "Ataxia," http://www.merriam-webster.com/medical/ataxia (accessed April 2, 2012).
40. Hadjivassiliou et al., "Autoantibodies in Gluten Ataxia."
41. Hadjivassiliou et al., "Autoantibody Targeting of Brain."
42. Hadjivassiliou et al., "Gluten Ataxia."
43. Hadjivassiliou et al., "Myopathy Associated with Gluten."
44. Hadjivassiliou et al., "Dietary Treatment of Gluten."
45. Hadjivassiliou et al., "Gluten Ataxia in Perspective."
46. Bürk et al., "Sporadic Cerebellar Ataxia."

47. Aszalós, "Neurological and Psychiatric."
48. MedlinePlus, s.v. "Peripheral Neuropathy," http://www.nlm.nih.gov/medlineplus/ency/article/000593.htm4/3/12 (accessed April 3, 2012).
49. Volta et al., "Clinical Findings."
50. Chin et al., "Celiac Neuropathy."
51. Hadjivassiliou et al., "Sensory Ganglionopathy."
52. Latov, "Celiac Disease and Peripheral."
53. Lewey, "Your Brain on Gluten."
54. Rigamonti et al., "Celiac Disease Presenting."
55. TheFreeDictionary, s.v. "Multiple Sclerosis," http://medical-dictionary.thefreedictionary.com/multiple+sclerosis (accessed December 1, 2011).
56. Hernández-Lahoz and Rodrigo, "Gluten Sensitivity."
57. Reichelt and Jensen, "IgA Antibodies against Gliadin."
58. Shor et al., "Gluten Sensitivity in Multiple."
59. Obeid, McCaddon, and Herrmann, "The Role."
60. Miller et al., "Vitamin B12, Demyelination."
61. Sandyk and Awerbuch, "Vitamin B12."
62. Ricotta et al., "Physio-pathological Roles."
63. Bushara, "Neurologic Presentation."
64. Bushara, Nance, and Gomez, "Antigliadin Antibodies in Huntington's."
65. Karpuj, Becher, and Steinman, "Evidence for a Role."
66. Vermes et al., "Elevated Concentration of Cerebrospinal."
67. Brown et al., "White Matter Lesions."
68. Turner et al., "A Case of Celiac Disease."
69. Black's, s.v. "Mitochondria," 437.
70. Kidd, "Neurodegeneration from Mitochondrial."
71. Fine, "About EnteroLab."
72. Maniar, Yadav, and Gokhale, "Intractable Seizures and Metabolic."
73. TheFreeDictionary, s.v. "Hippocampal Sclerosis," http://www.ncbi.nlm.nih.gov/pubmed/16366737?dopt=Citation (accessed November 14, 2010).
74. Peltola et al., "Hippocampal Sclerosis in Refractory."
75. Canales et al., "Epilepsy and Celiac Disease."
76. Díaz, González-Rabelino, and Delfino, "Epilepsy, Cerebral Calcifications."
77. Mavroudi et al., "Successful Treatment of Epilepsy."
78. Pfaender et al., "Visual Disturbances Representing."
79. Kieslich et al., "Brain White-matter Lesions."
80. Gobbi et al., "Celiac Disease, Posterior."
81. Gobbi, "Coeliac Disease, Epilepsy."
82. TheFreeDictionary, s.v. "Paroxysmal Nonkinesigenic Dyskinesia," http://encyclopedia.thefreedictionary.com/Paroxysmal+Nonkinesigenic+Dyskinesia (accessed December 1, 2011).
83. Hall, Parsons, and Benke, "Paroxysmal Nonkinesigenic Dystonia."
84. TheFreeDictionary, s.v. "Chorea," http://www.thefreedictionary.com/chorea (accessed April 3, 2012).
85. Pereira et al., "Choreic Syndrome and Coeliac."
86. Hadjivassiliou et al., "Neuromuscular Disorder."
87. TheFreeDictionary, s.v. "Rhabdomyolysis," http://medical-dictionary.thefreedictionary.com/rhabdomyolysis (accessed April 3, 2012).
88. Meini et al., "An Unusual Association."
89. Bhatia et al., "Progressive Myoclonic Ataxia."
90. Kalaydjian et al., "The Gluten Connection."
91. Cascella et al., "Prevalence of Celiac Disease."
92. Dickerson et al., "Markers of Gluten Sensitivity."
93. Eaton et al., "Association of Schizophrenia."
94. Dohan et al., "Is Schizophrenia Rare."
95. Dohan, "Genetic Hypothesis of Idiopathic."
96. Singh and Kay, "Wheat Gluten."

97. Cade et al., "Autism and Schizophrenia."
98. Kraft and Westman, "Schizophrenia, Gluten."
99. Bürk et al., "Neurological Symptoms in Patients."
100. *NHS, "NICE Clinical Guidelines* 86: Coeliac Disease," 1.1.3.
101. Cicarelli et al., "Clinical and Neurological Abnormalities."
102. Pynnönen et al., "Mental Disorders in Adolescents."
103. Hernanz and Polanco, "Plasma Precursor Amino Acids."
104. Carta et al., "Association between Panic Disorder."
105. Weisbrot et al., "Psychiatric Comorbidity."
106. Corvaglia et al., "Depression in Adult."
107. Garakani et al., "Comorbidity of Irritable Bowel."
108. Lydiard, "Irritable Bowel Syndrome."
109. Coppen and Bolander-Gouaille, "Treatment of Depression."
110. Durand et al., "Psychiatric Manifestations of Vitamin."
111. Stabler, Lindenbaum, and Allen, "Vitamin B-12 Deficiency."
112. Addolorato et al., "Anxiety but Not Depression."
113. *National Center for Complementary*, "Headaches and Complementary."
114. Bürk et al., "Neurological."
115. Lionetti et al., "Headache in Pediatric."
116. Roche Herrero et al., "The Prevalence of Headache."
117. Benito Conejero et al., "Cerebral Calcifications."
118. Lionetti et al., "Headache in Pediatric."
119. *Black's, s.v.* "Restless Legs Syndrome," 575.
120. Weinstock et al., "Celiac Disease is Associated."
121. Manchanda, Davies, and Picchietti, "Celiac Disease as a Possible."
122. Sun et al., "Iron and the Restless."
123. Oner et al., "Association between Low Serum."

Chapter 10 – Autoimmune Disease

1. *National Institute of Arthritis*, "Understanding Autoimmune Diseases."
2. *American Autoimmune Related*, "A Question to Explore."
3. *National Institute of Allergy*, "Autoimmune Diseases."
4. Kumar, Rajadhyaksha, and Wortsman, "Celiac Disease-Associated."
5. Ventura, Magazzù, and Greco. "Duration of Exposure."
6. *University of Chicago*, "Celiac Disease Facts."
7. Vojdani, "The Role of Mucosal Immunity," slide 66.
8. Bizzaro, "The Predictive Significance."
9. Visser et al., "Tight Junctions, Intestinal Permeability."
10. Forsgren, "NeuroImmunology: From Leaky."
11. American Diabetes Association, "National Diabetes Fact Sheet."
12. Barera et al., "Occurrence of Celiac Disease."
13. Barker, "Clinical Review."
14. Nóvoa Medina, "Impact of Diagnosis."
15. Ziegler, "Early Infant Feeding."
16. Kumar, Rajadhyaksha, and Wortsman, "Celiac Disease-Associated."
17. Ch'ng, Jones, and Kingham, "Celiac Disease and Autoimmune."
18. Kumar, Rajadhyaksha, and Wortsman, "Celiac Disease-Associated."
19. Holmes, "Screening for Coeliac."
20. Stanford School of Medicine, "Type-2 Diabetes Linked."
21. Syed et al., "Is Type 2 Diabetes?"
22. Cervin et al., "Genetic Similarities between Latent."
23. Libonati, "Recognizing Celiac Disease," 104.
24. Daher et al., "Consequences of Dysthyroidism."
25. *MedicineNet*, s.v. "Thyroid Peroxidase," http://www.medterms.com/script/main/art.asp?articlekey=19048 (accessed April 17, 2012).
26. Iuorio et al., "Prevalence of Celiac Disease."

27. Ch'ng et al., "Prospective Screening for Coeliac."
28. Ch'ng, Jones, and Kingham, "Celiac Disease and Autoimmune."
29. Spadaccino et al., "Celiac Disease in North."
30. Ventura et al., "Gluten-dependent Diabetes-related."
31. Toscano et al., "Importance of Gluten."
32. Sategna-Guidetti et al., "Prevalence of Thyroid."
33. Valentino et al., "Unusual Association of Thyroiditis."
34. Saito et al., "A Case of Hashimoto's Encephalopathy."
35. Trbojević and Djurica, "Diagnosis of Autoimmune."
36. Black's, s.v. "Vitiligo," 715.
37. Birlea, Fain, and Spritz, "A Romanian Population."
38. Spritz, "Shared Genetic Relationships."
39. Seyhan et al., "The Mucocutaneous Manifestations."
40. Alkhateeb et al., "Epidemiology of Vitiligo."
41. Laberge et al., "Early Disease Onset."
42. Coenen et al., "Common and Different Genetic."
43. Zhernakova et al., "Meta-analysis of Genome-wide."
44. Hafström et al., "A Vegan Diet Free."
45. Ferrell, "47 – The Shatin Research," 28–29.
46. Binder et al., "Gluten and the Small."
47. Al-Mayouf, Al-Mehaidib, and Alkaff, "Significance of Elevated."
48. Stagi et al., "Thyroid Function."
49. Falcini et al., "Recurrent Monoarthritis."
50. Lindqvist et al., "IgA Antibodies to Gliadin."
51. Cottafava and Cosso, "Psoriatic Arthritis and Celiac."
52. Prignano et al., "Juvenile Psoriatic Arthritis."
53. Ozyemisci-Taskiran, Cengiz, and Atalay, "Celiac Disease."
54. Elkan et al., "Gluten-free Vegan Diet."
55. Podas et al., "Is Rheumatoid Arthritis."
56. Mouyis et al., "Hypovitaminosis D."
57. MedlinePlus, "Healthy Joints."
58. Ibid.
59. Stark et al., "Genetics in Neuroendocrine."
60. Vereckei et al., "Back Pain and Sacroiliitis."
61. Liossis and Tsokos, "Cellular Immunity in Osteoarthritis."
62. Goel, McBane, and Kamath, "Cardiomyopathy Associated."
63. Curione et al., "Idiopathic Dilated Cardiomyopathy."
64. Winter Del et al., "Dilated Cardiomyopathy."
65. Uslu et al., "Dilated Cardiomyopathy."
66. Braly and Hoggan, Dangerous Grains; iron deficiency anemia 53, idiopathic thrombocytopenia purpura 118, Grave's disease 123, osteoporosis 134–143, and Appendix D.
67. Hatting et al., "Anemia and Severe Thrombocytopenia."
68. Dogan et al., "Concurrent Celiac Disease."
69. Halfdanarson, Litzow, and Murray, "Hematologic Manifestations."
70. Williams, Mincey, and Calamia, "Inclusion Body Myositis."
71. Kahn, Fiel, and Janowitz, "Celiac Sprue, Idiopathic."
72. Duggan and Duggan, "Systematic Review: The Liver."
73. Volta, "Pathogenesis and Clinical Significance."
74. Freeman, "Hepatobiliary and Pancreatic."
75. Caprai et al., "Autoimmune Liver Disease."
76. Barbero Villares et al., "Hepatic Involvement."
77. Casswall et al., "Severe Liver Damage."
78. Duggan, "The Great Imitator."
79. Ertem et al., "The Response to Hepatitis."
80. Kaukinen et al., "Celiac Disease in Patients."
81. Ludvigsson, Montgomery, and Ekbom, "Risk of Pancreatitis."

82. Carroccio et al., "Unexplained Elevated Serum."
83. Halabi, "Coeliac Disease Presenting."
84. Patel, Johlin, and Murray, "Celiac Disease and Recurrent."
85. Barera et al., "Macroamylasemia Attributable."
86. Rodrigo et al., "Relapsing Acute Pancreatitis."
87. Tattersall, "Hypoadrenia."
88. Collin et al., "Endocrinological Disorders."
89. Elfström et al., "Risk of Primary Adrenal."
90. Betterle et al., "Celiac Disease in North."
91. Valentino et al., "Unusual Association of Thyroiditis."
92. Fasano and Counts, "Editorial: Commentary on 'Anti-Pituitary.' "
93. Delvecchio et al., "Anti-pituitary Antibodies."
94. De Bellis et al., "Autoimmunity as a Possible."
95. Meazza et al., "Short Stature in Children."
96. Donaldson, Speight, and Loomis, "Fibromyalgia Syndrome."
97. Petersen and Petersen, The Gluten Effect, 281.
98. Zipser et al., "Presentations of Adult."
99. Wallace and Hallegua, "Fibromyalgia."
100. Kurland et al., "Prevalence of Irritable."
101. Veale et al., "Primary Fibromyalgia."
102. *National Institute of Neurological Disorders,* "What Is Stiff-person?"
103. Hadjivassiliou et al., "GAD Antibody-associated."
104. O'Sullivan et al., "A Case of Stiff-person."
105. Hijazi, Bedat-Millet, and D. Hannequin, "Stiff-person Syndrome."
106. Bilic et al., "Stiff-person Syndrome."
107. *Black's* s.vv. "Scleroderma," 399; "Lupus," 591.
108. Rosato et al., "High Incidence of Celiac."
109. Trucco Aguirre et al., "Celiac Disease Associated."
110. Marguerie et al., "Malabsorption Caused by Coeliac."
111. Hadjivassiliou et al., "Gluten Sensitivity Masquerading."
112. Mavragani and Moutsopoulos, "The Geoepidemiology of Sjögren's."
113. Lidén et al.,"Gluten Sensitivity."
114. Prochorec-Sobieszek and Wagner, "Lymphoproliferative Disorders."
115. Delalande et al., "Neurologic Manifestations."
116. Iltanen et al., "Celiac Disease and Markers."
117. Teppo and Maury, "Antibodies to Gliadin."
118. Song et al., "Dermatomyositis Associated with Celiac."
119. Evron et al., "Polymyositis, Arthritis, and Proteinuria."
120. Farber and Bitton, "Dermatomyositis and Adult."
121. Marie et al., "An Uncommon Association."
122. *Merck Manuals Online Medical Library,* "Skin Manifestations."
123. Selva-O'Callaghan et al., "Celiac Disease in Patients.
124. Hadjivassiliou et al., "Myopathy Associated."
125. Kleopa et al., "Reversible Inflammatory."
126. Hadjivassiliou et al., "Neuromuscular Disorder."
127. Corazza et al., "Celiac Disease and Alopecia."
128. Dreifus, "Living and Studying Alopecia."
129. Haque, Mir, and Hsu, "Vogt-Koyanagi-Harada Syndrome."
130. Vañó-Galván et al., "Sudden Hair Loss."
131. Fessatou, Kostaki, and Karpathios, "Coeliac Disease and Alopecia."
132. Storm, "Celiac Disease and Alopecia."
133. Naveh et al., "Celiac Disease-associated Alopecia."
134. Corazza et al., "Celiac Disease and Alopecia."
135. Cooper et al., "The Association of Lichen."
136. *Merriam-Webster, s.v.* "Cystic Fibrosis," http://www.merriam-webster.com/medical/cystic+fibrosis?show=0&t=1323015692 (accessed December 4, 2011).

137. Fluge et al., "Co-morbidity of Cystic Fibrosis."
138. Walkowiak et al., "Cystic Fibrosis."
139. Chiaravalloti et al., "Celiac Disease and Cystic Fibrosis."
140. Venuta et al., "Coexistence of Cystic Fibrosis."
141. Gastroenterology, 131, no. 4.

Chapter 11 – The Skin You're In

1. Katz et al., "HL-A8: A Genetic Link."
2. Collin and Reunala, "Recognition and Management."
3. Mustalahti, "Unusual Manifestations."
4. Pfeiffer, "Dermatitis Herpetiformis."
5. Ibid.
6. Lioger, Machet, and Machet, "Dermatitis Herpetiformis."
7. Collin, Pukkala, and Reunala, "Malignancy and Survival."
8. Reunala and Collin, "Diseases Associated with Dermatitis."
9. Powell, Bruckner, and Weston, "Dermatitis Herpetiformis Presenting."
10. Woollons et al., "Childhood Dermatitis Herpetiformis."
11. Abenavoli et al., "Cutaneous Manifestations."
12. Singh et al., "Celiac Disease-associated Antibodies."
13. Michaëlsson et al., "Psoriasis Patients with Antibodies."
14. Addolorato et al., "Rapid Regression of Psoriasis."
15. Montalto et al., "Atypical Mole Syndrome."
16. Meyers et al., "Cutaneous Vasculitis."
17. Oosterheert et al., "Blue Rubber Bleb Nevus."
18. Abenavoli et al., "Cutaneous Manifestations."

Chapter 12 – Our Children Are Our Future

1. Martinelli et al., "Coeliac Disease and Unfavourable."
2. Ibid.
3. *Celiac Sprue Association*, "Celiac Disease Facts."
4. Pellicano et al., "Women and Celiac Disease."
5. Anjum et al., "Maternal Celiac Disease."
6. Martinelli et al., "Reproductive Life."
7. Ibid.
8. Ozgör and Selimoğlu, "Coeliac Disease and Reproductive."
9. Soni and Badawy, "Celiac Disease and Its Effect."
10. Martinelli et al., "Reproductive Life."
11. Di Simone et al., "Anti-tissue Transglutaminase."
12. Martinelli et al., "Reproductive Life."
13. Stazi and Trinti, "Reproductive Aspects."
14. Karagiannis and Harsoulis, "Gonadal Dysfunction."
15. Sher et al., "Infertility, Obstetric and Gynaecological."
16. Nowowiejska, Kaczmarski, and Dabrowska, "A Long-term Study."
17. Stazi and Montovanni, "Celiac Disease and Its Endocrine."
18. Merriam-Webster, s.v. "Preeclampsia," http://www.merriam-webster.com/medical/preeclampsia (accessed April 4, 2012).
19. Weil, "How to Handle."
20. Jorge, Jorge, and Camus, "Celiac Disease Associated."
21. Holmes, "Menopause & Perimenopause."
22. Stephansson, Falconer, and Ludvigsson, "Risk of Endometriosis."
23. Aguiar et al., "Serological Testing."
24. Endometriosis.org. "Dietary Modification."
25. Sinaii et al., "High Rates of Autoimmune."
26. Radetti et al., "Foetal and Neonatal Thyroid."
27. Stazi and Mantovani, "Celiac Disease. Risk Factors."

28. Nørgård et al., "Birth Outcomes of Women."
29. Lozoff, "Iron Deficiency."

Chapter 13 – Gluten Indicted: An "Enhancer to Cancer"

1. *Celiac Sprue Association, "Celiac Disease Facts."*
2. Braly, *Gluten Sensitivity, Coeliac Disease,* slide 10.
3. Ibid, slide 9.
4. Holmes et al., "Coeliac Disease, Gluten-free."
5. Holmes et al., "Malignancy in Coeliac."
6. Marsch et al., "Adenocarcinoma of the Small."
7. Straker, Gunasekaran, and Brady, "Adenocarcinoma of the Jejunum."
8. Sahin et al., "The Patient Presenting," quoted in Green et al., "Risk of Malignancy," and Smedby et al., "Malignant Lymphomas."
9. Schweizer, Oren, and Mearin, "Cancer in Children."
10. Silano et al., "Delayed Diagnosis of Coeliac."
11. Brottveit and Lundin. "Cancer Risk."
12. Sahin et al., "The Patient Presenting," quoted in Gogos et al., "Autoimmune Cholangitis," and Green and Jabri, "Celiac Disease and Other."
13. Kolacek et al., "Gluten-free Diet."
14. Jabri and Sollid, "Tissue-mediated Control."
15. Caputo et al., "Tissue Transglutaminase in Celiac."
16. Griffin, Casadio, and Bergamini, "Transglutaminases: Nature's."
17. Holmes, "Coeliac Disease and Malignancy."
18. Smedby et al., "Malignant Lymphomas in Coeliac."
19. Ahluwalia et al., "Aggressive Burkitt-like Lymphoma."
20. Howell, Calder, and Grimble, "Gene Polymorphisms, Inflammatory."
21. Elfström et al., "Risk of Lymphoproliferative Malignancy."
22. Sonet et al., "Clinical and Pathological Features."
23. Catassi, Bearzi, and Holmes, "Association of Celiac Disease."
24. Wright, "The Major Complications."
25. Silano et al., "Effect of a Gluten-free."
26. Green et al., "Risk of Malignancy."
27. Prochorec-Sobieszek and Wagner, "Lymphoproliferative Disorders."
28. Collin, Pukkala, and Reunala, "Malignancy and Survival."
29. Holmes, "Coeliac Disease and Malignancy."
30. Collin, Pukkala, and Reunala, "Malignancy and Survival."
31. Anderson et al., "Risks of Myeloid Malignancies."
32. Carroccio et al., "Extreme Thrombocytosis."
33. Potter et al., "The Role of Defective."
34. Wright, "The Major Complications."
35. Juranić et al., "Humoral Immunoreactivity to Gliadin."
36. Juranić et al., "Antibodies Contained in 'M' Component."
37. Verbeek et al., "Aberrant T-lymphocytes in Refractory."
38. Weizman et al., "Treatment Failure in Celiac."
39. Regan and DiMagno, "Exocrine Pancreatic Insufficiency."
40. Evans et al., "Pancreatic Insufficiency in Adult."
41. Reddymasu, Sostarich, and McCallum, "Small Intestinal Bacterial."
42. Tursi, Brandimarte, and Giorgetti, "High Prevalence of Small."
43. Lin and Pimentel, "Bacterial Concepts in Irritable."
44. Bures et al., "Small Intestinal Bacterial."
45. Reddymasu, Sostarich, and McCallum, "Small Intestinal."
46. Ghoshal et al., "Partially Responsive Celiac Disease."
47. Ciacci et al., "Hereditary Fructose Intolerance."
48. Kasper et al., "Lambliasis As Differential Diagnosis."
49. Davis, *Wheat Belly, 89.*
50. West et al., "Malignancy and Mortality."

Chapter 14 – Organ Malfunction: A Medical Masquerade

1. da Silva, "Micronutrient Support in Heart."
2. Mavroudis et al., "Irreversible End-stage Heart."
3. Hurley and Baggs, "Hypocalcemic Cardiac Failure."
4. Hoţoleanu et al., "Hyperhomocysteinemia: Clinical."
5. Emilsson et al., "Increased Risk of Atrial."
6. Vojdani, O'Bryan, and Kellermann, "The Immunology of Gluten."
7. Ludvigsson et al., "Nationwide Cohort Study."
8. Polat et al., "Cardiac Functions in Children."
9. Callejas Rubio et al., "Celiac Disease Presenting."
10. Weil, "How to Handle."
11. Baryshnikov et al., "Lower Extremity Deep Vein."
12. Dillmann, "Cardiac Hypertrophy and Thyroid."
13. Patanè and Marte, "Atrial Fibrillation Associated."
14. Fater-Debska et al., "Thyrometabolic Disorders."
15. Duggal et al., "Cardiovascular Risk."
16. Yoon, Ostchega, and Louis, "Recent Trends."
17. Ibid, quoted in Whitworth, "2003 World Health Organization."
18. MedlinePlus, s.v. "Hypertension," http://www.nlm.nih.gov/medlineplus/ency/article/000468.htm (accessed July 25, 2012).
19. Lim et al., "Reversible Hypertension Following."
20. Kara and Sandikci, "Successful Treatment of Portal."
21. Zamani et al., "Celiac Disease as a Potential."
22. Dickey et al., "Homocysteine and Related."
23. Audia et al., "Stroke in Young Adults."
24. Obeid, McCaddon, and Herrmann, "The Role."
25. Dickey et al., "Homocysteine and Related."
26. Doğan et al., "Stroke and Dilated Cardiomyopathy."
27. El Moutawakil et al., "Celiac Disease and Ischemic."
28. Millen et al., "Vitamin D Status."
29. Ludvigsson et al., "Celiac Disease Confers."
30. Raina et al., "Bilateral Total Cataract."
31. Jacob et al., "Gluten Sensitivity and Neuromyelitis."
32. Black's, s.v. "Uveitis," 701.
33. Krifa et al., "Uveitis Responding on Gluten."
34. Merriam-Webster, s.v. "Keratoconus," http://www.merriam-webster.com/medical/keratoconus (accessed February 15, 2011).
35. Nemet et al., "The Association of Keratoconus."
36. Tuncer, Yeniad, and Peksayar, "Regression of Conjunctival Tumor."
37. Black's, s.v. "Opthalmoplegia," 480.
38. Freeman, "Neurological Disorders."
39. Lowder et al., "Macular and Paramacular."
40. Hadjivassiliou et al., "Gluten Ataxia in Perspective."
41. Danese et al., "Extraintestinal Manifestations in Inflammatory."
42. Tezel and Wax, "Glaucoma."
43. New York Times, "Health Guide: Glaucoma."
44. Wax, "The Case for Autoimmunity"; Shazly et al., "Autoimmune Basis."
45. Tezel and Wax, "Glaucoma."
46. Libonati, Recognizing Celiac Disease, 213.
47. Sadowski et al., "Corneal Manifestations in Vitamin."
48. Libonati, Recognizing Celiac Disease, 213–14.
49. Tarlo et al., "Association between Celiac Disease."
50. Wright, "The Major Complications."
51. Birring et al., "Airway Function and Markers."
52. Brightling et al., "A Case of Cough."
53. Kallel-Sellami et al., "Recurrent Rhinitis and Pulmonary."

54. Ludvigsson et al., "A Nationwide Cohort."
55. Tsiligianni and van der Molen, "A Systematic Review."
56. Smit, "Chronic Obstructive Pulmonary."
57. Romieu and Trenga, "Diet and Obstructive."
58. Hwang et al., "Sarcoidosis in Patients."
59. Ludvigsson et al., "Risk of Sarcoidosis."
60. Rutherford et al., "Prevalence of Coeliac Disease."
61. Papadopoulos et al., "Evidence of Gastrointestinal Immune."
62. Loche and Bazex, "Celiac Disease Associated."
63. TheFreeDictionary s.v. "Idiopathic Pulmonary Hemosiderosis," http://medical-dictionary.thefreedictionary.com/idiopathic+pulmonary+hemosiderosis (accessed January 23, 2012).
64. Malhotra et al., "Coeliac Disease as a Cause."
65. Perelman, Dupuy, and Bourrillon, "The Association of Pulmonary."
66. Pacheco et al., "Long-term Clinical Follow-up."
67. Hoca, Dayioglu, and Ogretensoy, "Pulmonary Hemosiderosis."
68. Fraquelli et al., "Gallbladder Motility in Obesity."
69. Deprez et al., "Expression of Cholecystokinin."
70. Hoggan, "Gall Bladder Disease."
71. Croese, Harris, and Bain, "Coeliac Disease."
72. Wright, "The Major Complications."
73. O'Grady et al., "Hyposplenism and Gluten-sensitive."
74. Corazza et al., "Effect of Gluten-free."
75. Biyikli et al., "The Co-existence of Membranoproliferative."
76. Jhaveri et al., "Coeliac Sprue-associated Membranoproliferative."
77. Welander et al., "Increased Risk of End-stage."
78. Smerud et al., "Gluten Sensitivity in Patients."
79. Rabsztyn et al., "Macroamylasemia in Patients."
80. Barera et al., "Macroamylasemia Attributable."
81. Cohan, *The Better Bladder Book*.

Chapter 15 – A Commodity of Oddities

1. Mäki et al., "Prevalence of Celiac Disease."
2. Lapid, "Eating Disorder or Celiac"; based on a study by Leffler et al., "Interaction between Eating Disorders."
3. Karwautz et al., "Eating Pathology in Adolescents."
4. NHS. *"NICE Clinical Guidelines: Coeliac Disease,"* 2.4.1.
5. Yucel et al., "Eating Disorders and Celiac."
6. Jost et al., "Very Severe Iron-Deficiency."
7. Cheng et al., "The Association between Celiac."
8. Bilello, Ciulla, and Caradonna, "Celiac Disease and Malocclusion."
9. Shakeri et al., "Gluten Sensitivity Enteropathy."
10. Campisi et al., "Coeliac Disease: Oral Ulcer."
11. Hizli et al., "Sensorineural Hearing Loss."
12. Hajas et al., "Sensorineural Hearing Loss."
13. Leggio et al., "Coeliac Disease and Hearing."
14. Arroyave, "Recurrent Otitis Media."
15. St. Clair et al., "Celiac Disease Presenting."
16. Stagi et al., "Coeliac Disease in Patients."
17. Fawcett, Linford, and Stulberg, "Nail Abnormalities."
18. Yeruham, Avidar, and Perl, "An Apparently Gluten-induced."
19. Korman, "Pica as a Presenting."
20. Béchade et al., "Common Variable Immunodeficiency."

Chapter 16 – Gluten 102: Traditional Blood Testing

1. Treem, "Emerging Concepts."

2. Hill et al., "Guideline for the Diagnosis."
3. Zermeno, Phyllis , email to author, October 8, 2008.
4. Lewis and Scott, "Meta-analysis: Deamidated"; Volta et al., "Old and New Serological."
5. Hoggan and Adams, *Cereal Killers*, 186.
6. *MedlinePlus*, s.v. "Antibody," http://www.nlm.nih.gov/medlineplus/ency/article/002223.htm (accessed July 2, 2012).
7. *MedlinePlus*, s.v. "Autoimmune Disorders," http://www.nlm.nih.gov/medlineplus/ency/article/000816.htm (accessed July 2, 2012).
8. Mäki et al., "Prevalence of Celiac Disease."
9. West et al., "The Iceberg of Celiac."
10. Alaedini and Green, "Autoantibodies in Celiac."
11. Koskinen et al., "Gluten-dependent Small Bowel."
12. Rostami et al., "Autoantibodies and Histogenesis."
13. Ibid.
14. Green, "Where Are All Those."
15. Mäki et al., ""Prevalence of Celiac Disease."
16. Kurppa et al., "Diagnosing Mild Enteropathy."
17. Dickey, Hughes, and McMillan, "Reliance on Serum Endomysial."
18. Rostami et al., "Autoantibodies."
19. Hadjivassiliou and Grünewald, "The Neurology of Gluten."
20. Zermeno, Phyllis , email message to author, November 18, 2011.
21. Wauters et al., "Serum IgG and IgA."
22. Aszalós, "Neurological and Psychiatric."
23. Villalta et al., "Diagnostic Accuracy of IgA."
24. Reddick, Crowell, and Fu, "Clinical Inquiries."
25. Henker et al., "Pitfalls in Diagnosis."
26. Korponay-Szabó et al., "Elevation of IgG Antibodies."
27. Kurppa et al., "Antibodies Against Deamidated."
28. Volta et al., "Deamidated Gliadin Peptide."
29. Mothes, Uhlig, and Richter, "Recent Aspects of Antibody."
30. Liu et al., "Natural History of Antibodies."
31. Bonamico et al., "First Salivary Screening."
32. Kotze et al., "A Brazilian Experience."
33. Carroccio et al., "IgA Anti-actin Antibodies"; Clemente et al., "Immune Reaction Against."
34. Volta et al., "Anti-ganglioside Antibodies."
35. Westerholm-Ormio et al., "Inflammatory Cytokines."
36. Drago et al., "Gliadin, Zonulin and Gut."
37. Fasano, "Zonulin and Its Regulation."
38. Duerksen et al., "A Comparison of Antibody."
39. Lagerqvist et al., "Antigliadin Immunoglobulin."
40. Basso et al., "Antibodies Against Synthetic."
41. Agardh, "Antibodies Against Synthetic."
42. Lagerqvist et al., "Antigliadin Immunoglobulin."
43. Zermeno, Phyllis , email to author, November 20, 2008.
44. Dickey and Hughes, "Prevalence of Celiac Disease."
45. Hoggan and Adams, *Cereal Killers*, 113–14.
46. Rostami et al., "Autoantibodies and Histogenesis."

Chapter 17 – Gluten 103: Progressive Stool Testing

1. Fine, "Do I Have?"
2. Fine, "Welcome to EnteroLab: About Enterolab."
3. Fine, "Early Diagnosis of Gluten Sensitivity."
4. Koskinen et al., "Gluten-dependent Small Bowel."
5. Not et al., "Cryptic Genetic Gluten Intolerance."
6. Carroccio et al., "Fecal Assays Detect Hypersensitivity."
7. Kaukinen, Collin, and Mäki, "Natural History of Celiac."

8. Kaukinen et al., "Small-bowel Mucosal Transglutaminase."
9. Halblaub et al., "Comparison of Different Salivary."
10. Picarelli et al., "Antiendomysial Antibody Detection."
11. Zermeno, Phyllis (via Dr. Fine), email to author, November 20, 2008.
12. Zermeno, Phyllis , email to author, May 3, 2012.
13. Fine, "Early Diagnosis."

Chapter 18 – A Lousy Inheritance

1. *Black's*, s.v. "Human Leukocyte Antigens," 314.
2. Treem, "Emerging Concepts."
3. Kaukinen et al., "HLA-DQ Typing."
4. *University of Chicago,* "Of Mice and Men."
5. Trynka, Wijmenga, and van Heel, "A Genetic Perspective."
6. Coenen et al., "Common and Different Genetic."
7. Plenge, "Unlocking the Pathogenesis."
8. Bürk et al., "Neurological Symptoms in Patients."

Chapter 19 – The Gluten-Free Lifestyle: Say It with a Smile

1. Fine, "Can I Have Gluten?"
2. Biagi et al., "A Milligram of Gluten."
3. Waldo, "Iron-deficiency Anemia," quoted in Annibale et al., "Efficacy of Gluten-free."
4. Holmes et al., "Malignancy in Coeliac."
5. Jones, D'Souza, and Habouri, "Patterns of Clinical Presentation."
6. See and Murray, "Gluten-free Diet."
7. Pietzak, "Follow-up of Patients."
8. Vahedi et al., "Reliability of Antitransglutaminase Antibodies."
9. Purnak et al., "Mean Platelet Volume."
10. Yachha and Poddar, "Celiac Disease in India."
11. Lee et al., "Duodenal Histology in Patients."

Chapter 20 – One Bite at a Time

1. Gluten Intolerance Group, "Gluten-Free Food Service."

Chapter 21 – Dairy, Dairy, Quite Contrary

1. Volta et al., "Antibodies to Dietary Antigens."
2. Watt, Pincott, and Harries, "Combined Cow's Milk."
3. Ibid.
4. Caffarelli et al., "Cow's Milk Protein Allergy."
5. Smerud et al., "Gastrointestinal Sensitivity to Soy."
6. Konic-Ristic et al., "Different Levels of Humoral."
7. Crowley et al., "Evidence for a Role."
8. Lidén et al., "Cow's Milk Protein Sensitivity."
9. Kristjánsson, Venge, and Hällgren, "Mucosal Reactivity to Cow's."
10. Kagalwalla et al., "Cow's Milk Protein-induced."
11. Kuitunen et al., "Malabsorption Syndrome."
12. Muscari et al., "Association of Serum IgA."
13. Leffler, "Celiac Disease Management," 10.

Bibliography

Abenavoli, L., I. Proietti, L. Leggio, A. Ferrulli, L. Vonghia, R. Capizzi, M. Rotoli, P. L. Amerio, G. Gasbarrini, and G. Addolorato. "Cutaneous Manifestations in Celiac Disease." *World Journal Gastroenterology* 12, no. 6 (2006): 843–52.

Acquaviva, A., G. Municchi, S. Marconcini, A. D'Ambrosio, and G. Morgese. "Celiac Disease in a Patient with [beta]-Thalassemia Major." *Journal of Pediatric Gastroenterology and Nutrition* 36, no. 4 (2003): 489–91.

Addolorato, G., E. Capristo, G. Ghittoni, C. Valeri, R. Mascianà, C. Ancona, and G. Gasbarrini. "Anxiety but Not Depression Decreases in Coeliac Patients after One-year Gluten-free Diet: A Longitudinal Study." *Scandinavian Journal of Gastroenterology* 36, no. 5 (2001): 502–6.

Addolorato, G., A. Parente, G. de Lorenzi, M. E. D'angelo Di Paola, L. Abenavoli, L. Leggio, E. Capristo et al. "Rapid Regression of Psoriasis in a Coeliac Patient After Gluten-free Diet. A Case Report and Review of the Literature." *Digestion* 68, no. 1 (2003): 9–12.

Agardh, D. "Antibodies Against Synthetic Deamidated Gliadin Peptides and Tissue Transglutaminase for the Identification of Childhood Celiac Disease." *Clinical Gastroenterology and Hepatology* 5, no. 11 (2007): 1276–81.

Aguiar, F. M., S. B. Melo, L. C. Galvão, J. C. Rosa-e-Silva, R. M. dos Reis, and R. A. Ferriani. "Serological Testing for Celiac Disease in Women with Endometriosis. A Pilot Study." *Clinical and Experimental Obstetrics and Gynecology* 36, no. 1 (2009): 23–25.

Ahluwalia, M., V. Gotlieb, V. Damerla, and M. W. Saif. "Aggressive Burkitt-like Lymphoma of Colon in a Patient with Prior Celiac Disease." *Yale Journal of Biology and Medicine* 79, no. 3–4 (2006): 173–75.

Al Furaikh, S., and A. A. Al Zaben. "Recurrent Small Bowel Intussusceptions: An Uncommon Presentation of Celiac Disease in an Arab Child." *Tropical Gastroenterology* 26, no. 1 (2005): 38–39.

Al-Mayouf, S. M., A. I. Al-Mehaidib, and M. A. Alkaff. "The Significance of Elevated Serologic Markers of Celiac Disease in Children with Juvenile Rheumatoid Arthritis." *Saudi Journal of Gastroenterology* 9, no. 2 (2003): 75–78.

Alaedini, A., and P. H. Green. "Autoantibodies in Celiac Disease." *Autoimmunity* 41, no. 1 (2008): 19–26.

Alkhateeb, A., P. R. Fain, A. Thody, D. C. Bennett, and R. A. Spritz. "Epidemiology of Vitiligo and Associated Autoimmune Diseases in Caucasian Probands and Their Families." *Pigment Cell Research* 16, no. 3 (2003): 208–14.

American Autoimmune Related Disease Association, Inc. "A Question to Explore: How Do We Count the Cost of Autoimmune Disease? What are Some Numbers?" http://www.aarda.org/infocus_article.php?ID=74 (accessed April 10, 2012).

American Diabetes Association. "Diabetes Statistics: Data from the 2011 National Diabetes Fact Sheet." (released Jan. 26, 2011). http://www.diabetes.org/diabetes-basics/diabetes-statistics/ (accessed April 11, 2012).

Anderson, L. A., R. M. Pfeiffer, O. Landgren, S. Gadalla, S. I. Berndt, and E. A. Engels. "Risks of Myeloid Malignancies in Patients with Autoimmune Conditions." *British Journal of Cancer* 100, no. 5 (2009): 822–28.

Anjum, N., P. N. Baker, N. J. Robinson, and J. D. Aplin. "Maternal Celiac Disease Autoantibodies Bind Directly to Syncytiotrophoblast and Inhibit Placental Tissue Transglutaminase Activity." *Reproductive Biology and Endocrinology* 7 (2009): 16.

Annibale, B., C. Severi, A. Chistolini, G. Antonelli, E. Lahner, A. Marcheggiano, C. Iannoni, B. Monarca, and G. Delle Fave. "Efficacy of Gluten-free Diet Alone on Recovery from Iron Deficiency Anemia in Adult Celiac Patients." *American Journal of Gastroenterology* 96, no. 1 (2001): 132–37.

Arroyave, C. M. [Recurrent Otitis Media with Effusion and Food Allergy in Pediatric Patients.] [In Spanish.] *Revista Alergia Mexico* 48, no. 5 (2001): 141–44.

Aszalós, Z. [Neurological and Psychiatric Aspects of Some Gastrointestinal Diseases.] [In Hungarian.] *Orvosi Hetilap* 149, no. 44 (2008): 2079–86.

Atikou, A., M. Rabhi, H. Hidani, M. El Alaoui Faris, and F. Toloune. [Celiac Crisis with Quadriplegia Due to Potassium Depletion as Presenting Feature of Celiac Disease.] [In French.] *Revue de Medecine Interne* 30, no. 6 (2009): 516–18.

Atladóttir, H.O., M. G. Pedersen, P. Thorsen, P. B. Mortensen, B. Deleuran, W. W. Eaton, and E. T. Parner. "Association of Family History of Autoimmune Diseases and Autism Spectrum Disorders." *Pediatrics* 124, no. 2 (2009): 687–94.

Audia, S., C. Duchêne, M. Samson, G. Muller, P. Bielefeld, F. Ricolfi, M. Giroud, and J. F. Besancenot. [Stroke in Young Adults with Celiac Disease.] [In French.] *Revue of Medecine Interne* 29, no. 3 (2008): 228–31.

Barbero Villares, A., J. A. Moreno Monteagudo, R. Moreno Borque, and R. Moreno Otero. [Hepatic Involvement in Celiac Disease.] [In Spanish.] *Journal of Gastroenterology and Hepatology* 31, no. 1 (2008): 25–28.

Bardella, M. T., L. Elli, P. Velio, C. Fredella, L. Prampolini, and B. Cesana. "Silent Celiac Disease is Frequent in the Siblings of Newly Diagnosed Celiac Patients." *Digestion* 75, no. 4 (2007): 182–87.

Barera, G., E. Bazzigaluppi, M. Viscardi, F. Renzetti, C. Bianchi, G. Chiumello, and E. Bosi. "Macroamylasemia Attributable to Gluten-related Amylase Autoantibodies: A Case Report." *Pediatrics* 107, no. 6 (2001): E93.

Barera, G., R. Bonfanti, M. Viscardi, E. Bazzigaluppi, G. Calori, F. Meschi, C. Bianchi, and G. Chiumello. "Occurrence of Celiac Disease After Onset of Type 1 Diabetes: A 6-year Prospective Longitudinal Study." *Pediatrics* 109, no. 5 (2002): 833–38.

Barker, J.M. "Clinical Review: Type 1 Diabetes-associated Autoimmunity: Natural History, Genetic Associations, and Screening." *Journal of Clinical Endocrinology and Metabolism* 91, no. 4 (2006): 1210–17.

Baryshnikov, E. N., L. M. Krums, N. N. Vorob'eva, and A. I. Parfenov. [Lower Extremity Deep Vein Thrombosis Associated with Gluten-sensitivity Celiac Disease.] [In Russian.] *Terapevticheskii ArkhivTerapevticheskii Arkhiv* 82, no. 2 (2010): 52–54.

Basso, D., G. Guariso, P. Fogar, A. Meneghel, C. F. Zambon, F. Navaglia, E. Greco, S. Schiavon, M. Rugge, and M. Plebani. "Antibodies Against Synthetic Deamidated Gliadin Peptides for Celiac Disease Diagnosis and Follow-up in Children." *Clinical Chemistry* 55, no. 1 (2009): 150–57.

Beck, Melinda. *Wall Street Journal.* "Clues to Gluten Sensitivity." March 15, 2011. http://online.wsj.com/article/SB10001424052748704893604576200393522456636.html#articleTabs%3Darticle (accessed March 18, 2011).

Benito Conejero, S., C. Díaz Espejo, J. M. López Domínguez, and E. Pujol de la Llave. [Cerebral Calcifications: A Clue for a Diagnostic Process in a Nonspecific Clinical Case.] [In Spanish.] *Anales de Medicina Interna* 23, no. 3 (2006): 127–29.

Béchade, D., J. Desramé, G. De Fuentès, P. Camparo, J. J. Raynaud, and J. P. Algayres. [Common Variable Immunodeficiency and Celiac Disease.] [In French.] *Gastroenterologie Clinique et Biologique* 28, no. 10 pt. 1 (2004): 909–12.

Berni Canani, R., S. Ruotolo, V. Discepolo, and R. Troncone. "The Diagnosis of Food Allergy in Children." *Current Opinion in Pediatrics* 20, no. 5 (2008): 584–89.

Betterle, C., F. Lazzarotto, A. C. Spadaccino, D. Basso, M. Plebani, B. Pedini, S. Chiarelli, and M. Albergoni. "Celiac Disease in North Italian Patients with Autoimmune Addison's Disease." *European Journal of Endocrinology* 154, no. 2 (2006): 275–79.

Bhatia, K. P., P. Brown, R. Gregory, G. G. Lennox, H. Manji, P. D. Thompson, D. W. Ellison, and C. D. Marsden. "Progressive Myoclonic Ataxia Associated with Coeliac Disease. The Myoclonus Is of Cortical Origin, but the Pathology Is in the Cerebellum." *Brain* 118, pt. 5 (1995): 1087–93.

Biagi, F., J. Campanella, S. Martucci, D. Pezzimenti, P. J. Ciclitira, H. J. Ellis, and G. R. Corazza. "A Milligram of Gluten a Day Keeps the Mucosal Recovery Away: A Case Report." *Nutrition Review* 62, no. 9 (2004): 360–63.

Biagi, F., O. Luinetti, J. Campanella, C. Klersy, C. Zambelli, V. Villanacci, A. Lanzini, and G. R. Corazza. "Intraepithelial Lymphocytes in the Villous Tip: Do They Indicate Potential Coeliac Disease?" *Journal of Clinical Pathology* 57, no. 8 (2004): 835–39.

Bianchi, M. L., and M. T. Bardella. "Bone in Celiac Disease. Review" *Osteoporosis International* 19, no. 12 (2008): 1705–16.

Bilello, G., C. Ciulla, and C. Caradonna. [Celiac Disease and Malocclusion.] [In Italian.] *Recenti Progressi in Medicina* 101, no. 4 (2010): 159–62.

Bilic, E., E. Bilic, B. I. Sepec, D. Vranjes, M. Zagar, V. Butorac, and D. Cerimagic. "Stiff-person Syndrome in a Female Patient with Type 1 Diabetes, Dermatitis Herpetiformis, Celiac Disease, Microcytic Anemia and Copper Deficiency. Just a Coincidence or an Additional Shared Pathophysiological Mechanism?" *Clinical Neurology and Neurosurgery* 111, no. 7 (2009): 644–45.

Binder, H. J., W. M. O'Brien, H. M. Spiro, and J. W. Hollingsworth. "Gluten and the Small Intestine in Rheumatoid Arthritis." *Journal of American Medical Association* 195, no. 10 (1966): 857–58.

Birlea, S. A., P. R. Fain, and R. A. Spritz. "A Romanian Population Isolate with High Frequency of Vitiligo and Associated Autoimmune Diseases." *Archives of Dermatology* 144, no. 3 (2008): 310–16.

Birring, S., R. Patel, D. Parker, S. Mckenna, B. Hargadon, W. Monteiro, S. Falconer, and I. Pavord. "Airway Function and Markers of Airway Inflammation in Patients with Treated Hypothyroidism." *Thorax* 60, no. 3 (2005): 249–53.

Bittner, C., B. Grassau, K. Frenzel, and X. Baur. "Identification of Wheat Gliadins as an Allergen Family Related to Baker's Asthma." *Journal of Allergy and Clinical Immunology* 121, no. 3 (2008): 744–49.

Biyikli, N. K., I. Gökçe, F. Cakalağoğlu, S. Arbak, and H. Alpay. "The Co-existence of Membranoproliferative Glomerulonephritis Type 1 and Coeliac Disease: A Case Report." *Pediatric Nephrology* 24, no. 6 (2009): 1247–50.

Bizzaro, N. "The Predictive Significance of Autoantibodies in Organ-specific Autoimmune Diseases." *Clinical Reviews in Allergy and Immunology* 34, no. 3 (2008): 326–31.

Black's Medical Dictionary. 42nd edition edited by Dr. Harvey Marcovitch. London: A & C Black Publishers, 2010.

Bonamico, M., R. Nenna, M. Montuori, R. P. Luparia, A. Turchetti, M. Mennini, F. Lucantoni et al. "First Salivary Screening of Celiac Disease by Detection of Anti-transglutaminase Autoantibody Radioimmunoassay in 5000 Italian Primary Schoolchildren." *Journal of Pediatric Gastroenterology and Nutrition* 52, no. 1 (2011): 17–20.

Braly, James, and Ron Hoggan. *Dangerous Grains: Why Gluten Cereal Grains May Be Hazardous To Your Health.* New York: Avery, 2002.

Braly, James. *Gluten Sensitivity, Coeliac Disease and Chronic Brain Syndromes.* http://www.scribd.com/amy_henderson_22/d/54268450-Celiac (accessed January 21, 2012).

Brandimarte, G., A. Tursi, and G. M. Giorgetti. "Changing Trends in Clinical Form of Celiac Disease. Which is Now the Main Form of Celiac Disease in Clinical Practice?" *Minerva Gastroenterologica e Dietologica* 48, no. 2 (2002): 121–30.

Brightling, C. E., F. A. Symon, S. S. Birring, A. J. Wardlaw, R. Robinson, and I. D. Pavord. "A Case of Cough, Lymphocytic Bronchoalveolitis and Coeliac Disease with Improvement Following a Gluten Free Diet." *Thorax* 57, no. 1 (2002): 91–92.

Brottveit, M., and K. E. Lundin. [Cancer Risk in Coeliac Disease.] [In Norweigen.] *Tidsskrift For Den Norske Laegeforening* 128, no. 20 (2008): 2312–15.

Brown, K. J., V. Jewells, H. Herfarth, and M. Castillo. "White Matter Lesions Suggestive of Amyotrophic Lateral Sclerosis Attributed to Celiac Disease." *American Journal of Neuroradiology* 31, no. 5 (2010): 880–81.

Bürk, K., S. Bösch, C. A. Müller, A. Melms, C. Zühlke, M. Stern, I. Besenthal et al. "Sporadic Cerebellar Ataxia Associated with Gluten Sensitivity." *Brain* 124, pt. 5 (2001): 1013–19.

Bürk, K., M. L. Farecki, G. Lamprecht, G. Roth, P. Decker, M. Weller, H. G. Rammensee, and W. Oertel. "Neurological Symptoms in Patients with Biopsy Proven Celiac Disease." *Movement Disorders* 24, no. 16 (2009): 2358–62.

Bures, J., J. Cyrany, D. Kohoutova, M. Förstl, S. Rejchrt, J. Kvetina, V. Vorisek, and M. Kopacova. "Small Intestinal Bacterial Overgrowth Syndrome." *World Journal of Gastroenterology* 16, no. 24 (2010): 2978–90.

Bushara, K. O. "Neurologic Presentation of Celiac Disease." *Gastroenterology* 128, no. 4 suppl. no. 1 (2005): S92–97.

Bushara, K. O., M. Nance, and C. M. Gomez. "Antigliadin Antibodies in Huntington's Disease." *Neurology* 62, no. 1 (2004): 132–33.

Byrne, M. F., A. R. Razak, M. B. Leader, K. M. Sheehan, and S. E. Patchett. "Disabling Osteomalacic Myopathy as the Only Presenting Feature of Coeliac Disease." *European Journal of Gastroenterology and Hepatology* 14, no. 11 (2002): 1271–74.

Cade, R., M. Privette, M. Fregly, N. Rowland, Z. Sun, V. Zele, H. Wagemaker, and C. Edelstein. "Autism and Schizophrenia: Intestinal Disorders." *Nutritional Neuroscience* 3, no. 1 (2000): 57–72.

Caffarelli, C., F. Baldi, B. Bendandi, L. Calzone, M. Marani, and P. Pasquinelli. "Cow's Milk Protein Allergy in Children: A Practical Guide." *Italian Journal of Pediatrics* 36 (2010): 5.

Caja, S., M. Mäki, K. Kaukinen, and K. Lindfors. "Antibodies in Celiac Disease: Implications Beyond Diagnostics." *Cellular and Molecular Immunology* 8 (2011): 103–9.

Callejas Rubio, J. L., N. Ortego, A. Diez-Ruiz, J. Guilarte, and J. De la Higuera-Iorres. "Celiac Disease Presenting as Chronic Anemia Associated with Heart Block." *American Journal of Gastroenterology* 93 (1998): 1391–92.

Cameron, E. A., J. A. Stewart, K. P. West, and B. J. Rathbone. "Coeliac Disease Presenting with Intraperitoneal Haemorrhage." *European Journal of Gastroenterology and Hepatology* 10, no. 7 (1998): 619–20.

Campisi, G., C. Di Liberto, A. Carroccio, D. Compilato, G. Iacono, M. Procaccini, G. Di Fede et al. "Coeliac Disease: Oral Ulcer Prevalence, Assessment of Risk and Association with Gluten-free Diet in Children." *Digestive and Liver Diseases* 40, no. 2 (2008): 104–7.

Canales, P., V. P. Mery, F. J. Larrondo, F. L. Bravo, and J. Godoy. "Epilepsy and Celiac Disease: Favorable Outcome with a Gluten-free Diet in a Patient Refractory to Antiepileptic Drugs." *Neurologist* 12, no. 6 (2006): 318–21.

Caprai, S., P. Vajro, A. Ventura, M. Sciveres, and G. Maggiore. "Autoimmune Liver Disease Associated with Celiac Disease in Childhood: A Multicenter Study." *Clinical Gastroenterology and Hepatology* 6, no. 7 (2008): 803–6.

Capriles, V. D., L. A. Martini, and J. A. Arêas. "Metabolic Osteopathy in Celiac Disease: Importance of a Gluten-free Diet." *Nutrition Reviews* 67, no. 10 (2009): 599–606.

Caputo, I., M. V. Barone, S Martucciello, M. Lepretti, and C. Esposito. "Transglutaminase in Celiac Disease: Role of Autoantibodies." *Amino Acids* 36, no. 4 (2009): 693–99.

Carroccio, A., I. Brusca, G. Iacono, M. G. Alessio, A. Sonzogni, L. Di Prima, M. Barrale et al. "IgA Anti-actin Antibodies ELISA in Coeliac Disease: A Multicentre Study." *Digestive and Liver Disease* 39, no. 9 (2007): 818–23.

Carroccio, A., I. Brusca, P. Mansueto, M. Soresi, A. D'Alcamo, G. Ambrosiano, I Pepe et al., "Fecal Assays Detect Hypersensitivity to Cow's Milk Protein and Gluten in Adults with Irritable Bowel Syndrome." *Clinical Gastroenterology and Hepatology* 9, no. 11 (2011): 965–71.

Carroccio, A., L. Di Prima, C. Scalici, M. Soresi, A. B. Cefalù, D. Noto, M. R. Averna, G. Montalto, and G. Iacono. "Unexplained Elevated Serum Pancreatic Enzymes: A Reason to Suspect Celiac Disease." *Clinical Gastroenterology and Hepatology* 4, no. 4 (2006): 455–59.

Carroccio, A., L. Giannitrapani, L. Di Prima, E. Iannitto, G. Montalto, and A. Notarbartolo. "Extreme Thrombocytosis as a Sign of Coeliac Disease in the Elderly: Case Report." *European Journal of Gastroenterology and Hepatology* 14, no. 8 (2002): 897–900.

Carta, M. G., M. C. Hardoy, M. F. Boi, S. Mariotti, B. Carpiniello, and P. Usai. "Association between Panic Disorder, Major Depressive Disorder and Celiac Disease: A Possible Role of Thyroid Autoimmunity." *Journal of Psychosomatic Research* 55, no. 6 (2003): 573–74.

Cascella, N. G., D. Kryszak, B. Bhatti, P. Gregory, D. L. Kelly, J. P. McEvoy, A. Fasano, and W. W. Eaton. "Prevalence of Celiac Disease and Gluten Sensitivity in the United States Clinical Antipsychotic Trials of Intervention Effectiveness Study Population." *Schizophrenia Bulletin* 37, no. 1 (2011): 94–100.

Casswall, T. H., N. Papadogiannakis, S. Ghazi, and A. Németh. "Severe Liver Damage Associated with Celiac Disease: Findings in Six Toddler-aged Girls." *European Journal of Gastroenterology and Hepatology* 21, no. 4 (2009): 452–59.

Catassi, C., I. Bearzi, and G. K. Holmes. "Association of Celiac Disease and Intestinal Lymphomas and Other Cancers." *Gastroenterology* 128, no. 4 suppl. no. 1 (2005): S79–86.

Catassi, C., and A. Fasano. "Celiac Disease Diagnosis: Simple Rules are Better Than Complicated Algorithms." *American Journal of Medicine* 123, no. 8 (2010): 691–93.

Catassi, C., D. Kryszak, O. Louis-Jacques, D. R. Duerksen, I. Hill, S. E. Crowe, A. R. Brown et al. "Detection of Celiac Disease in Primary Care: A Multicenter Case-finding Study in North America." *American Journal of Gastroenterology* 102, no. 7 (2007): 1456–60.

Celiac Sprue Association. "Celiac Disease Facts: What Is the Impact of Celiac Disease?" http://www.csaceliacs.info/diagnosis_of_celiac_disease_fact_sheet.jsp (accessed February 2, 2012). Extracted from "Canadian Celiac Health Survey" published in 2007.

Cervin, C., V. Lyssenko, E. Bakhtadze, E. Lindholm, P. Nilsson, T. Tuomi, C. M. Cilio, and L. Groop. "Genetic Similarities between Latent Autoimmune Diabetes in Adults, Type 1 Diabetes, and Type 2 Diabetes." *Diabetes* 57, no. 5 (2008): 1433–37.

Cheng, J., P. S. Brar, A. R. Lee, and P. H. Green. "Body Mass Index in Celiac Disease: Beneficial Effect of a Gluten-free Diet." *Journal of Clinical Gastroenterology* 44, no. 4 (2010): 267–71.

Cheng, J., T. Malahias, P. Brar, M. T. Minaya, and P. H. Green. "The Association between Celiac Disease, Dental Enamel Defects, and Aphthous Ulcers in a United States Cohort." *Journal of Clinical Gastroenterology* 44, no. 3 (2010): 191–94.

Chiaravalloti, G., A. Baracchini, V. Rossomando, C. Ughi, and M. Ceccarelli. [Celiac Disease and Cystic Fibrosis: Casual Association?] [In Italian.]*Minerva Pediatrica* 47, nos. 1-2 (1995): 23–26.

Chin, R. L., H. W. Sander, T. H. Brannagan, P. H. Green, A. P. Hays, A. Alaedini, and N. Latov. "Celiac Neuropathy." *Neurology* 60, no. 10 (2003): 1581–85.

Ch'ng, C. L., M. Biswas, A. Benton, M. K. Jones, and J. G. Kingham. "Prospective Screening for Coeliac Disease in Patients with Graves' Hyperthyroidism Using Anti-gliadin and Tissue Transglutaminase Antibodies." *Clinical Endocrinology* 62, no. 3 (2005): 303–6.

Ch'ng, C. L., M. K. Jones, and J. G. Kingham. "Celiac Disease and Autoimmune Thyroid Disease." *Clinical Medicine and Research* 5, no. 3 (2007): 184–92.

Ciacci, C., D. Gennarelli, G. Esposito, R. Tortora, F. Salvatore, and L. Sacchetti. "Hereditary Fructose Intolerance and Celiac Disease: A Novel Genetic Association." *Clinical Gastroenterology and Hepatology* 4, no. 5 (2006): 635–38.

Cicarelli, G., G. Della Rocca, M. Amboni, C. Ciacci, G. Mazzacca, A. Filla, and P. Baron. "Clinical and Neurological Abnormalities in Adult Celiac Disease." *Neurological Science* 24, no. 5 (2003): 311–17.

Clemente, M. G., M. P. Musu, F. Frau, G. Brusco, G. Sole, G. R. Corazza, and S. De Virgiliis. "Immune Reaction Against the Cytoskeleton in Coeliac Disease." *Gut* 2000 47, no. 4 (2000): 520–26.

Coenen, M. J., G. Trynka, S. Heskamp, B. Franke, C.C. van Diemen, J. Smolonska, M. van Leeuwen et al. "Common and Different Genetic Background for Rheumatoid Arthritis and Coeliac Disease." *Human Molecular Genetics* 18, no. 21 (2009): 4195–4203.

Cohan, Wendy. *The Better Bladder Book: A Holistic Approach to Healing Interstitial Cystitis and Chronic Pelvic Pain.* Alameda, California: Hunter House Publishing, 2010.

Collin, P., K. Kaukinen, M. Välimäki, and J. Salmi. "Endocrinological Disorders and Celiac Disease." *Endocrine Reviews* 23, no. 4 (2002): 464–83.

Collin, P., E. Pukkala, and T. Reunala. "Malignancy and Survival in Dermatitis Herpetiformis: A Comparison with Coeliac Disease." *Gut* 38, no. 4 (1996): 528–30.

Collin, P., and T. Reunala. "Recognition and Management of the Cutaneous Manifestations of Celiac Disease: A Guide for Dermatologists." *American Journal of Clinical Dermatology* 4, no. 1 (2003): 13–20.

Cooper, S. M., I. Ali, M. Baldo, and F. Wojnarowska. "The Association of Lichen Sclerosus and Erosive Lichen Planus of the Vulva with Autoimmune Disease: A Case-control Study." *Archives of Dermatology* 144, no. 11 (2008): 1432–35.

Coppen, A., and C. Bolander-Gouaille. "Treatment of Depression: Time to Consider Folic Acid and Vitamin B12." *Journal of Psychopharmacology* 19, no. 1 (2005): 59–65.

Corazza, G. R., M. L. Andreani, N. Venturo, M. Bernardi, A. Tosti, and G. Gasbarrini. "Celiac Disease and Alopecia Areata: Report of a New Association." *Gastroenterology* 109, no. 4 (1995): 1333–37.

Corazza, G. R., M. Frisoni, D. Vaira, and G. Gasbarrini. "Effect of Gluten-free Diet on Splenic Hypofunction of Adult Coeliac Disease." *Gut* 24, no. 3 (1983): 228–30.

Corvaglia L., R. Catamo, G. Pepe, R. Lazzari, and E. Corvaglia. "Depression in Adult Untreated Celiac Subjects: Diagnosis by the Pediatrician." *American Journal of Gastroenterology* 94, no. 3 (1999): 839–43.

Cottafava, F., and D. Cosso. [Psoriatic Arthritis and Celiac Disease in Childhood. A Case Report.] [In Italian.] *Pediatria Medica e Chirurgica* 13, no. 4 (1991): 431–33.

Cottone M., C. Marrone, A. Casà, L. Oliva, A. Orlando, E. Calabrese, G. Martorana, and L. Pagliaro. "Familial Occurrence of Inflammatory Bowel Disease in Celiac Disease." *Inflammatory Bowel Diseases* 9, no. 5 (2003): 321–23.

Croese, J., O. Harris, and B. Bain. "Coeliac Disease. Haematological Features, and Delay in Diagnosis." *Medical Journal of Australia* 2, no. 7 (1979): 335–38.

Crowley, E., L. Williams, T. Roberts, P. Jones, and R. Dustan. "Evidence for a Role of Cow's Milk Consumption in Chronic Functional Constipation in Children: Systematic Review of the Literature from 1980 to 2006." *Nutrition and Dietetics* 65, no. 1 (2008): 29–35.

Cuoco, L., G. Cammarota, R. A. Jorizzo, L. Santarelli, R. Cianci, M. Montalto, A. Gasbarrini, and G. Gasbarrini. "Link between Helicobacter Pylori Infection and Iron-deficiency Anaemia in Patients with Coeliac Disease." *Scandinavian Journal of Gastroenterology* 36, no. 12 (2001): 1284–88.

Curione, M., M. Barbato, F. Viola, P. Francia, L. De Biase, and S. Cucchiara. "Idiopathic Dilated Cardiomyopathy Associated with Coeliac Disease: The Effect of a Gluten-free Diet on Cardiac Performance." *Digestive and Liver Disease* 34, no. 12 (2002): 866–69.

Daher, R., T. Yazbeck, J. B. Jaoude, and B. Abboud. "Consequences of Dysthyroidism on the Digestive Tract and Viscera." *World Journal of Gastroenterology* 15, no. 23 (2009): 2834–38.

Danese, S., S. Semeraro, A. Papa, I. Roberto, F. Scaldaferri, G. Fedeli, G. Gasbarrini, and A. Gasbarrini. "Extraintestinal Manifestations in Inflammatory Bowel Disease." *World Journal of Gastroenterology* 11, no. 46 (2005): 7227–36.

Davis, William. *Wheat Belly: Lose the Wheat, Lose the Weight, and Find Your Path Back to Health.* New York: Rodale, 2011.

De Bellis, A., A. Colao, G. Tirelli, G. Ruocco, C. Di Somma, M. Battaglia, E. Pane et al. "Autoimmunity As a Possible Cause of Growth Hormone Deficiency." *Journal of Endocrinological Investigation* 31, no. 12 (2008): 1132–44.

Delalande, S., J. de Seze, A. L. Fauchais, E. Hachulla, T. Stojkovic, D. Ferriby, S. Dubucquoi, J. P. Pruvo, P. Vermersch, and P. Y. Hatron. "Neurologic Manifestations in Primary Sjögren Syndrome: A Study of 82 Patients." *Medicine* 83, no. 5 (2004): 280–91.

Delvecchio, M., A. De Bellis, R. Francavilla, V. Rutigliano, B. Predieri, F. Indrio, D. De Venuto et al. "Anti-pituitary Antibodies in Children with Newly Diagnosed Celiac Disease: A Novel Finding Contributing to Linear-growth Impairment." *American Journal of Gastroenterology* 105, no. 3 (2010): 691–96.

Deprez, P. H., C. Sempoux, C. De Saeger, J. Rahier, P. Mainguet, S. Pauwels, and A. Geubel. "Expression of Cholecystokinin in the Duodenum of Patients with Coeliac Disease: Respective Role of Atrophy and Lymphocytic Infiltration." Clinical Science 103, no. 2 (2002): 171–77.

Di Simone, N., M. Silano, R. Castellani, F. Di Nicuolo, M. C. D'Alessio, F. Franceschi, A. Tritarelli et al. "Anti-tissue Transglutaminase Antibodies from Celiac Patients are Responsible for Trophoblast Damage Via Apoptosis in Vitro." *American Journal of Gastroenterology* 105, no. 10 (2010): 2254–61.

Di Tola, M., L. Sabbatella, M. C. Anania, A. Viscido, R. Caprilli, R. Pica, and P. Paoluzi. "Anti-tissue Transglutaminase Antibodies in Inflammatory Bowel Disease: New Evidence." *Clinical Chemistry and Laboratory Medicine* 42, no. 10 (2004): 1092–97.

Díaz, R. M., G. González-Rabelino, and A. Delfino. [Epilepsy, Cerebral Calcifications and Coeliac Disease. The Importance of an Early Diagnosis.] [In Spanish.] *Revue Neurologique* 40, no. 7 (2005): 417–20.

Dickerson F., C. Stallings, A. Origoni, C. Vaughan, S. Khushalani, F. Leister, S. Yang, B. Krivogorsky, A. Alaedini, and R. Yolken. "Markers of Gluten Sensitivity and Celiac Disease in Recent-onset Psychosis and Multi-episode Schizophrenia." *Biological Psychiatry* 68, no. 1 (2010): 100–104.

Dickey, W., and D. Hughes. "Prevalence of Celiac Disease and Its Endoscopic Markers among Patients Having Routine Upper Gastrointestinal Endoscopy." *American Journal of Gastroenterology* 94, no. 8 (1999): 2182–86.

Dickey, W., D. F. Hughes, and S. A. McMillan. "Reliance on Serum Endomysial Antibody Testing Underestimates the True Prevalence of Coeliac Disease by One Fifth." *Scandinavian Journal of Gastroenterology* 35, no. 2 (2000): 181–83.

Dickey, W., M. Ward, C. R. Whittle, M. T. Kelly, K. Pentieva, G. Horigan, S. Patton, and H. McNulty. "Homocysteine and Related B-vitamin Status in Coeliac Disease: Effects of Gluten Exclusion and Histological Recovery." *Scandinavian Journal of Gastroenterology* 43, no. 6 (2008): 682–88.

Dietrich W., and F. Erbguth. [Neurological Complications of Inflammatory Intestinal Diseases.] [In German.] *Fortschritte der Neurologie-Psychiatrie* 71, no. 8 (2003): 406–14.

Dillmann, W. "Cardiac Hypertrophy and Thyroid Hormone Signaling." *Heart Failure Reviews* 15, no. 2 (2010): 125–32.

Djuric, Z., B. Kamenov, and V. Katic. "Celiac Disease Manifested by Polyneuropathy and Swollen Ankles." *World Journal of Gastroenterology* 13, no. 18 (2007): 2636–38.

Djuric, Z., S. Zivic, and V. Katic. "Celiac Disease with Diffuse Cutaneous Vitamin K-deficiency Bleeding." *Advances in Therapy* 24, no. 6 (2007): 1286–89.

Dogan, M., E. Sal, S. Akbayram, E. Peker, Y. Cesur, and A. F. Oner. "Concurrent Celiac Disease, Idiopathic Thrombocytopenic Purpura and Autoimmune Thyroiditis: A Case Report." *Clinical and Applied Thrombosis/Hemostasis* 17, no.6 (2011): E13–16.

Dohan, F. C., "Genetic Hypothesis of Idiopathic Schizophrenia: Its Exorphin Connection." *Schizophrenia Bulletin* 14, no. 4 (1988): 489–94.

Dohan, F. C., E. H. Harper, M. H. Clark, R. B. Rodrigue, and V. Zigas. "Is Schizophrenia Rare If Grain Is Rare?" *Biological Psychiatry* 19, no. 3 (1984): 385–99.

Donaldson, M. S., N. Speight, and S. Loomis. "Fibromyalgia Syndrome Improved Using a Mostly Raw Vegetarian Diet: An Observational Study." *BioMedCentral Complementary and Alternative Medicine* 1 (2001): 7.

Drago, S., R. El Asmar, M. Di Pierro, M. Grazia Clemente, A. Tripathi, A. Sapone, M. Thakari et al. "Gliadin, Zonulin and Gut Permeability: Effects on Celiac and Non-celiac Intestinal Mucosa and Intestinal Cell Lines." *Scandinavian Journal of Gastroenterology* 41 (2006): 408–19.

Dreifus, Claudia. "Living and Studying Alopecia." *New York Times,* December 27, 2010. http://www.nytimes.com/2010/12/28/science/28conversation.html?_r=2 (accessed February 22, 2011).

Drut, R., and R. M. Drut. "Lymphocytic Gastritis in Pediatric Celiac Disease – Immunohistochemical Study of the Intraepithelial Lymphocytic Component." *Medical Science Monitor* 10, no. 1 (2004): CR38–42.

Duerksen, D. R., C. Wilhelm-Boyles, R. Veitch, D. Kryszak, and D. M. Parry. "A Comparison of Antibody Testing, Permeability Testing, and Zonulin Levels with Small-bowel Biopsy in Celiac Disease Patients on a Gluten-free Diet." *Digestive Diseases and Sciences* 55, no. 4 (2010): 1026–31.

Duggal, J., S. Singh, C. P. Barsano, and R. Arora. "Cardiovascular Risk with Subclinical Hyperthyroidism and Hypothyroidism: Pathophysiology and Management." *Journal of Cardiometabolic Syndrome* 2, no. 3 (2007): 198–206.

Duggan, J. M. "Coeliac Disease: The Great Imitator." *Medical Journal of Australia* 180, no. 10 (2004): 524–26.

Duggan, J. M., and A. E. Duggan. "Systematic Review: The Liver in Coeliac Disease." *Alimentary Pharmacology and Therapeutics* 21, no. 5 (2005): 515–18.

Dupond, J. L., B. de Wazières, F. Flausse-Parrot, T. Fest, G. Morin, F. Closs, and D.Vuitton. "Thrombocytosis of Celiac Disease in Adults: A Diagnostic and Prognostic Marker?" *La Presse Médicale* 22, no. 29 (1993): 1344–46.

Durand, C., S. Mary, P. Brazo, and S. Dollfus. [Psychiatric Manifestations of Vitamin B12 Deficiency: A Case Report.] [In French.] *Encephale* 29, no. 6 (2003): 560–65.

Eaton, W.W., M. Byrne, H. Ewald, O. Mors, C. Y. Chen, E. Agerbo, and P. B. Mortensen. "Association of Schizophrenia and Autoimmune Diseases: Linkage of Danish National Registers." *American Journal of Psychiatry* 163, no. 3 (2006): 521–28.

El Moutawakil, B., N. Chourkani, M. Sibai, F. Moutaouakil, M. Rafai, M. Bourezgui, and I. Slassi. [Celiac Disease and Ischemic Stroke.] [In French.] *Revue Neurologique* 165, no. 11 (2009): 962–66.

Elder, J. H. "The Gluten-free, Casein-free Diet in Autism: An Overview with Clinical Implications." *Nutrition in Clinical Practice* 23, no. 6 (2008): 583–88.

Elfström, P., F. Granath, K. Ekström Smedby, S. M. Montgomery, J Askling, A. Ekbom, and J. F. Ludvigsson. "Risk of Lymphoproliferative Malignancy in Relation to Small Intestinal Histopathology Among Patients With Celiac Disease." *Journal of the National Cancer Institute* 103, no. 5 (2011): 436–44.

Elfström, P., S. M. Montgomery, O. Kämpe, A. Ekbom, and J. F. Ludvigsson. "Risk of Primary Adrenal Insufficiency in Patients with Celiac Disease." *Journal of Clinical Endocrinology and Metabolism* 92, no. 9 (2007): 3595–98.

Elkan, A. C., B. Sjöberg, B. Kolsrud, B. Ringertz, I. Hafström, and J. Frostegård. "Gluten-free Vegan Diet Induces Decreased LDL and Oxidized LDL Levels and Raised Atheroprotective Natural Antibodies against Phosphorylcholine in Patients with Rheumatoid Arthritis: A Randomized Study." *Arthritis Research and Therapy* 10, no. 2 (2008): R34.

Emilsson, L., J. G. Smith, J. West, O. Melander, and J. F. Ludvigsson. "Increased Risk of Atrial Fibrillation in Patients with Coeliac Disease: A Nationwide Cohort Study." *European Heart Journal* 32, no. 19 (2011): 2430–37.

Endometriosis.org. "Dietary Modification to Alleviate Endometriosis Symptoms." http://endometriosis.org/resource/articles/dietary-modification/ (accessed March 9, 2011). Interview between nutritionist Dian Shepperson Mills and Dr. Mark Perloe.

Ertem, D., I. Gonen, C. Tanidir, M. Ugras, A. Yildiz, E. Pehlivanoğlu, and E. Eksioglu-Demiralp. "The Response to Hepatitis B Vaccine: Does It Differ in Celiac Disease?" *European Journal of Gastroenterology and Hepatology* 22, no. 7 (2009): 787–93.

Evans, K. E., J. S. Leeds, S. Morley, and D. S. Sanders. "Pancreatic Insufficiency in Adult Celiac Disease: Do Patients Require Long-term Enzyme Supplementation?" *Digestive Diseases and Sciences* 55, no. 10 (2010): 2999–3004.

Evron, E., J. M. Abarbanel, D. Branski, and Z. M. Sthoeger. "Polymyositis, Arthritis, and Proteinuria in a Patient with Adult Celiac Disease." *Journal of Rheumatology* 23, no. 4 (1996): 782–83.

Falcini, F., R. Ferrari, G. Simonini, G. B. Calabri, A. Pazzaglia, and P. Lionetti. "Recurrent Monoarthritis in an 11-year-old Boy with Occult Coeliac Disease. Successful and Stable Remission After Gluten-free Diet." *Clinical and Experimental Rheumatology* 17, no. 4 (1999): 509–11.

Farber, D., and A. Bitton. "Dermatomyositis and Adult Celiac Disease." *Canadian Journal of Gastroenterology: Canadian Digestive Diseases Week* March 5–12, 2000, no. 061.

Farkas, H., B. Visy, B. Fekete, I. Karádi, J. B. Kovács, I. B. Kovács, L. Kalmár, A. Tordai, and L. Varga. "Association of Celiac Disease and Hereditary Angioneurotic Edema." *American Journal of Gastroenterology* 97, no. 10 (2002): 2682–83.

Fasano, A. "Clinical Presentation of Celiac Disease in the Pediatric Population." *Gastroenterology* 128, no. 4 suppl. no. 1 (2005): S68–73.

Fasano, A. "Zonulin and Its Regulation of Intestinal Barrier Function: The Biological Door to Inflammation, Autoimmunity, and Cancer." *Physiological Reviews* 91, no.1 (2011): 151–75.

Fasano A., I. Berti, T. Gerarduzzi, T. Not, R. B. Colletti, S. Drago, Y. Elitsur et al. "Prevalence of Celiac Disease in At-risk and Not-at-risk Groups in the United States: A Large Multicenter Study." *Archives of Internal Medicine* 163, no. 3 (2003): 286–92.

Fasano, A., and D. Counts. "*Editorial:* Commentary on 'Anti-Pituitary Antibodies in Children With Newly Diagnosed Celiac Disease: A Novel Finding Contributing to Linear Growth.' " *American Journal of Gastroenterology* 105 (2010): 697–98.

Fater-Debska, A., P. Gworys, J. Brzeziński, and Z. Gawor. [Thyrometabolic Disorders and Heart Failure.] [In Polish.] *Endokrynologia Polska* 58, no. 3 (2007): 228–35.

Fawcett, R. S., S. Linford, and D. L. Stulberg. "Nail Abnormalities: Clues to Systemic Disease." *American Family Physician* 69, no. 6 (2004): 1417–24.

Fayed, S.B., M. I. Aref, H. M. Fathy, S. M. Abd El Dayem, N. A. Emara, A. Maklof, and A. Shafik. "Prevalence of Celiac Disease, Helicobacter Pylori and Gastroesophageal Reflux in Patients with Refractory Iron Deficiency Anemia." *Journal of Tropical Pediatrics* 54, no. 1 (2008): 43–53.

Ferrell, Vance. *Arthritis and Rheumaticism.* "47 – The Shatin Research." Harvestime E-Book ed. 28-29 http://www.sdadefend.com/MINDEXResource%20Library/Arthritis.pdf (accessed April 17, 2012).

Fessatou, S., M. Kostaki, and T. Karpathios. "Coeliac Disease and Alopecia Areata in Childhood." *Journal of Paediatrics and Child Health* 39, no. 2 (2003): 152–54.

Fine, Kenneth. "Early Diagnosis of Gluten Sensitivity: Before the Villi are Gone." *EnteroLab.com. FinerHealth.com.*

Fine, Kenneth. "Frequently Asked Questions: Can I Be Tested if I Am Already on a Gluten-free Diet?" *EnteroLab.com.*

Fine, Kenneth. "Frequently Asked Questions: Can I Have Gluten Sensitivity if Screening Blood Tests for Celiac Sprue Are Negative or Indeterminate?" *EnteroLab.com.*

Fine, Kenneth. "Frequently Asked Questions: Do I Have to Be Eating Gluten for a Gluten Antibody Test to Be Positive?" *EnteroLab.com*

Fine, Kenneth. "Welcome to EnteroLab: About Enterolab." *EnteroLab.com.*

Fluge, G., H. V. Olesen, M. Gilljam, P. Meyer, T. Pressler, O. T. Storrösten, F. Karpati, and L. Hjelte. "Co-morbidity of Cystic Fibrosis and Celiac Disease in Scandinavian Cystic Fibrosis Patients." *Journal of Cystic Fibrosis* 8, no. 3 (2009): 198–202.

Ford, Rodney. *The Gluten Syndrome: Is Wheat Causing You Harm?* Christchurch, NZ: RRS Global Ltd., 2007.

Forsgren, Scott. "NeuroImmunology: From Leaky Gut to Leaky Brain." *Public Health Alert.* http://www.publichealthalert.org/Articles/scottforsgren/neuroimmunology.htm (accessed August 1, 2011).

Fraquelli, M., M. Pagliarulo, A. Colucci, S. Paggi, and D. Conte. "Gallbladder Motility in Obesity, Diabetes Mellitus and Coeliac Disease." *Digestive and Liver Disease* 35, suppl. no. 3 (2003): S12–16.

Freeman, H. J., "Hepatobiliary and Pancreatic Disorders in Celiac Disease." *World Journal of Gastroenterology* 12, no. 10 (2006): 1503–8.

Freeman, H. J. "Neurological Disorders in Adult Celiac Disease." *Canadian Journal of Gastroenterology* 22, no. 11 (2008): 909–11.

Freeman, H. J. "Risk Factors in Familial Forms of Celiac Disease." *World Journal of Gastroenterology* 16, no.15 (2010): 1828–31.

Garakani. A., T. Win, S. Virk, S. Gupta, D. Kaplan, and P. S. Masand. "Comorbidity of Irritable Bowel Syndrome in Psychiatric Patients: A Review." *American Journal of Therapy* 10, no. 1 (2003): 61–67.

Gasbarrini, G., N. Malandrino, V. Giorgio, C. Fundarò, G. Cammarota, G. Merra, D. Roccarina, A. Gasbarrini, and E. Capristo. "Celiac Disease: What's New About It?" *Digestive Diseases* 26, no. 2 (2008): 121–27.

Gastroenterology 131, no. 4 (2006). A Journal of the American Gastroenterological Association Institute.

Genuis, S. J., and T. P. Bouchard. "Celiac Disease Presenting as Autism." *Journal of Child Neurology* 25, no. 1 (2010): 114–19.

Ghezzi, A., and M. Ghezzi. "Neurological Manifestations of Gastrointestinal Disorders, with Particular Reference to the Differential Diagnosis of Multiple Sclerosis." *Neurological Science* 22, suppl. 2 (2001): S117–22.

Ghoshal, U. C., U. Ghoshal, A. Misra, and G. Choudhuri. "Partially Responsive Celiac. Disease Resulting from Small Intestinal Bacterial Overgrowth and Lactose Intolerance." *BioMedCentral Gastroenterology* 4 (2004): 10.

Glas, J., J. Stallhofer, S. Ripke, M. Wetzke, S. Pfenning, W. Klein, J. T. Epplen et al. "Novel Genetic Risk Markers for Ulcerative Colitis in the IL2/IL21 Region are in Epistasis with IL23R and Suggest a Common Genetic Background for Ulcerative Colitis and Celiac Disease." *American Journal of Gastroenterology* 104, no. 7 (2009): 1737–44.

Gluten Intolerance Group of North America (GIG). "Gluten-Free Food Service Training & Management Certification (GFFS)." http://www.glutenfree.net/ (accessed September 27, 2013).

Gobbi G. "Coeliac Disease, Epilepsy and Cerebral Calcifications." *Brain and Development* 27, no. 3 (2005): 189–200.

Gobbi, G., P. Ambrosetto, M. G. Zaniboni, A. Lambertini, G. Ambrosioni, and C. A. Tassinari. "Celiac Disease, Posterior Cerebral Calcifications and Epilepsy." *Brain and Development* 14, no. 1 (1992): 23–29.

Goel, N. K., R. D. McBane, and P.S. Kamath. "Cardiomyopathy Associated with Celiac Disease." *Mayo Clinic Proceedings* 80, no. 5 (2005): 674–76.

Gogos, C. A., V. Nikolopoulou, V. Zolota, V. Siampi, and A. Vagenakis. "Autoimmune Cholangitis in a Patient with Celiac Disease: A Case Report and Review of the Literature." *Journal of Hepatology* 30 (1999): 321–24.

Green, P. H. "The Many Faces of Celiac Disease: Clinical Presentation of Celiac Disease in the Adult Population." *Gastroenterology* 128, no. 4 suppl. no. 1 (2005): S74–78.

Green, P. H. "Where are All Those Patients with Celiac Disease?." *American Journal of Gastroenterology* 102 (2007): 1461–63.

Green, P. H., A. T. Fleischauer, G. Bhagat, R. Goyal, B. Jabri, and A. I. Neugut. "Risk of Malignancy in Patients with Celiac Disease." *American Journal of Medicine* 115, no. 3 (2003): 191–95.

Green, P. H., and B. Jabri. "Celiac Disease and Other Precursors to Small Bowel Malignancy. *Gastroenterology Clinics of North America* 31 (2002): 625–39.

Green, P. H., and B. Jabri. "Coeliac Disease." *Lancet* 362, no. 9381 (2003): 383–91.

Green, P. H., and Rory Jones. *Celiac Disease: A Hidden Epidemic.* New York: HarperCollins, 2006.

Green, P. H., S. N. Stavropoulos, S. G. Panagi, S. L. Goldstein, D. J. McMahon, H. Absan, and A. I. Neugut. "Characteristics of Adult Celiac Disease in the USA: Results of a National Survey." *American Journal of Gastroenterology* 96, no. 1 (2001): 126–27.

Green, P. H., J. Yang, J. Cheng, A. R. Lee, J. W. Harper, and G. Bhagat. "An Association between Microscopic Colitis and Celiac Disease." *Clinical Gastroenterology and Hepatology* 7, no. 11 (2009): 1210–16.

Grey-Davies, E., J. M. Hows, and J. C. Marsh. "Aplastic Anaemia in Association with Coeliac Disease: A Series of Three Cases." *British Journal of Haematology* 143, no. 2 (2008): 258–60.

Griffin, M., R. Casadio, and C. M. Bergamini. "Transglutaminases: Nature's Biological Glues." *Biochemical Journal* 368, pt. 2 (2002): 377–96.

Hadithi, M., C. J. Mulder, F. Stam, J. Azizi, J. B. Crusius, A. S. Peña, C. D. A. Stehouwer, and Y. M. Smulders. "Effect of B Vitamin Supplementation on Plasma Homocysteine Levels in Celiac Disease." *World Journal of Gastroenterology* 15, no 8 (2009): 955–60.

Hadjivassiliou, M., D. Aeschlimann, R. A. Grünewald, D. S. Sanders, B. Sharrack, and N. Woodroofe. "GAD Antibody-associated Neurological Illness and Its Relationship to Gluten Sensitivity." ACTA Neurologica Scandinavica 123, no. 3 (2011): 175–80.

Hadjivassiliou, M., P. Aeschlimann, A. Strigun, D. S. Sanders, N. Woodroofe, and D. Aeschlimann. "Autoantibodies in Gluten Ataxia Recognize a Novel Neuronal Transglutaminase." *Annals of Neurology* 64, no. 3 (2008): 332–43.

Hadjivassiliou, M., A. Chattopadhyay, G. Davies-Jones, A. Gibson, R. Grunewald, and A. Lobo. "Neuromuscular Disorder as a Presenting Feature of Coeliac Disease." *Journal of Neurology, Neurosurgery and Psychiatry* 63, no. 6 (1997): 770–75.

Hadjivassiliou, M., A. K. Chattopadhyay, R. A. Grünewald, J. A. Jarratt, R. H. Kandler, D. G. Rao, D. S. Sanders, S. B. Wharton, and G. A. Davies-Jones. "Myopathy Associated with Gluten Sensitivity." *Muscle Nerve* 35, no. 4 (2007): 443–50.

Hadjivassiliou, M., G. A. Davies-Jones, D. S. Sanders, and R. A. Grünewald. "Dietary Treatment of Gluten Ataxia." *Journal of Neurology, Neurosurgery and Psychiatry* 74, no. 9 (2003): 1221–24.

Hadjivassiliou, M., and R. Grünewald. "The Neurology of Gluten Sensitivity: Science vs. Conviction." *Practical Neurology* 4 (2004): 124–26.

Hadjivassiliou, M., R. Grünewald, B. Sharrack, D. Sanders, A. Lobo, C. Williamson, N. Woodroofe, N. Wood, and A. Davies-Jones. "Gluten Ataxia in Perspective: Epidemiology, Genetic Susceptibility and Clinical Characteristics." *Brain* 126, pt. 3 (2003): 685–91.

Hadjivassiliou, M., M. Mäki, D. S. Sanders, C. A. Williamson, R. A. Grünewald, N. M. Woodroofe, and I. R. Korponay-Szabó. "Autoantibody Targeting of Brain and Intestinal Transglutaminase in Gluten Ataxia." *Neurology* 66, no. 3 (2006): 373–77.

Hadjivassiliou, M., D. G. Rao, S. B. Wharton, D. S. Sanders, R. A. Grünewald, and A. G. Davies-Jones. "Sensory Ganglionopathy Due to Gluten Sensitivity." *Neurology* 75, no. 11 (2010): 1003–8.

Hadjivassiliou, M., D. S. Sanders, R. A. Grünewald, and M. Akil. "Gluten Sensitivity Masquerading as Systemic Lupus Erythematosus." *Annals of the Rheumatic Diseases* 63, no. 11 (2004): 1501–3.

Hadjivassiliou, M., D. S. Sanders, R. A. Grünewald, N. Woodroofe, S. Boscolo, and D. Aeschlimann. "Gluten Sensitivity: From Gut to Brain." *Lancet Neurology* 9, no. 3 (2010): 318–30.

Hadjivassiliou, M., D. S. Sanders, N. Woodroofe, C. Williamson, and R. A. Grünewald. "Gluten Ataxia." *Cerebellum* 7, no. 3 (2008): 494–98.

Hafström, I., B. Ringertz, A. Spångberg, L. von Zweigbergk, S. Brannemark, I. Nylander, J. Rönnelid, L. Laasonen, and L. Klareskog. "A Vegan Diet Free of Gluten Improves the Signs and Symptoms of Rheumatoid Arthritis: The Effects on Arthritis Correlate with a Reduction in Antibodies to Food Antigens." *Rheumatology* 40, no. 10 (2001): 1175–79.

Hagen, E. M., I. O. Gjerde, C. Vedeler, and N. Hovdenak. [Neurological Diseases Associated with Celiac Disease.] [In Norwegian.] *Tidsskrift For Den Norske Laegeforening* 120, no. 4 (2000): 439–42.

Hajas, A., P. Szodoray, S. Barath, S. Sipka, S. Rezes, M. Zeher, I. Sziklai, G. Szegedi, and E. Bodolay. "Sensorineural Hearing Loss in Patients with Mixed Connective Tissue Disease: Immunological Markers and Cytokine Levels." *Journal of Rheumatology* 36, no. 9 (2009): 1930–36.

Halabi, I. M. "Coeliac Disease Presenting as Acute Pancreatitis in a 3-year-old." *Annals of Tropical Paediatrics* 30, no. 3 (2010): 255–57.

Halblaub, J. M., J. Renno, A. Kempf, J. Bartel, and H. Schmidt-Gayk. "Comparison of Different Salivary and Fecal Antibodies for the Diagnosis of Celiac Disease." *Clinical Laboratory* 50, no. 9–10 (2004): 551–57.

Halfdanarson, T.R., M. R. Litzow, and J. A. Murray. "Hematologic Manifestations of Celiac Disease." *Blood* 109, no. 2 (2007): 412–21.

Hall, D. A., J. Parsons, and T. Benke. "Paroxysmal Nonkinesigenic Dystonia and Celiac Disease." *Movement Disorders* 22, no. 5 (2007): 708–10.

Hamilton, David P. "Gut Check: Belatedly, an Illness Of the Intestines Gets Notice in U.S." *Wall Street Journal*, December 9, 2005. http://online.wsj.com/article/SB113408786563817920-search.html (accessed November 23, 2011).

Haque, W. M., M. R. Mir, and S. Hsu. "Vogt-Koyanagi-Harada Syndrome: Association with Alopecia Areata." *Dermatology Online Journal* 15, no.12 (2009).

Harvard Medical School. Harvard Health Publications. Stampfer, M. J., ed. Dadoly, A. M. *A Special Health Report from Harvard Medical School.* "The Benefits and Risks of Vitamins and Minerals: What You Need to Know." 2003.

Hatting, M., O. Galm, M. Meyer, C. Trautwein, and J. J. Tischendorf. [Anemia and Severe Thrombocytopenia in Celiac Disease.] [In German.] *Medizinische Klinik* 105, no. 4 (2010): 249–52.

He, S.-W., L.-X. Wang. "The Impact of Anemia on the Prognosis of Chronic Heart Failure: A Meta-Analysis and Systemic Review." *Congestive Heart Failure* 15, no. 3 (2009): 123–30.

Heap, G. A., and D. A. van Heel. "The Genetics of Chronic Inflammatory Diseases." *Human Molecular Genetics* 18, no.1 (2009): R101–6.

Henker, J., M. Laass, G. Baretton, R. Fischer, and D. Aust. [Pitfalls in Diagnosis of Celiac Disease.] [In German.] *Zeitschrift fur Gastroenterologie* 46, no. 7 (2008): 675–80.

Hernández-Lahoz, C., and L. Rodrigo. "Gluten Sensitivity and the CNS: Diagnosis and Treatment." *The Lancet Neurology* 9, no. 7 (2010): 653–54.

Hernanz, A., and I. Polanco. "Plasma Precursor Amino Acids of Central Nervous System Monoamines in Children with Coeliac Disease." *Gut* 32, no.12 (1991): 1478–81.

Hijazi, J., A. L. Bedat-Millet, and D. Hannequin. [Stiff-person Syndrome and Other Neurological Disorders Associated with Anti-GAD Antibodies.] [In French.] *Revue de Medecine Interne* 31, no. 1 (2010): 23–28.

Hill, I. D., M. H. Dirks, G. S. Liptak, R. B. Colletti, A. Fasano, S. Guandalini, E. J. Hoffenberg et al. "Guideline for the Diagnosis and Treatment of Celiac Disease in Children: Recommendations of the North American Society for Pediatric Gastroenterology, Hepatology and Nutrition." *Journal of Pediatrics Gastroenterology and Nutrition* 40, no. 1 (2005): 1–19.

Hizli, S., H. Karabulut, O. Ozdemir, B. Acar, A. Abaci, M. Dağli, and R. M. Karaşen. "Sensorineural Hearing Loss in Pediatric Celiac Patients." *International Journal of Pediatric Otorhinolaryngology* 75, no. 1 (2011): 65–68.

Hoca, N. T., D. Dayioglu, and M. Ogretensoy. "Pulmonary Hemosiderosis in Association with Celiac Disease." *Lung* 184, no. 5 (2006): 297–300.

Hogberg L., L. Stenhammar, K. Falth-Magnusson, and E. Grodzinsky, "Anti-endomysium and Anti-gliadin Antibodies as Serological Markers for a Very Late Mucosal Relapse in a Coeliac Girl." *ACTA Paediatrica* 86, no. 3 (1997): 335–36.

Hoggan, Ron. "Gall Bladder Disease and Celiac Disease." *Celiac.com* July 26, 1996. http://www.celiac.com/articles/119/1/Gall-Bladder-Disease-and-Celiac-Disease---By-Ronald-Hoggan/Page1.html (accessed February 12, 2011).

Hoggan, Ron. "Gluten Intolerant, Gluten Sensitive & Celiac– Explained by Ron Hoggan, Ed. D." August 27, 2010. *GlutenFreeHelp.info.*

Hoggan, Ron, and Scott Adams. *Cereal Killers: Celiac Disease and Gluten-Free A to Z.* Charleston: Watersideworks and Celiac.com, *2010 (from essay by Dr. Scott Lewey).*

Holmes, G. K. "Coeliac Disease and Malignancy." *Digestive and Liver Disease* 34, no. 3 (2002): 229–37.

Holmes, G. K. "Screening for Coeliac Disease in Type 1 Diabetes." *Archives of Disease in Childhood* 87 (2002): 495–98.

Holmes, G. K., P. Prior, M. R. Lane, D. Pope, and R. N. Allan. "Malignancy in Coeliac Disease: Effect of a Gluten Free Diet." *Gut* 30, no. 3 (1989): 333–38.

Holmes, G. K., P. L. Stokes, T. M. Sorahan, P. Prior, J. A. Waterhouse, and W. T. Cooke. "Coeliac Disease, Gluten-free Diet, and Malignancy." *Gut* 17, no. 8 (1976): 612–19.

Holmes, Marcy. "Menopause and Perimenopause: Endometrial Hyperplasia of the Uterus." http://www.womentowomen.com/menopause/uterinehyperplasia.aspx#medicalandsurgicaloptions (accessed March 19, 2011).

Horvath, K., and J. A. Perman. "Autistic Disorder and Gastrointestinal Disease." *Current Opinion in Pediatrics* 14, no. 5 (2002): 583–87.

Howell, W. M., P. C. Calder, and R. F. Grimble. "Gene Polymorphisms, Inflammatory Diseases and Cancer." *Proceedings of the Nutrition Society* 61, no. 4 (2002): 447–56.

Hungin, A. P. S., L. Chang, G. R. Locke, E. H. Dennis, and V. Barghout. "Irritable Bowel Syndrome in the United States: Prevalence, Symptom Patterns and Impact." *Alimentary Pharmacology and Therapeutics* 21, no. 11 (2005): 1365–75.

Hurley, K., and D. Baggs. "Hypocalcemic Cardiac Failure in the Emergency Department." *Journal of Emergency Medicine* 28, no. 2 (2005): 155–59.

Hwang, E., R. McBride, A. I. Neugut, and P. H. Green. "Sarcoidosis in Patients with Celiac Disease." *Digestive Diseases and Sciences* 53, no. 4 (2008): 977–81.

Il Messaggero.it (*The Messenger*, an Italian newspaper based in Rome). "The False Discovery [of] Celiac Disease: Hit Three Million in Italy," *Last updated: March 15.* http://www.ilmessaggero.it%2Farticolo.php%3Fid%3D141914%26sez%3DHOME_SCIENZA (accessed March 18, 2011).

Iltanen, S., P. Collin, M. Korpela, K. Holm, J. Partanen, A. Polvi, and M. Mäki. "Celiac Disease and Markers of Celiac Disease Latency in Patients with Primary Sjögren's Syndrome." *American Journal of Gastroenterology* 94, no. 4 (1999): 1042–46.

Iuorio, R., V. Mercuri, F. Barbarulo, T. D'Amico, N. Mecca, G. Bassotti, D. Pietrobono, P. Gargiulo, and A. Picarelli. "Prevalence of Celiac Disease in Patients with Autoimmune Thyroiditis." *Minerva Endocrinologica* 32, no. 4 (2007): 239–43.

Ivanovski, P., D. Nikolić, N. Dimitrijević, I. Ivanovski, and V. Perišić. "Erythrocytic Transglutaminase Inhibition Hemolysis at Presentation of Celiac Disease." *World Journal of Gastroenterology* 16, no. 44 (2010): 5647–50.

Jabri, B., and L. M. Sollid. "Tissue-mediated Control of Immunopathology in Coeliac Disease." *Nature Reviews Immunology* 9, no. 12 (2009): 858–70.

Jacob, S., M. Zarei, A. Kenton, and H. Allroggen. "Gluten Sensitivity and Neuromyelitis Optica: Two Case Reports." *Journal of Neurology, Neurosurgery and Psychiatry* 76, no. 7 (2005): 1028–30.

Jankowiak, C., and D. Ludwig. "Frequent Causes of Diarrhea: Celiac Disease and Lactose Intolerance." *Medizinische Klinik* 103, no. 6 (2008): 413–22.

Järvinen, T.T., P. Collin, M. Rasmussen, S. Kyrönpalo, M. Mäki, J. Partanen, T. Reunala, and K. Kaukinen. "Villous Tip Intraepithelial Lymphocytes as Markers of Early-stage Coeliac Disease." *Scandinavian Journal of Gastroenterology* 39, no. 5 (2004): 428–33.

Jhaveri, K. D., V. D. D'Agati, R. Pursell, and D. Serur. "Coeliac Sprue-associated Membranoproliferative Glomerulonephritis (MPGN)." *Nephrology Dialysis Transplantation* 24, no. 11 (2009): 3545–48.

Jones, S., C. D'Souza, and N. Y. Haboubi. "Patterns of Clinical Presentation of Adult Coeliac Disease in a Rural Setting." *Nutrition Journal* 14, no. 5 (2006): 24.

Jordá, F. C., and J. López Vivancos. "Fatigue as a Determinant of Health in Patients with Celiac Disease." *Journal of Clinical Gastroenterology* 44, no. 6 (2010): 423–27.

Jorge, O., A. Jorge, and G. Camus. [Celiac Disease Associated with Antiphospholipid Syndrome.] [In Spanish.] *Revista Espanola de Enfermedades Digestivas* 100, no. 2 (2008): 102–3.

Jost, P. J., S. M. Stengel, W. Huber, M. Sarbia, C. Peschel, and J. Duyster. "Very Severe Iron-Deficiency Anemia in a Patient with Celiac Disease and Bulimia Nervosa: A Case Report." *International Journal of Hematology* 82, no. 4 (2005): 310–11.

Juranić, Z., J. Radic, A. Konic-Ristic, S. Jelic, I. Besu, and B. Mihaljevic. "Antibodies Contained in 'M' Component of Some Patients with Multiple Myeloma Are Directed to Food Antigens?" *Leukemia Research* 30, no. 12 (2006): 1585–86.

Juranic, Z., J. Radic, A. Konic-Ristic, S. Jelic, B. Mihaljevic, I. Stankovic, S. Matkovic, I. Besu, and D. Gavrilović. "Humoral Immunoreactivity to Gliadin and to Tissue Transglutaminase is Present in Some Patients with Multiple Myeloma." *BioMedCentral Immunology* 9 (2008): 22.

Kagalwalla, A. F., A. Shah, S. Ritz, H. Melin-Aldana, and B. U. Li. "Cow's Milk Protein-induced Eosinophilic Esophagitis in a Child with Gluten-sensitive Enteropathy." *Journal of Pediatric Gastroenterology and Nutrition* 44, no. 3 (2007): 386–88.

Kahn, O., M. I. Fiel, and H. D. Janowitz. "Celiac Sprue, Idiopathic Thrombocytopenic Purpura, and Hepatic Granulomatous Disease. An Autoimmune Linkage?" *Journal of Clinical Gastroenterology* 23, no. 3 (1996): 214–16.

Kalaydjian, A. E., W. Eaton, N. Cascella, and A. Fasano. "The Gluten Connection: The Association between Schizophrenia and Celiac Disease." *Acta Psychiatrica Scandinavica* 113, no. 2 (2006): 82–90.

Kallel-Sellami, M., L. Laadhar, M. Zitouni, and S. Makni. [Recurrent Rhinitis and Pulmonary Infections Revealing Celiac Disease: Case Report.] [In French.] *Revue de Pneumologie Clinique* 64, no. 1 (2008): 27–29.

Kapur, G., A. K. Patwari, S. Narayan, and V. K. Anand. "Iron Supplementation in Children with Celiac Disease." *Indian Journal of Pediatrics* 70, no. 12 (2003): 955–58.

Kara, B., and M. Sandikci. "Successful Treatment of Portal Hypertension and Hypoparathyroidism with a Gluten-free Diet." *Journal of Clinical Gastroenterology* 41, no. 7 (2007): 724–25.

Karagiannis, A., and F. Harsoulis. "Gonadal Dysfunction in Systemic Diseases." *European Journal of Endocrinology* 152, no. 4 (2005): 501-13

Karpuj, M. V., M. W. Becher, and L. Steinman. "Evidence for a Role for Transglutaminase in Huntington's Disease and the Potential Therapeutic Implications." *Neurochemistry International* 40, no. 1 (2002): 31–36.

Karwautz, A., G. Wagner, G. Berger, U. Sinnreich, V. Grylli, and W. D. Huber. "Eating Pathology in Adolescents with Celiac Disease." *Psychosomatics* 49, no. 5 (2008): 399–406.

Kasper, H. U., M. Kemper, F. Siebert, and C. Langner. [Lambliasis As Differential Diagnosis of MARSH Type 3b.] [In German.] *Zeitschrift fur Gastroenterologie* 48, no. 8 (2010): 829–32.

Katz, S. I., Z. M. Falchuk, M. V. Dahl, G. N. Rogentine, and W. Strober. "HL-A8: A Genetic Link between Dermatitis Herpetiformis and Gluten-sensitive Enteropathy." *Journal of Clinical Investigation* 51, no. 11 (1972): 2977–80.

Kaukinen, K., P. Collin, and M. Mäki. "Latent Coeliac Disease or Coeliac Disease Beyond Villous Atrophy." *Gut* 56, no. 10 (2007): 1339–40.

Kaukinen, K., P. Collin, and M. Mäki. "Natural History of Celiac Disease." *Fasano A., Troncone R., Branski D. (eds):* "Frontiers in Celiac Disease." *Pediatric and Adolescent Medicine. Basel, Karger*, 2008, 12 (2008): 12–17.

Kaukinen, K., L. Halme, P. Collin, M. Färkkilä, M. Mäki, P. Vehmanen, J. Partanen, and K. Höckerstedt. "Celiac Disease in Patients with Severe Liver Disease: Gluten-free Diet May Reverse Hepatic Failure." *Gastroenterology* 122, no. 4 (2002): 881–88.

Kaukinen, K., J. Partanen, M. Mäki, and P. Collin. "HLA-DQ Typing in the Diagnosis of Celiac Disease." *American Journal of Gastroenterolgy* 97, no. 3 (2002): 695–99.

Kaukinen K., M. Peräaho, P. Collin, J. Partanen, N. Woolley, T. Kaartinen, T. Nuutinen, T. Halttunen, M. Mäki, and I. Korponay-Szabo. "Small-bowel Mucosal Transglutaminase 2-specific IgA Deposits in Coeliac Disease without Villous Atrophy: A Prospective and Randomized Clinical Study." *Scandinavian Journal of Gastroenterology* 40, no. 5 (2005): 564–72.

Kero, J., M. Gissler, E. Hemminki, and E. Isolauri. "Could TH1 and TH2 Diseases Coexist? Evaluation of Asthma Incidence in Children with Coeliac Disease, Type 1 Diabetes, or Rheumatoid Arthritis: A Register Study." *Journal of Allergy and Clinical Immunology* 108, no. 5 (2001): 781–83.

Khazai, N., S. E. Judd, and V. Tangpricha. "Calcium and Vitamin D: Skeletal and Extraskeletal Health." *Current Rheumatology Reports* 10, no. 2 (2008): 110–17.

Khemiri M., M. Ouederni, F. Khaldi, and S. Barsaoui. "Screening for Celiac Disease in Idiopathic Pulmonary Hemosiderosis." *Gastroenterologie Clinique et Biologique* 32, no. 8–9 (2010): 745–48.

Kidd, P. M. "Neurodegeneration from Mitochondrial Insufficiency: Nutrients, Stem Cells, Growth Factors, and Prospects for Brain Rebuilding Using Integrative Management." *Alternative Medicine Review* 10, no. 4 (2005): 268–93.

Kiefte-de Jong, J. C., J. C. Escher, L. R. Arends, V. W. Jaddoe, A. Hofman, H. Raat, and H. A. Moll. "Infant Nutritional Factors and Functional Constipation in Childhood: The Generation R Study." *American Journal of Gastroenterology* 105, no. 4 (2010): 940–45.

Kieslich, M., G. Errázuriz, H. G. Posselt, W. Moeller-Hartmann, F. Zanella, and H. Boehles. "Brain White-Matter Lesions in Celiac Disease: A Prospective Study of 75 Diet-Treated Patients." *Pediatrics* 108, no. 2 (2001): 1–4.

Kleopa, K. A., K. Kyriacou, E. Zamba-Papanicolaou, and T. Kyriakides. "Reversible Inflammatory and Vacuolar Myopathy with Vitamin E Deficiency in Celiac Disease." *Muscle and Nerve* 31, no. 2 (2005): 260–65.

Kolacek, S., O. Jadresin, I. Petković, Z. Misak, Z. Sonicki, and I. W. Booth. "Gluten-free Diet Has a Beneficial Effect on Chromosome Instability in Lymphocytes of Children with Coeliac Disease." *Journal of Pediatrics Gastroenterology and Nutrition* 38, no. 2 (2004): 177–80.

Konic-Ristic A., D. Dodig, R. Krstic, S. Jelic, I. Stankovic, A. Ninkovic, J. Radic et al. "Different Levels of Humoral Immunoreactivity to Different Wheat Cultivars Gliadin are Present in Patients with Celiac Disease and in Patients with Multiple Myeloma." *BioMedCentral Immunology* 10 (2009): 32.

Konofal, E., M. Lecendreux, I. Arnulf, and M. C. Mouren. "Iron Deficiency in Children with Attention-deficit/hyperactivity Disorder." *Archives of Pediatrics and Adolescent Medicine* 158, no. 12 (2004): 1113–15.

Korkut, E., M. Bektas, E. Oztas, M. Kurt, H. Cetinkaya, and A. Ozden. "The Prevalence of Celiac Disease in Patients Fulfilling Rome III Criteria for Irritable Bowel Syndrome." *European Journal of Internal Medicine* 21, no. 5 (2010): 389–92.

Korman, S. H. "Pica as a Presenting Symptom in Childhood Celiac Disease." *American Journal of Clinical Nutrition* 51, no. 2 (1990): 139–41.

Korn, Danna. *Wheat-Free, Worry-Free: The Art of Happy, Healthy Gluten-free Living.* Carlsbad, CA: Hay House, 2002.

Korponay-Szabó, I. R., I. Dahlbom, K. Laurila, S. Koskinen, N. Woolley, J. Partanen, J. B. Kovács, M. Mäki, and T. Hansson. "Elevation of IgG Antibodies Against Tissue Transglutaminase as a Diagnostic Tool for Coeliac Disease in Selective IgA Deficiency." *Gut* 52, 11 (2003): 1567–71.

Koskinen, O., P. Collin, I. Korponay-Szabo, T. Salmi, S. Iltanen, K. Haimila, J. Partanen, M. Mäki, and K. Kaukinen. "Gluten-dependent Small Bowel Mucosal Transglutaminase 2-Specific IgA Deposits in Overt and Mild Enteropathy Coeliac Disease." *Journal of Pediatric Gastroenterology and Nutrition* 47, no. 4 (2008): 436–42.

Kostopoulou, O., C. Devereaux-Walsh, and B. C. Delaney, "Missing Celiac Disease in Family Medicine: The Importance of Hypothesis Generation." *Medical Decision Making* 29, no. 3 (2009): 282–90.

Kotze, L. M., A. P. Brambila Rodrigues, L. R. Kotze, and R. M. Nisihara. "A Brazilian Experience of the Self Transglutaminase-based Test for Celiac Disease Case Finding and Diet Monitoring." *World Journal of Gastroenterology* 15, no. 35 (2009): 4423–28.

Kozłowska, Z. E. [Evaluation of Mental Status of Children with Malabsorption Syndrome after Long-term Treatment with Gluten-free Diet (Preliminary Report).] [In Polish.] *Psychiatria Polska* 25, no. 2 (1991): 130–34. Translated by Jerry Lazkowski. Email from Ron Hoggan, EdD. April 14, 2010.

Kraft, B. D., and E. C. Westman. "Schizophrenia, Gluten, and Low-carbohydrate, Ketogenic Diets: A Case Report and Review of the Literature. *Nutrition and Metabolism* 6 (2009): 10.

Krifa, F., L. Knani, W. Sakly, I. Ghedira, A. S. Essoussi, J. Boukadida, and F. Ben Hadj Hamida. "Uveitis Responding on Gluten Free Diet in a Girl with Celiac Disease and Diabetes Mellitus Type 1." *Gastroenterologie Clinique et Biologique* 34, no. 4-5 (2010): 319–20.

Kristjánsson, G., P. Venge, and R. Hällgren. "Mucosal Reactivity to Cow's Milk Protein in Coeliac Disease." *Clinical and Experimental Immunology* 147, no. 3 (2007): 449–55.

Kuitunen P., E. Savilahti, and M. Verkasalo. "Late Mucosal Relapse in a Boy with Coeliac Disease and Cow's Milk Allergy." *ACTA Paediatrica Scandinavica* 75, no. 2 (1986): 340–42.

Kuitunen, P., J. K. Visakorpi, E. Savilahti, and P. Pelkonen. "Malabsorption Syndrome with Cow's Milk Intolerance. Clinical Findings and Course in 54 Cases." *Archives of Disease in Childhood* 50, no. 5 (1975): 351–56.

Kuloğlu Z., C. T. Kirsaçlioğlu, A. Kansu, A. Ensari, and N. Girgin. "Celiac Disease: Presentation of 109 Children." *Yonsei Medical Journal* 50, no. 5 (2009): 617–23.

Kumar, V., M. Rajadhyaksha, and J. Wortsman. "Celiac Disease-Associated Autoimmune Endocrinopathies." *Clinical and Diagnostic Laboratory Immunology* 8, no. 4 (2001): 678–85.

Kurland, J. E., W. J. Coyle, A. Winkler, and E. Zable. "Prevalence of Irritable Bowel Syndrome and Depression in Fibromyalgia." *Digestive Diseases and Sciences* 51, no. 3 (2006): 454–60.

Kurppa, K., P. Collin, M. Viljamaa, K. Haimila, P. Saavalainen, J. Partanen, K. Laurila et al. "Diagnosing Mild Enteropathy Celiac Disease: A Randomized, Controlled Clinical Study." *Gastroenterology* 136, no. 3 (2009): 816–23.

Kurppa, K., K. Lindfors, P. Collin, P. Saavalainen, J. Partanen, K. Haimila, H. Huhtala, K. Laurila, M. Mäki, and K. Kaukinen. "Antibodies Against Deamidated Gliadin Peptides in Early-stage Celiac Disease." *Journal of Clinical Gastroenterology* 45, no. 8 (2011): 673–78.

Laberge, G., C. M. Mailloux, K. Gowan, P. Holland, D. C. Bennett, P. R. Fain, and R. A. Spritz. "Early Disease Onset and Increased Risk of Other Autoimmune Diseases in Familial Generalized Vitiligo." *Pigment Cell Research* 18, no. 4 (2005): 300–305.

Lagerqvist, C., I. Dahlbom, T. Hansson, E. Jidell, P. Juto, P. Olcén, H. Stenlund, O. Hernell, and A. Ivarsson. "Antigliadin Immunoglobulin A Best in Finding Celiac Disease in Children Younger Than 18 Months of Age." *Journal of Pediatrics Gastroenterology and Nutrition* 47, no. 4 (2008): 428–35.

Lapid, Nancy, "Celiac Disease & Gluten Sensitivity: Eating Disorder or Celiac Disease?...Or Both?" *About.com* updated August 04, 2010. http://celiacdisease.about.com/od/medicalguidelines/a/EatingDisorders.htm (accessed April 5, 2011).

Latov, Norman. "Celiac Disease and Peripheral Neuropathy." February 3, 2002. Presentation to Westchester Celiac Sprue Support Group. Summarized by Sue Goldstein. http://beepdf.com/doc/65023/celiac_disease_and_peripheral_neuropathy.html (accessed April20, 2011).

Lazzari, R., A. Collina, G. Arena, A. Bochicchio, L. Corvaglia, M. Vallini, M. Marzatico, L. Forchielli, A. Pasetti, and S. Frassineti. [Sideropenic Anemia and Celiac Disease.] [In Italian.] *La Pediatria Medica e Chirurgica* 16, no. 6 (1994): 549–50.

Lee, S. K., and P. H. Green. "Celiac Sprue (The Great Modern-day Imposter)." *Current Opinion in Rheumatology* 18, no. 1 (2006): 101–7.

Lee, S. K., W. Lo, L. Memeo, H. Rotterdam, and P. H. Green. "Duodenal Histology in Patients with Celiac Disease after Treatment with a Gluten-free Diet." *Gastrointestinal Endoscopy* 57, no. 2 (2003): 187–91.

Leeds, J. S., B. S. Höroldt, R. Sidhu, A. D. Hopper, K. Robinson, B. Toulson, L. Dixon et al. "Is There an Association between Coeliac Disease and Inflammatory Bowel Diseases? A Study of Relative Prevalence in Comparison with Population Controls." *Scandinavian Journal of Gastroenterology* 42, no. 10 (2007): 1214–20.

Leffler, D. A... *Defining, Diagnosing, and Managing Celiac Disease in Primary Care.* "Celiac Disease Management Recommendations." *Celiac CME Newsletter* 1: 10. http://www.celiaccmecentral.com/getstarted.html (accessed February 4, 2012).

Leffler, D. A., M. Dennis, J. B. Edwards George, and C. P. Kelly. "The Interaction between Eating Disorders and Celiac Disease: An Exploration of 10 Cases." *European Journal of Gastroenterology and Hepatology* 19, no. 3 (2007):251–55.

Leggio, L., G. Cadoni, C. D'Angelo, A. Mirijello, S. Scipione, A. Ferrulli, S. Agostino, G. Paludetti, G. Gasbarrini, and G. Addolorato. "Coeliac Disease and Hearing Loss: Preliminary Data on a New Possible Association." *Scandinavian Journal of Gastroenterology* 42, no. 10 (2007): 1209–13.

Leslie, C., C. Mews, A. Charles, and M. Ravikumara. "Celiac Disease and Eosinophilic Esophagitis: A True Association." *Journal of Pediatric Gastroenterology and Nutrition* 50, no. 4 (2010): 397–99.

Lewey, Scot. *The Food Doc Journal.* "Your Brain on Gluten: Should You Lay Off the Gluten Before It's Too Late?" http://thefooddoc.blogspot.com/2007/12/your-brain-on-gluten-should-you-lay-off.html (accessed June 21, 2010).

Lewis, N. R., and B. B. Scott. "Meta-analysis: Deamidated Gliadin Peptide Antibody and Tissue Transglutaminase Antibody Compared as Screening Tests for Coeliac Disease." *Alimentary Pharmacology and Therapeutics* 31, no. 1 (2010): 73–81.

Libonati, Cleo J. *Recognizing Celiac Disease: Signs, Symptoms, Associated Disorders & Complications.* Fort Washington, PA: Gluten Free Works Publishing, 2007.

Lidén, M., G. Kristjánsson, S. Valtysdottir, P. Venge, and R. Hällgren. "Cow's Milk Protein Sensitivity Assessed by the Mucosal Patch Technique is Related to Irritable Bowel Syndrome in Patients with Primary Sjögren's Syndrome." *Clinical and Experimental Allergy* 38, no. 6 (2008): 929–35.

Lim, P. O., N. Tzemos, C. A. Farquharson, J. E. Anderson, P. Deegan, R. S. MacWalter, A. D. Struthers, and T. M. MacDonald. "Reversible Hypertension Following Coeliac Disease Treatment: The Role of Moderate Hyperhomocysteinaemia and Vascular Endothelial Dysfunction." *Journal of Human Hypertension* 16, no. 6 (2002): 411–15.

Lin, H. C., and M. Pimentel. "Bacterial Concepts in Irritable Bowel Syndrome." *Reviews in Gastroenterological Disorders* 5, suppl. no. 3 (2005): S3–9.

Lindqvist, U., A. Rudsander, A. Boström, B. Nilsson, and G. Michaëlsson. "IgA Antibodies to Gliadin and Coeliac Disease in Psoriatic Arthritis." *Rheumatology (Oxford)* 41, no. 1 (2002): 31–37.

Lioger, B., M. C. Machet, and L. Machet. [Dermatitis Herpetiformis.] [In French.] *Presse Medicale* 39, no. 10 (2010): 1042–48.

Lionetti, E., R. Francavilla, L. Maiuri, M. Ruggieri, M. Spina, P. Pavone, T. Francavilla, A. M. Magistà, and L. Pavone. "Headache in Pediatric Patients with Celiac Disease and Its Prevalence as a Diagnostic Clue." *Journal of Pediatrics Gastroenterology and Nutrition* 49, no. 2 (2009): 202–7.

Liossis, S. N., and G. C. Tsokos. "Cellular Immunity in Osteoarthritis: Novel Concepts for an Old Disease." *Clinical and Diagnostic Laboratory Immunology* 5, no. 4 (1998): 427–29.

Liu, E., M. Li, L. Emery, I Taki, K. Barriga, C. Tiberti, G. S. Eisenbarth, M. J. Rewers, and E. J. Hoffenberg. "Natural History of Antibodies to Deamidated Gliadin Peptides and Transglutaminase in Early Childhood Celiac Disease." *Journal of Pediatric Gastroenterology and Nutrition* 45, no. 3 (2007): 293–300.

Loche, F., and J. Bazex. [Celiac Disease Associated with Cutaneous Sarcoidosic Granuloma.] [In French.] *Revue de Medecine Interne* 18, no. 12 (1997): 975–78.

Lohi, S., K. Mustalahti, K. Kaukinen, K. Laurila, P. Collin, H. Rissanen, O. Lohi et al., "Increasing Prevalence of Coeliac Disease Over Time." *Alimentary Pharmacology and Theraputics* 26 (2007): 1217–1225.

Lomer, M. C., G. C. Parkes, and J. D. Sanderson. "Review Article: Lactose Intolerance in Clinical Practice–Myths and Realities." *Alimentary Pharmacology and Therapeutics* 27, no. 2 (2008): 93–103.

Lowder, C. Y., F. A. Gutman, H. Zegarra, Z. N. Zakov, J. N. Lowder, and J. D. Clough. "Macular and Paramacular Detachment of the Neurosensory Retina Associated with Systemic Diseases." *Transactions of the American Ophthalmological Society* 79 (1981): 347–70.

Lozoff, B. "Iron Deficiency and Child Development." *Food and Nutrition Bulletin* 28, suppl. no. 4 (2007): S560–71.

Ludvigsson, J. F., L. Brandt, and S. M. Montgomery. "Symptoms and Signs in Individuals with Serology Positive for Celiac Disease but Normal Mucosa." *BioMedCentral Gastroenterology* 9 (2009): 57.

Ludvigsson, J. F., K. Hemminki, J. Wahlström, and C. Almqvist. "Celiac Disease Confers a 1.6-fold Increased Risk of Asthma: A Nationwide Population-based Cohort Study." *Journal of Allergy and Clinical Immunology* 127, no. 4 (2011): 1071–73.

Ludvigsson, J. F., M. Inghammar, M. Ekberg, and A. Egesten. "A Nationwide Cohort Study of the Risk of Chronic Obstructive Pulmonary Disease in Coeliac Disease." *Journal of Internal Medicine* 271, no. 5 (2012): 481–89.

Ludvigsson, J. F., S. James, J. Askling, U. Stenestrand, and E. Ingelsson. "Nationwide Cohort Study of Risk of Ischemic Heart Disease in Patients with Celiac Disease." *Circulation* 123, no. 5 (2011): 483–90.

Ludvigsson, J. F., K. Michaelsson, A. Ekbom, and S. M. Montgomery. "Coeliac Disease and the Risk of Fractures– General Population-based Cohort Study." *Alimentary Pharmacology and Therapeutics* 25, no. 3 (2007): 273–85.

Ludvigsson, J. F., S. M. Montgomery, and A. Ekbom. "Risk of Pancreatitis in 14,000 Individuals with Celiac Disease." *Clinical Gastroenterology and Hepatology* 5, no. 11 (2007): 1347–53.

Ludvigsson, J. F., J. Wahlstrom, J. Grunewald, A. Ekbom, and S. M. Montgomery. "Coeliac Disease and Risk of Sarcoidosis." *Sarcoidosis, Vasculitis and Diffuse Lung Diseases* 24, no. 2 (2007): 121–26.

Lukowski, A. F., M. Koss, M. J. Burden, J. Jonides, C. A. Nelson, N. Kaciroti, E. Jimenez, and B. Lozoff. "Iron Deficiency in Infancy and Neurocognitive Functioning at 19 Years: Evidence of Long-term Deficits in Executive Function and Recognition Memory." *Nutritional Neuroscience* 13, no. 2 (2010): 54–70.

Lydiard, R. B. "Irritable Bowel Syndrome, Anxiety, and Depression: What Are the Links?" *Journal of Clinical Psychiatry* 62, suppl. no. 8 (2001): 38–45.

Maieron, R., L. Elli, M. Marino, I. Floriani, F. Minerva, C. Avellini, G. Falconieri, S. Pizzolitto, and M. Zilli. "Celiac Disease and Intestinal Metaplasia of the Esophagus (Barrett's Esophagus)." *Digestive Diseases and Sciences* 50, no.1 (2005): 126–29.

Mäki, M., K. Mustalahti, J. Kokkonen, P. Kulmala, M. Haapalahti, T. Karttunen, J. Ilonen et al, "Prevalence of Celiac Disease among Children in Finland." *New England Journal of Medicine* 348 (2003): 2517–24.

Malhotra, P., R. Aggarwal, A. N. Aggarwal, S. K. Jindal, A. Awasthi, and B. D. Radotra. "Coeliac Disease as a Cause of Unusually Severe Anaemia in a Young Man with Idiopathic Pulmonary Haemosiderosis." *Respiratory Medicine* 99, no. 4 (2005): 451–53.

Manchanda, S., C. R. Davies, and D. Picchietti. "Celiac Disease as a Possible Cause for Low Serum Ferritin in Patients with Restless Legs Syndrome." *Sleep Medicine* 10, no. 7 (2009): 763–65.

Maniar, V. P., S. S. Yadav, and Y. A. Gokhale. "Intractable Seizures and Metabolic Bone Disease Secondary to Celiac Disease." *Journal of the Association of Physicians India* 58 (2010): 512–15.

Marconi, G., E. Radice, S. Greco, C. Bezzio, and G. Bianchi Porro. "Transient Small-bowel Intussusceptions in Adults: Significance of Ultrasonographic Detection." *Clinical Radiology* 62 (2007): 792–97.

Marcovitch, Dr. Harvey. *Black's Medical Dictionary* 42nd. London: A & C Black Publishers, 2010.

Marguerie, C., S. Kaye, T. Vyse, C. Mackworth-Young, M. J. Walport, and C. Black. "Malabsorption Caused by Coeliac Disease in Patients Who Have Scleroderma." *British Journal of Rheumatology* 34, no. 9 (1995): 858–61.

Marie, I., F. Lecomte, E. Hachulla, M. Antonietti, A. François, H. Levesque, and H. Courtois. "An Uncommon Association: Celiac Disease and Dermatomyositis in Adults." *Clinical and Experimental Rheumatology* 19, no. 2 (2001): 201–3.

Mark, J. D. "Pediatric Asthma: An Integrative Approach to Care." *Nutrition in Clinical Practice* 24, no. 5 (2009): 578–88.

Marsch, S. C., M. Heer, H. Sulser, and A. Hany. [Adenocarcinoma of the Small Intestine in Celiac Disease. Case Report and Literature Review.] [In German.] *Schweizerische Medizinische Wochenschrift. Journal Suisse de Medecine* 120, no. 5 (1990): 135–41.

Martinelli, D., F. Fortunato, S. Tafuri, C. A. Germinario, and R. Prato. "Reproductive Life Disorders in Italian Celiac Women. A Case-control Study." *BioMedCentral Gastroenterology* 10 (2010): 89.

Martinelli, P., R. Troncone, F. Paparo, P. Torre, E. Trapanese, C. Fasano, A. Lamberti, G. Budillon, G. Nardone, and L. Greco. "Coeliac Disease and Unfavourable Outcome of Pregnancy." *Gut* 46, no. 3 (2000): 332–35.

Martinez, G., N. R. B. Israel, and J. J. White. "Celiac Disease Presenting as Entero-enteral Intussusception." *Pediatric Surgical International* 17, no. 1 (2001): 68–70.

Matteoni, C. A., J. R. Goldblum, N. Wang, A. Brzezinski, E. Achkar, and E. E. Soffer. "Celiac Disease is Highly Prevalent in Lymphocytic Colitis." *Journal of Clinical Gastroenterology* 32, no. 3 (2001): 225–27.

Mavragani, C. P., and H. M. Moutsopoulos. "The Geoepidemiology of Sjögren's Syndrome." *Autoimmunity Reviews* 9, no. 5 (2010): A305–10.

Mavroudi, A., E. Karatza, T. Papastavrou, C. Panteliadis, and .K. Spiroglou. "Successful Treatment of Epilepsy and Celiac Disease with a Gluten-free Diet." *Pediatric Neurology* 33, no. 4 (2005): 292–95.

Mavroudis, K., K. Aloumanis, P. Stamatis, G. Antonakoudis, K. Kifnidis, and C. Antonakoudis. "Irreversible End-stage Heart Failure in a Young Patient Due to Severe Chronic Hypocalcemia Associated with Primary Hypoparathyroidism and Celiac Disease." *Clinical Cardiology* 33, no. 2 (2010): E72–75.

Mayberry, J. F., H. L. Smart, and P. J. Toghill. "Familial Association between Coeliac Disease and Ulcerative Colitis: Preliminary Communication." *Journal of the Royal Society of Medicine* 79, no. 4 (1986): 204–5.

Mayo Clinic. "Mayo Clinic Discovers Potential Link Between Celiac Disease And Cognitive Decline." October 10, 2006. *ScienceDaily*. Retrieved March 30, 2012. http://www.sciencedaily.com / releases/2006/10/061010022602.htm (accessed November 9, 2010).

Mayo Clinic. "Mayo Clinic Study Finds Celiac Disease Four Times More Common than in 1950s." July 1, 2009. *MayoClinic.org*. Study lead by J. Murray and colleagues.

McCashland, T. M., J. P. Donovan, R. S. Strobach, J. Linder, and E. M. Quigley. "Collagenous Enterocolitis: A Manifestation of Gluten-sensitive Enteropathy." *Journal of Clinical Gastroenterology* 15, no. 1 (1992): 45–51.

McGowan, K. E., D. A. Castiglione, and J. D. Butzner. "The Changing Face of Childhood Celiac Disease in North America: Impact of Serological Testing." *Pediatrics* 124, no. 6 (2009): 1572–78.

Meazza, C., S. Pagani, K. Laarej, F. Cantoni, P. Civallero, A. Boncimino, and M. Bozzola. "Short Stature in Children with Coeliac Disease." *Pediatric Endocrinological Reviews* 6, no. 4 (2009): 457–63.

Medical News Today. "What Is Edema? What Causes Edema?" July 29, 2009. http://www.medicalnewstoday.com/articles/159111.php (accessed February 1, 2011).

MedlinePlus, "Food Allergy." http://www.nlm.nih.gov/medlineplus/ency/article/000817.htm (accessed September 14, 2011).

MedlinePlus. "Healthy Joints for a Lifetime." Spring 2009. Fast Facts. http://www.nlm.nih.gov/medlineplus/magazine/issues/spring09/articles/spring09pg10-11.html (accessed November 17, 2012).

Meini, A., L. Morandi, M. Mora, P. Bernasconi, V. Monafo, M. N. Pillan, A. G. Ugazio, and A. Plebani. "An Unusual Association: Celiac Disease and Becker Muscular Dystrophy." *American Journal of Gastroenterology* 91, no. 7 (1996): 1459–60.

Merck Manuals Online Medical Library. "Skin Manifestations of Internal Disease." http://www.merckmanuals.com/professional/sec10/ch109/ch109f.html (accessed March 9, 2011).

Meyers, S., S. Dikman, H. Spiera, N. Schultz, and H. D. Janowitz. "Cutaneous Vasculitis Complicating Coeliac Disease." *Gut* 22, no. 1 (1981): 61–64.

Michaëlsson, G., B. Gerdén, E. Hagforsen, B. Nilsson, I. Pihl-Lundin, W. Kraaz, G. Hjelmquist, and L. Lööf. "Psoriasis Patients with Antibodies to Gliadin Can Be Improved by a Gluten-free Diet." *British Journal of Dermatology* 142, no. 1 (2000): 44–51.

Millen, A. E., R. Voland, S. A. Sondel, N. Parekh, R. L. Horst, R. B. Wallace, G. S. Hageman et al. "Vitamin D Status and Early Age-related Macular Degeneration in Postmenopausal Women." *Archives of Opthalmology* 129, no. 4 (2011): 481–89.

Miller, A., M. Korem, R. Almog, and Y. Galboiz. "Vitamin B12, Demyelination, Remyelination and Repair in Multiple Sclerosis." *Journal of Neurological Sciences* 233, no. 1–2 (2005): 93–97.

Millward, C., M. Ferriter, S. Calver, and G. Connell-Jones. "Gluten- and Casein-free Diets for Autistic Spectrum Disorder." *Cochrane Database of Systemmatic Reviews* 16, no. 2 (2008): CD003498.

Mody, R. J., P. I. Brown, and D. S. Wechsler. "Refractory Iron Deficiency Anemia as the Primary Clinical Manifestation of Celiac Disease." *Journal of Pediatric Hematology and Oncology* 25, no. 2 (2003): 169–72.

Montalto, M., A. Diociaiuti, G. Alvaro, R. Manna, P. L. Amerio, and G. Gasbarrini. "Atypical Mole Syndrome and Congenital Giant Naevus in a Patient with Celiac Disease." *Panminerva Medica* 45, no. 3 (2003): 219–21.

Mora, S., G. Barera, A. Ricotti, G. Weber, C. Bianchi, and G. Chiumello. "Reversal of Low Bone Density with a Gluten-free Diet in Children and Adolescents with Celiac Disease." *American Journal of Clinical Nutrition* 67, no. 3 (1998): 477–81.

Morris, C. R., and M. C. Agin. "Syndrome of Allergy, Apraxia, and Malabsorption: Characterization of a Neurodevelopmental Phenotype that Responds to Omega 3 and Vitamin E Supplementation." *Alternative Therapies in Health and Medicine* 15, no. 4 (2009): 34–43.

Mothes, T., H. H. Uhlig, and T. Richter. [Recent Aspects of Antibody Determination for the Diagnosis of Coeliac Disease.] [In German.] *Deutsche Tierarztliche Wochenschrift* 134, no. 30 (2009): 1525–28.

Mousain-Bosc, M., M. Roche, A. Polge, D. Pradal-Prat, J. Rapin, and J. P. Bali. "Improvement of Neurobehavioral Disorders in Children Supplemented with Magnesium-vitamin B6. I. Attention Deficit Hyperactivity Disorders." *Magnesium Research* 19, no. 1 (2006): 46–52.

Mouyis, M., A. J. Ostor, A. J. Crisp, A. Ginawi, D. J. Halsall, N. Shenker, and K. E. Poole. "Hypovitaminosis D among Rheumatology Outpatients in Clinical Practice." *Rheumatology: Oxford Journals* 47, no. 9 (2008): 1348–51.

Murray, J. A., "The Widening Spectrum of Celiac Disease." *American Journal of Clinical Nutrition* 69, no. 3 (1999): 354–65.

Murray, J. A., T. Watson, B. Clearman, and F. Mitros. "Effect of a Gluten-free Diet on Gastrointestinal Symptoms in Celiac Disease." *American Journal of Clinical Nutrition* 79, no. 4 (2004): 669–73.

Muscari, A., U. Volta, C. Bonazzi, G.M. Puddu, C. Bozzoli, C. Gerratana, F.B. Bianchi, and P. Puddu. "Association of Serum IgA Antibodies to Milk Antigens with Severe Atherosclerosis." *Atherosclerosis* 77, nos. 2-3 (1989): 251–56.

Mushtaq, N., S. Marven, J. Walker, J. W. Puntis, M. Rudolf, and M. D. Stringer. "Small Bowel Intussusception in Celiac Disease." *Journal of Pediatric Surgery* 34, no. 12 (1999): 1833–35.

Mustalahti, K. "Unusual Manifestations of Celiac Disease." *Indian Journal of Pediatrics* 73, no. 8 (2006): 711–16.

Nachman, F., H. Vázquez, A. González, P. Andrenacci, L. Compagni, H. Reyes, E. Sugai et al. "Gastroesophageal Reflux Symptoms in Patients with Celiac Disease and the Effects of a Gluten-free Diet." *Clinical Gastroenterology and Hepatology* 9, no. 3 (2011): 214–19.

National Center for Complementary and Alternative Medicine. "Headaches and Complementary Health Practices," November 2011. http://nccam.nih.gov/health/providers/digest/headaches.htm (accessed 3/10/13).

National Digestive Diseases Information Clearinghouse. Celiac Disease. "How is Celiac Disease Diagnosed?" http://digestive.niddk.nih.gov/ddiseases/pubs/celiac/ (accessed January 8, 2011).

National Foundation of Celiac Awareness. "Defining, Diagnosing, and Managing Celiac Disease." CeliacCentral.org. http://www.celiaccentral.org/SiteData/docs/Celiac%20CME/722dd759b09fe971/Celiac%20CME%20Postcard.pdf (accessed March 18, 2013).

National Heart Lung and Blood Institute. "National Asthma Guidelines Updated." August 29, 2007. http://public.nhlbi.nih.gov/newsroom/home/GetPressRelease.aspx?id=2442 (accessed September 20, 2011).

National Institute of Allergy and Infectious Diseases. "Autoimmune Diseases." http://www.niaid.nih.gov/topics/autoimmune/Pages/default.aspx (accessed December 27, 2011).

National Institute of Arthritis and Musculoskeletal and Skin Diseases. "Autoimmune Diseases: Understanding Autoimmune Diseases." September 2010. http://www.niams.nih.gov/Health_Info/Autoimmune/default.asp (accessed April 10, 2012).

National Institutes of Health: Office of Dietary Supplements. "Vitamin B12: Groups at Risk for B12 Deficiency." http://ods.od.nih.gov/factsheets/vitaminb12.asp (accessed March 25, 2012).

National Institute of Neurological Disorders and Stroke. "What Is Stiff-person Syndrome?" http://www.ninds.nih.gov/disorders/stiffperson/stiffperson.htm (accessed December 3, 2011).

Naveh, Y., E. Rosenthal, Y. Ben-Arieh, and A. Etzioni. "Celiac Disease-associated Alopecia in Childhood." *Journal of Pediatrics* 134, no. 3 (1999): 362–64.

Neffati, S., B. Charfeddine, M. A. Smach, L. Ben Othmen, A. Ltaief , I. Brahem, H. Dridi, and K. Limem. [Hypocholesterolemia and Celiac Disease: About One Case.] [In French.] *Annales de Biologie Clinique* 67, no. 3 (2009): 359–61.

Nelson, E. W., A. Ertan, F. P. Brooks, and J. J. Cerda. "Thrombocytosis in Patients with Celiac Sprue." *Gastroenterology* 70, no. 6 (1976): 1042–44.

Nemet, A. Y., S. Vinker, I. Bahar, and I. Kaiserman. "The Association of Keratoconus with Immune Disorders." *Cornea* 29, no. 11 (2010): 1261–64.

New York Times. "Health Guide: Glaucoma." http://health.nytimes.com/health/guides/disease/glaucoma/causes.html (accessed January 11, 2012).

NHS National Institute for Health and Clinical Excellence. "NICE Clinical Guidelines 86: Coeliac Disease: Recognition and Assessment of Coeliac Disease." May 2009. http://publications.nice.org.uk/coeliac-disease-cg86/patient-centred-care (accessed November 17, 2012).

Niederhofer, H., and K. Pittschieler. "A Preliminary Investigation of ADHD Symptoms in Persons with Celiac Disease." *Journal of Attention Disorders* 10, no. 2 (2006): 200–204.

Nørgård, B., K. Fonager, H. T. Sørensen, and J. Olsen. "Birth Outcomes of Women with Celiac Disease: A Nationwide Historical Cohort Study." *American Journal of Gastroenterology* 94, no. 9 (1999): 2435–40.

Not, T., F. Ziberna, S. Vatta, S. Quaglia, S. Martelossi, V. Villanacci, and R. Marzari. "Cryptic Genetic Gluten Intolerance Revealed by Intestinal Antitransglutaminase Antibodies and Response to Gluten-free Diet." *Gut* 60, no. 11 (2011): 1487–93.

Nóvoa Medina, Y., M. López-Capapé, E. Lara Orejas, M. Alonso Blanco, C. Camarero Salces, and R. Barrio Castellanos. [Impact of Diagnosis of Celiac Disease on Metabolic Control of Type 1 Diabetes.] [In Spanish.] *Anales de Pediatría* 68, no. 1 (2008): 13–17.

Nowowiejska, B., M. Kaczmarski, and E. J. Dabrowska. "A Long-term Study in Children with a Recognized Gluten Intolerance." *Roczniki Akademii Medycznej W Bialymstoku* 40, no. 3 (1995): 580–87.

Obeid, R., A. McCaddon, and W. Herrmann. "The Role of Hyperhomocysteinemia and B-vitamin Deficiency in Neurological and Psychiatric Diseases." *Clinical Chemistry and Laboratory Medicine* 45, no. 12 (2007): 1590–1606.

O'Grady, J. G., F. M. Stevens, B. Harding, T. A. O'Gorman, B. McNicholl, and C. F. McCarthy. "Hyposplenism and Gluten-sensitive Enteropathy. Natural History, Incidence, and Relationship to Diet and Small Bowel Morphology." *Gastroenterology* 87, no. 6 (1984): 1326–31.

Ojetti, V., G. Nucera, A. Migneco, M. Gabrielli, C. Lauritano, S. Danese, M. A. Zocco et al. "High Prevalence of Celiac Disease in Patients with Lactose Intolerance." *Digestion* 71, no. 2 (2005): 106–10.

Oner, P., E. B. Dirik, Y. Taner, A. Caykoylu, and O. Anlar. "Association between Low Serum Ferritin and Restless Legs Syndrome in Patients with Attention Deficit Hyperactivity Disorder." *Tohoku Journal of Experimental Medicine* 213, no. 3 (2007): 269–76.

Oosterheert, J. J., M. T. Bousema, J. Lagendijk, and M. H. Kramer. "Blue Rubber Bleb Nevus Syndrome Co-existing with Celiac Disease." *Netherlands Journal of Medicine* 64, no. 11 (2006): 431–34.

Oregon State University: Linus Pauling Institute. "Micronutrient Information Center: Vitamin K: Deficiency." http://lpi.oregonstate.edu/infocenter/vitamins/vitaminK/ (accessed March 27, 2012).

O'Sullivan, E. P., L. A. Behan, T. F. King, O. Hardiman, and D. Smith. "A Case of Stiff-person Syndrome, Type 1 Diabetes, Celiac Disease and Dermatitis Herpetiformis." *Clinical Neurology and Neurosurgery* 111, no. 4 (2009): 384–86.

Ozgör, B., and M. A. Selimoğlu. "Coeliac Disease and Reproductive Disorders." *Scandinavian Journal of Gastroenterology* 45, no. 4 (2010): 395–402.

Ozyemisci-Taskiran, O., M. Cengiz, and F. Atalay. "Celiac Disease of the Joint." *Rheumatology International* 31, no. 5 (2011): 573–76.

Pacheco, A., C. Casanova, L. Fogue, and A. Sueiro. "Long-term Clinical Follow-up of Adult Idiopathic Pulmonary Hemosiderosis and Celiac Disease." *Chest* 99, no. 6 (1991): 1525–26.

Palosuo, K., "Update on Wheat Hypersensitivity." *Current Opinion in Allergy and Clinical Immunology* 3, no. 3 (2003): 205–9.

Palosuo, K., H. Alenius, E. Varjonen, M. Koivuluhta, J. Mikkola, H. Keskinen, N. Kalkkinen, and T. Reunala. "A Novel Wheat Gliadin as a Cause of Exercise-induced Anaphylaxis." *Journal of Allergy and Clinical Immunology* 103, no. 5 pt. 1 (1999): 912–17.

Papadopoulos, K. I., K. Sjöberg, S. Lindgren, and B. Hallengren. "Evidence of Gastrointestinal Immune Reactivity in Patients with Sarcoidosis." *Internal Medicine* 245, no. 5 (1999): 525–31.

Patanè, S., and F. Marte. "Atrial Fibrillation Associated with Subclinical Hyperthyroidism." *International Journal of Cardiology* 134 no. 3 (2009): e155–58.

Patel, R. S., F. C. Johlin, Jr., and J. A. Murray. "Celiac Disease and Recurrent Pancreatitis." *Gastrointestinal Endoscopy* 50, no. 6 (1999): 823–27.

Patwari, A. K., V. K. Anand, G. Kapur, and S. Narayan. "Clinical and Nutritional Profile of Children with Celiac Disease." *Indian Pediatrics* 40, no. 4 (2003): 337–42.

Pellicano, R., M. Astegiano, M. Bruno, S. Fagoonee, and M. Rizzetto. "Women and Celiac Disease: Association with Unexplained Infertility." *Minerva Medica* 98, no. 3 (2007): 217–19.

Peltola, M., K. Kaukinen, P. Dastidar, K. Haimila, J. Partanen, A. M. Haapala, M. Mäki, T. Keränen, and J. Peltola. "Hippocampal Sclerosis in Refractory Temporal Lobe Epilepsy is Associated with Gluten Sensitivity." *Journal of Neurology, Neurosurgery and Psychiatry* 80, no. 6 (2009): 626–30.

Peña Porta, J. M., E. Calvo Beguería, C. Vicente De Vera Floristán, and R. Oncins Torres. "Hypokalemic Rhabdomyolysis and Tetany as a Presentation of Celiac Disease in an Adult." *Nefrologie* 28, no. 3 (2008): 343–46.

Pereira, A. C., M. J. Edwards, P. C. Buttery, C. H. Hawkes, N. P. Quinn, G. Giovannoni, M. Hadjivassiliou, and K. P. Bhatia. "Choreic Syndrome and Coeliac Disease: A Hitherto Unrecognised Association." *Movement Disorders* 19, no. 4 (2004): 478–82.

Perelman, S., C. Dupuy, and A. Bourrillon. [The Association of Pulmonary Hemosiderosis and Celiac Disease. Apropos of a New Case in a Child.] [In French.] *Annales de Pediatrie* 39, no. 3 (1992): 185–88.

Petersen, Vikki, and Richard Peterson. *The Gluten Effect: How "Innocent" Wheat Is Ruining Your Health.* http://books.google.com/books?id=xxOuB1MV59EC&pg=PA281&lpg=PA281&dq (accessed February 15, 2011).

Pfaender, M., W. J. D'Souza, N. Trost, L. Litewka, M. Paine, and M. Cook. "Visual Disturbances Representing Occipital Lobe Epilepsy in Patients with Cerebral Calcifications and Coeliac Disease: A Case Series." *Journal of Neurology, Neurosurgery and Psychiatry* 75, no. 11 (2004): 1623–55.

Pfeiffer, C. [Dermatitis Herpetiformis. A Clinical Chameleon.] [In German.] *Hautarzt* 57, 11 (2006): 1021–28.

Picarelli, A., L. Sabbatella, T. M. Di, C. T. Di, S. Vetrano, and M. C. Anania. "Antiendomysial Antibody Detection in Fecal Supernatants: In Vivo Proof that Small Bowel Mucosa is the Site of Antiendomysial Antibody Production." *American Journal of Gastroenterology* 97, no. 1 (2002): 95–98.

Pietzak, M. M. "Follow-up of Patients with Celiac Disease: Achieving Compliance with Treatment." *Gastroenterology* 128, no. 4 suppl. no. 1 (2005): S135–41.

Pitner, J. K., and D. L. Bachman. "A Synopsis of the Practice Parameters on Dementia from the American Academy of Neurology on the Diagnosis of Dementia." *Consultant Pharmacist* 19, no. 1 (2004): 52–63.

Plenge, R. M. "Unlocking the Pathogenesis of Celiac Disease." *Nature Genetics* 42, no. 4 (2010): 281–82.

Podas, T., J. M. Nightingale, R. Oldham, S. Roy, N. J. Sheehan, and J. F. Mayberry. "Is Rheumatoid Arthritis a Disease That Starts in the Intestine? A Pilot Study Comparing an Elemental Diet with Oral Prednisolone." *Postgraduate Medical Journal* 83, no. 976 (2007): 128–31.

Polat, T. B., N. Urganci, Y. Yalcin, C. Zeybek, C. Akdeniz, A. Erdem, E. Imanov, and A. Celebi. "Cardiac Functions in Children with Coeliac Disease During Follow-up: Insights from Tissue Doppler Imaging." *Digestive and Liver Disease* 40, no. 3 (2008): 182–87.

Poloni, N., S. Vender, E. Bolla, P. Bortolaso, C. Costantini, and C. Callegari. "Gluten Encephalopathy with Psychiatric Onset: Case Report." *Clinical Practice and Epidemiology in Mental Health* 5 (2009): 16.

Potter, D. D., J. A. Murray, J. H. Donohue, L. J. Burgart, D. M. Nagorney, J. A. van Heerden, M. F. Plevak, A. R. Zinsmeister, and S. N. Thibodeau. "The Role of Defective Mismatch Repair in Small Bowel Adenocarcinoma in Celiac Disease." *Cancer Research* 64, no. 19 (2004): 7073–77.

Powell, G. R., A. L. Bruckner, and W. L. Weston. "Dermatitis Herpetiformis Presenting as Chronic Urticaria." *Pediatric Dermatology* 21, no. 5 (2004): 564–67.

Prignano, F., D. Bonciani, F. Bandinelli, M. Matucci Cerinic, and T. Lotti. "Juvenile Psoriatic Arthritis and Comorbidities: Report of a Case Associated with Enthesitis and Celiac Disease." *Dermatologic Therapy* 23, suppl. no. 2 (2010): S47–50.

Prochorec-Sobieszek, M., and T. Wagner. [Lymphoproliferative Disorders in Sjögren's Syndrome.] [In Polish.] *Otolaryngologia Polska* 59, no. 4 (2005): 559–64.

Purnak, T., C. Efe, O. Yuksel, Y. Beyazit, E. Ozaslan, and E. Altiparmak. "Mean Platelet Volume Could Be a Promising Biomarker to Monitor Dietary Compliance in Celiac Disease." *Upsala Journal of Medical Sciences* 116, no. 3 (2011): 208–11.

Pynnönen, P. A., E. T. Isometsä, E. T. Aronen, M. A. Verkasalo, E. Savilahti, and V. A. Aalberg. "Mental Disorders in Adolescents With Celiac Disease." *Psychosomatics* 45 (2004): 325–35.

Rabsztyn, A., P. H. Green, I. Berti, A. Fasano, J. A. Perman, and K. Horvath. "Macroamylasemia in Patients with Celiac Disease." *American Journal of Gastroenterology* 96, 4 (2001): 1096–1100.

Radetti, G., A. Zavallone, L. Gentili, P. Beck-Peccoz, and G. Bona. "Foetal and Neonatal Thyroid Disorders." *Minerva Pediatrica* 54, no. 5 (2002): 383–400.

Raina, U. K., N. Goel, R. Sud, M. Thakar, and B. Ghosh. "Bilateral Total Cataract as the Presenting Feature of Celiac Disease." International Ophthalmology 31, no. 1 (2011): 47–50.

Recognizing Celiac Disease. GFW Publishing. "Celiac Disease Symptoms." http://www.recognizingceliacdisease.com/21.html (accessed January 15, 2011).

Reddick, B. K., K. Crowell, and B. Fu. "Clinical Inquiries: What Blood Tests Help Diagnose Celiac Disease?" *Journal of Family Practice* 55, 12 (2006): 1088, 1090, 1093.

Reddymasu, S. C., S. Sostarich, and R. W. McCallum. "Small Intestinal Bacterial Overgrowth in Irritable Bowel Syndrome: Are There Any Predictors?" *BioMedCentral Gastroenterology* 10 (2010): 23.

Regan, P. T., and E. P. DiMagno. "Exocrine Pancreatic Insufficiency in Celiac Sprue: A Cause of Treatment Failure." *Gastroenterology* 78, no. 3 (1980): 484–87.

Reichelt, K. L., and D. Jensen. "IgA Antibodies against Gliadin and Gluten in Multiple Sclerosis." *Acta Neurologica Scandinavica* 110, no. 4 (2004): 239–41.

Reichlt, K. L., E. Sagedal, J. Landmark, B. T. Sangvik, O. Eggen, and H. Scott. "The Effect of [a] Gluten-Free Diet on Urinary Peptide Excretion and Clinical State in Schizophrenia" Journal of Orthomolecular Medicine 5, no. 4 (1990): 223–239.

Reunala, T., and P. Collin. "Diseases Associated with Dermatitis Herpetiformis." *British Journal of Dermatology* 136, no. 3 (1997): 315–18.

Ricotta, M., M. Iannuzzi, G. De Vivo, and V. Gentile. "Physio-pathological Roles of Transglutaminase-catalyzed Reactions." *World Journal of Biological Chemistry* 1, no. 5 (2010): 181–87.

Rigamonti, A., S. Magi, E. Venturini, L. Morandi, C. Ciano, and G. Lauria. "Celiac Disease Presenting with Motor Neuropathy: Effect of Gluten-free Diet." *Muscle Nerve* 35, no. 5 (2007): 675–77.

Roche Herrero, M. C., J. Arcas Martínez, A. Martínez-Bermejo, V. López Martín, I. Polanco, A. Tendero Gormaz, and A. Fernández Jaén. [The Prevalence of Headache in a Population of Patients with Coeliac Disease.][In Spanish.] *Revue Neurologique* 32, no. 4 (2001): 301–9.

Rodrigo, L., N. Alvarez, S. Riestra, R. de Francisco, O. González Bernardo, L. García Isidro, A. López Vázquez, and C. López Larrea. [Relapsing Acute Pancreatitis Associated with Gluten Enteropathy. Clinical, Laboratory, and Evolutive Characteristics in Thirty-four Patients.] [In Spanish.] *Revista Espanola de Enfermedades Digestivas* 100, no. 12 (2008): 746–51.

Romieu, I., and C. Trenga. "Diet and Obstructive Lung Diseases." *Epidemiologic Reviews* 23, no. 2 (2001): 268–87.

Rosato, E., D. De Nitto, C. Rossi, V. Libanori, G. Donato, M. Di Tola, S. Pisarri, F. Salsano, and A. Picarelli. "High Incidence of Celiac Disease in Patients with Systemic Sclerosis." *Journal of Rheumatology* 36, no. 5 (2009): 965–69.

Rostami, K., C. J. Mulder, S. Stapel, B. M. von Blomberg, J. Kerckhaert, J. W. Meijer, S. A. Peña, and H. S. Heymans. "Autoantibodies and Histogenesis of Celiac Disease." *Romanian Journal of Gastroenterology* 12, no. 2 (2003): 101–6.

Rutherford, R. M., M. H. Brutsche, M. Kearns, M. Bourke, F. Stevens, and J. J. Gilmartin. "Prevalence of Coeliac Disease in Patients with Sarcoidosis." *European Journal of Gastroenterology and Hepatology* 16, no. 9 (2004): 911–15.

Sadowski, B., J. M. Rohrbach, K. P. Steuhl, E. G. Weidle, and W. L. Castrillón-Oberndorfer. [Corneal Manifestations in Vitamin A Deficiency.] [In German.] *Klinische Monatsblätter für Augenheilkunde* 205, no. 2 (1994): 76–85.

Sahin, I., C. Demir, M. Alay, and L. Eminbeyli. "The Patient Presenting with Renal Failure Due to Multiple Myeloma Associated with Celiac Disease: Case Report." *International Journal of Hematology and Oncology* 21, no. 2 (2011): 131.

Saito, H., N. Fujita, M. Miyakoshi, A. Arai, and H. Nagai. [A Case of Hashimoto's Encephalopathy Associated with Graves' Disease.] [In Japanese.] *Rinsho Shinkeigaku (Clinical Neurology)* 42, no. 7 (2002): 619–22.

Sanders, D. S., K. E. Evans, and M. Hadjivassiliou. "Fatigue in Primary Care. Test for Coeliac Disease First?" *British Medical Journal* 2, no. 341 (2010): c5161.

Sandyk, R., and G. I. Awerbuch . "Vitamin B12 and Its Relationship to Age of Onset of Multiple Sclerosis." *International Journal of Neuroscience* 71, no. 1–4 (1993): 93–99.

Sategna-Guidetti, C., U. Volta, C. Ciacci, P. Usai, A. Carlino, L. De Franceschi, A. Camera, A. Pelli, and C. Brossa. "Prevalence of Thyroid Disorders in Untreated Adult Celiac Disease Patients and Effect of Gluten Withdrawal: An Italian Multicenter Study." *American Journal of Gastroenterology* 96, no. 3 (2001): 751–57.

Schedel, J., F. Rockmann, T. Bongartz, M. Woenckhaus, J. Schölmerich, and F. Kullmann. "Association of Crohn's Disease and Latent Celiac Disease: A Case Report and Review of the Literature." *International Journal of Colorectal Disease* 20, no. 4 (2005): 376–80.

Schreiber, F. S., T. Ziob, M. Vieth, and H. Elsbernd. [Atypical Celiac Disease in a Patient with Type 1 Diabetes Mellitus and Hashimoto's Thyreoiditis.] [In German.] *Deutsche Medizinische Wochenschriftr* 136, no. 3 (2011): 82–85.

Schweizer, J. J., A. Oren, and M. L. Mearin. "Cancer in Children with Celiac Disease: A Survey of the European Society of Paediatric Gastroenterology, Hepatology and Nutrition." *Journal of Pediatrics Gastroenterology and Nutrition* 33, no. 1 (2001): 97–100.

Science Daily. "Gluten-free Diet Alone Is Enough to Get Bones Healthy in Pediatric Patients with Celiac Disease." July 25, 2008. http://www.sciencedaily.com/releases/2008/07/080725105453.htm (accessed January 12, 2012).

Science Daily. "Scientists Characterize New Syndrome Of Allergy, Apraxia, Malabsorption." July 15, 2009. http://www.sciencedaily.com/releases/2009/07/090714104002.htm (accessed June 26, 2011).

See, J., and J. A. Murray. "Gluten-free Diet: The Medical and Nutrition Management of Celiac Disease." *Nutrition in Clinical Practice* 21, no. 1 (2006): 1–15.

Selva-O'Callaghan, A., F. Casellas, I. de Torres, E. Palou, J. M. Grau-Junyent, and M. Vilardell-Tarrés. "Celiac Disease in Patients with Inflammatory Myopathy." *Muscle and Nerve* 35, no. 1 (2007): 49–54.

Seyhan, M., T. Erdem, V. Ertekin, and M. A. Selimoğlu. "The Mucocutaneous Manifestations Associated with Celiac Disease in Childhood and Adolescence." *Pediatric Dermatology* 24, no. 1 (2007): 28–33.

Shakeri, R., F. Zamani, R. Sotoudehmanesh, A. Amiri, M. Mohamadnejad, F. Davatchi, A. M. Karakani, R. Malekzadeh, and F. Shahram. "Gluten Sensitivity Enteropathy in Patients with Recurrent Aphthous Atomatitis." *BioMedCentral Gastroenterology* 9 (2009): 44.

Shazly, T. A., M. Aljajeh, M. A. Latina. "Autoimmune Basis of Glaucoma." *Seminars in Ophthalmology* 26. no. 4–5 (2011): 278–81.

Sher, K. S., V. Jayanthi, C. S. Probert, C. R. Stewart, and J. F. Mayberry. "Infertility, Obstetric and Gynaecological Problems in Coeliac Sprue." *Digestive Diseases* 12, no. 3 (1994): 186–90.

Shor, D. B., O. Barzilai, M. Ram, D. Izhaky, B. S. Porat-Katz, J. Chapman, M. Blank, J. M. Anaya, and Y. Shoenfeld. "Gluten Sensitivity in Multiple Sclerosis: Experimental Myth or Clinical Truth?" *Annals of the New York Academy of Science* 1173 (2009): 343–49.

Silano, M., U. Volta, A. M. Mecchia, M. Dessì, R. Di Benedetto, and M. De Vincenzi. "Delayed Diagnosis of Coeliac Disease Increases Cancer Risk." *BioMedCentral Gastroenterology* 7 (2007): 8.

Silano, M., U. Volta, A. D. Vincenzi, M. Dessì, and M. D. Vincenzi. "Effect of a Gluten-free Diet on the Risk of Enteropathy-associated T-cell Lymphoma in Celiac Disease." *Digestive Diseases and Sciences* 53, no. 4 (2008): 972–76.

Sinaii, N., S. D. Cleary, M. L. Ballweg, L. K. Nieman, and P. Stratton. "High Rates of Autoimmune and Endocrine Disorders, Fibromyalgia, Chronic Fatigue Syndrome and Atopic Diseases among Women with Endometriosis: A Survey Analysis." *Human Reproduction* 17, no. 10 (2002): 2715–24.

Singh, M. M., and S. R. Kay. "Wheat Gluten as a Pathogenic Factor in Schizophrenia." *Science* 191, no. 4225 (1976): 401–2.

Singh, S., G. K. Sonkar, Usha, and S. Singh. "Celiac Disease-associated Antibodies in Patients with Psoriasis and Correlation with HLA Cw6." *Journal of Clinical Laboratory Analysis* 24, no. 4 (2010): 269–72.

Sinha, S. K., C. K. Nain, H. P. Udawat, K. K. Prasad, R. Das, B. Nagi, and K. Singh. "Cervical Esophageal Web and Celiac Disease." *Journal of Gastroenterology and Hepatology* 23, no. 7 pt. 1 (2008): 1149–52.

Sinn, N. "Nutritional and Dietary Influences on Attention Deficit Hyperactivity Disorder." *Nutrition Reviews* 66, no. 10 (2008): 558–68.

Smedby, K. E., M. Akerman, H. Hildebrand, B. Glimelius, A. Ekbom, and J. Askling. "Malignant Lymphomas in Coeliac Disease: Evidence of Increased Risks for Lymphoma Types Other Than Enteropathy-type T Cell Lymphoma." *Gut* 54, no. 1 (2005): 54–59.

Smerud, K. H., B. Fellström, R. Hällgren, S. Osagie, P. Venge, and G. Kristjánsson. "Gastrointestinal Sensitivity to Soy and Milk Proteins in Patients with IgA Nephropathy." *Clinical Nephrology* 74, no. 5 (2010): 364–71.

Smerud, H. K., B. Fellström, R. Hällgren, S. Osagie, P. Venge, and G. Kristjánsson. "Gluten Sensitivity in Patients with IgA Nephropathy." *Nephrology, Dialysis, Transplantation* 24, no. 8 (2009): 2476–81.

Smit, H. A. "Chronic Obstructive Pulmonary Disease, Asthma and Protective Effects of Food Intake: From Hypothesis to Evidence?" *Respiratory Research* 2, no. 5 (2001): 261–64.

Sonet, A., I. Théate, M. Delos, L. Montfort, P. Mineur, P. Driesschaert, L. Michaux, A. Ferrant, and A. Bosly. "Clinical and Pathological Features of 14 non-Hodgkin's Lymphomas Associated with Coeliac Disease." *ACTA Clinica Belgica* 59, no. 3 (2004): 143–51.

Song, M. S., D. Farber, A. Bitton, J. Jass, M. Singer, and G. Karpati. "Dermatomyositis Associated with Celiac Disease: Response to a Gluten-free Diet." *Cananadian Journal of Gastroenterology* 20, no. 6 (2006): 433–35.

Soni, S., and S. Z. Badawy. "Celiac Disease and Its Effect on Human Reproduction: A Review." *Journal of Reproductive Medicine* 55, nos. 1-2 (2010): 3–8.

Souroujon, M., A. Ashkenazi, M. Lupo, S. Levin, and E. Hegesh. "Serum Ferritin Levels in Celiac Disease." *American Journal of Clinical Pathology* 77, no. 1 (1982): 82–86.

Spadaccino, A. C., D. Basso, S. Chiarelli, M. P. Albergoni, A. D'Odorico, M. Plebani, B. Pedini, F. Lazzarotto, and C. Betterle. "Celiac Disease in North Italian Patients with Autoimmune Thyroid Diseases." *Autoimmunity* 41, no. 1 (2008): 116–21.

Spritz, R.A. "Shared Genetic Relationships Underlying Generalized Vitiligo and Autoimmune Thyroid Disease." *Thyroid* 20, no. 7 (2010): 745–54.

St. Clair, N. E., C. C. Kim, G. Semrin, A. L. Woodward, M. G. Liang, J. N. Glickman, A. M. Leichtner, and B. A. Binstadt. "Celiac Disease Presenting with Chilblains in an Adolescent Girl." *Pediatric Dermatology* 23, no. 5 (2006): 451–54.

Stabler, S. P., J. Lindenbaum, and R. H. Allen. "Vitamin B-12 Deficiency in the Elderly: Current Dilemmas." *American Journal of Clinical Nutrition* 66, no. 4 (1997): 741–49.

Stagi, S., T. Giani, G. Simonini, and F. Falcini. "Thyroid Function, Autoimmune Thyroiditis and Coeliac Disease in Juvenile Idiopathic Arthritis." *Rheumatology (Oxford)* 44, no. 4 (2005): 517–20.

Stagi, S., G. Simonini, L. Ricci, M. de Martino, and F. Falcini. "Coeliac Disease in Patients with Kawasaki Disease. Is There a Link?" *Rheumatology* 45, no. 7 (2006): 847–50.

Stancu, M., G. De Petris, T. P. Palumbo, and R. Lev. "Collagenous Gastritis Associated with Lymphocytic Gastritis and Celiac Disease." *Archives of Pathology and Laboratory Medicine* 125, no. 12 (2001): 1579–84.

Stanford School of Medicine. "Type-2 Diabetes Linked to Autoimmune Reaction in Study." April 17, 2011. Article by Krista Conger. http://med.stanford.edu/ism/2011/april/engleman.html (accessed July 31, 2011).

Stark, K., R. H. Straub, S. Blazicková, C. Hengstenberg, and J. Rovenský. "Genetics in Neuroendocrine Immunology: Implications for Rheumatoid Arthritis and Osteoarthritis." *Annals of the New York Academy of Sciences* 1193 (2010): 10–14.

Stazi, A. V., and A. Mantovani. [Celiac Disease and Its Endocrine and Nutritional Implications on Male Reproduction.] [In Italian.] *Minerva Medica* 95, no. 3 (2004): 243–54.

Stazi, A. V., and A. Mantovani. [Celiac Disease. Risk Factors for Women in Reproductive Age.] [In Italian.] *Minerva Ginecologica* 52, no. 5 (2000): 189–96.

Stazi, A. V., and B. Trinti. [Reproductive Aspects of Celiac Disease.] [In Italian.] *Annali Italiani di Medicina Interna* 20, no. 3 (2005): 143–57.

Stazi, A. V., B. Trinti. "Risk of Osteoporosis in Endocrine Disorders and Celiac Disease." *Annali dell'Istituto Superiore di Sanita* 43, no. 4 (2007): 430–33.

Stein, H. J., and J. R. Siewert. "Barrett's Esophagus: Pathogenesis, Epidemiology, Functional Abnormalities, Malignant Degeneration, and Surgical Management." *Dysphagia* 8, no. 3 (1993): 276–88.

Stenson, W. F., R. Newberry, R. Lorenz, C. Baldus, and R. Civitelli. "Increased Prevalence of Celiac Disease and Need for Routine Screening Among Patients with Osteoporosis." *Archives of Internal Medicine* 165, no. 4 (2005): 393–99.

Stephansson, O., H. Falconer, and J. F. Ludvigsson. "Risk of Endometriosis in 11,000 Women with Celiac Disease." *Human Reproduction* 26, no. 10 (2011): 2896–901.

Storm, W. "Celiac Disease and Alopecia Areata in a Child with Down's Syndrome." *Journal of Intellectual Disability Research* 44, pt. 5 (2000): 621–23.

Straker, R. J., S. Gunasekaran, and P. G. Brady. "Adenocarcinoma of the Jejunum in Association with Celiac Sprue." *Journal of Clinical Gastroenterology* 11, no. 3 (1989): 320–23.

Suares, N. C., and A. C. Ford. "Prevalence of, and Risk Factors for, Chronic Idiopathic Constipation in the Community: Systematic Review and Meta-analysis." *American Journal of Gastroenterology* 106, no. 9 (2011) 1582–91.

Suárez, T., M. Torrealba, N. Villegas, C. Osorio, and M. N. García-Casal. [Iron, Folic Acid and Vitamin B12 Deficiencies Related to Anemia in Adolescents from a Region with a High Incidence of Congenital Malformations in Venezuela.] [In Spanish.] *Archivos Latinoamericanos de Nutrición* 55, no. 2 (2005): 118–23.

Syed, M. A., E. Barinas-Mitchell, S. L. Pietropaolo, Y. J. Zhang, T. S. Henderson, D. E. Kelley, M. T. Korytkowski et al. "Is Type 2 Diabetes a Chronic Inflammatory/Autoimmune Disease?" *Diabetes Nutrition and Metabolism* 15, no. 2 (2002): 68–83.

Talley, N. J. "Pharmacologic Therapy for the Irritable Bowel Syndrome." *Amercian Journal of Gastroenterology* 98 (2003): 750–58.

Talley, N. J., M. Valdovinos, T. M. Petterson, H. A. Carpenter, and L. J. Melton, 3rd. "Epidemiology of Celiac Sprue: A Community-based Study." *American Journal of Gastroenterology* 89 (1994): 843–46.

Tarlo, S. M., I. Broder, E. J. Prokipchuk, L. Peress, and S. Mintz. "Association between Celiac Disease and Lung Disease." *Chest* 80, no. 6 (1981): 715–18.

Tattersall, R. B. "Hypoadrenia or 'A Bit of Addison's Disease.'" *Medical History* 43, no. 4 (1999): 450–67.

Teppo, A. M., and C. P. Maury. "Antibodies to Gliadin, Gluten and Reticulin Glycoprotein in Rheumatic Diseases: Elevated Levels in Sjögren's Syndrome." *Clinical and Experimental Immunology* 57, no. 1 (1984): 73–78.

Tezel, G., and M. B. Wax. "Glaucoma." *Chemical Immunology and Allergy* 92 (2007): 221–27.

Toscano, V., F. G. Conti, E. Anastasi, P. Mariani, C. Tiberti, M. Poggi, M. Montuori et al. "Importance of Gluten in the Induction of Endocrine Autoantibodies and Organ Dysfunction in Adolescent Celiac Patients." *American Journal of Gastroenterology* 95, no. 7 (2000): 1742–48.

Trbojević, B., and S. Djurica. [Diagnosis of Autoimmune Thyroid Disease.] [In Serbian] *Serbian Archives of Medicine* 133, suppl. no. 1 (2005): 25–33.

Treem, W. R. "Emerging Concepts in Celiac Disease." *Current Opinion in Pediatrics* 16, no. 5 (2004): 552–59.

Troncone, R., and B. Jabri. "Coeliac Disease and Gluten Sensitivity." *Journal of Internal Medicine* 269, no. 6 (2011): 582–90.

Tronconi, G. M., B. Parma, and G. Barera. [Celiac Disease and "Gluten Sensitivity."] [In Italian.] *Pediatria Medica e Chirurgica* 32, no. 5 (2010): 211–15.

Trucco Aguirre, E., C. Olano Gossweiler, C. Méndez Pereira, M. E. Isasi Capelo, E. S. Isasi Capelo, and M. Rondan Olivera. [Celiac Disease Associated with Systemic Sclerosis.] [In Spanish.] *Journal of Gastroenterology and Hepatology* 30, no. 9 (2007): 538–40.

Trynka, G., C. Wijmenga, and D. A. van Heel. "A Genetic Perspective on Coeliac Disease." *Trends in Molecular Medicine* 16, no. 11 (2010): 537–50.

Tsiligianni, I. G., and T. van der Molen. "A Systematic Review of the Role of Vitamin Insufficiencies and Supplementation in COPD." *Respiratory Research* 11 (2010): 171.

Tuncer, S., B.Yeniad, and G. Peksayar. "Regression of Conjunctival Tumor During Dietary Treatment of Celiac Disease." *Indian Journal of Ophthalmology* 58, no. 5 (2010): 433–4.

Turner, M.R., G. Chohan, G. Quaghebeur, R. C. Greenhall, M. Hadjivassiliou, and K. Talbot. "A Case of Celiac Disease Mimicking Amyotrophic Lateral Sclerosis." *Nature Clinical Practice Neurology* 3, no. 10 (2007): 581–84.

Tursi, A., G. Brandimarte, and G. Giorgetti. "High Prevalence of Small Intestinal Bacterial Overgrowth in Celiac Patients with Persistence of Gastrointestinal Symptoms After Gluten Withdrawal." *American Journal of Gastroenterology* 98, no. 4 (2003): 839–43.

Tursi, A., G. M. Giorgetti, G. Brandimarte, and W. Elisei. "High Prevalence of Celiac Disease among Patients Affected by Crohn's Disease." *Inflammatory Bowel Diseases* 11, no. 7 (2005): 662–66.

University of Chicago Celiac Disease Center. "Celiac Disease Facts and Figures." http://www.cureceliacdisease.org/wpcontent/uploads/2011/09/CDCFactSheets8_FactsFigures.pdf (accessed November 27, 2011).

University of Chicago Celiac Disease Center. Jabri, B. "Of Mice and Men: The Quest for a Mouse with Celiac Disease." *Impact*: Summer 2009.

University of Maryland Medical Center. "Researchers Find Increased Zonulin Levels Among Celiac Disease Patients." Last modified March 21, 2008 http://www.umm.edu/news/releases/zonulin.htm (accessed April 23, 2013).

University of Maryland School of Medicine. "News from the Center for Celiac Research: University of Maryland School of Medicine Researchers Identify Key Pathogenic Differences Between Celiac Disease & Gluten Sensitivity." March 10, 2011 http://somvweb.som.umaryland.edu/absolutenm/templates/?a=1474 (accessed April 23, 2013).

University of Maryland School of Medicine. "University of Maryland Study Shows Celiac Disease Is More Prevalent in U.S. Than Previously Thought." February 10, 2003 http://somvweb.som.umaryland.edu/absolutenm/templates/?a=53 (accessed April 23, 2013).

Usai, P., R. Manca, R. Cuomo, M. A. Lai, and M. F. Boi. "Effect of Gluten-free Diet and Co-morbidity of Irritable Bowel Syndrome-type Symptoms on Health-related Quality of Life in Adult Coeliac Patients." *Digestive and Liver Disease* 39, no. 9 (2007): 824–28.

Usai, P., R. Manca, R. Cuomo, M. A. Lai, L. Russo, and M. F. Boi. "Effect of Gluten-free Diet on Preventing Recurrence of Gastroesophageal Reflux Disease-related Symptoms in Adult Celiac Patients with Nonerosive Reflux Disease." *Journal of Gastroenterology and Hepatology* 23, no. 9 (2008): 1368–72.

Usai, P., A. Serra, B. Marini, S. Mariotti, L. Satta, M. F. Boi, A. Spanu, G. Loi, and M. Piga. "Frontal Cortical Perfusion Abnormalities Related to Gluten Intake and Associated Autoimmune Disease in Adult Coeliac Disease: 99mTc-ECD Brain SPECT Study." *Digestive and Liver Disease* 36, no. 8 (2004): 513–18.

Uslu, N., H. Demir, T. Karagöz, and I. N. Saltik-Temizel. "Dilated Cardiomyopathy in Celiac Disease: Role of Carnitine Deficiency." *ACTA Gastroenterologica Belgica* 73, no. 4 (2010): 530–31.

Vahedi, K., F. Mascart, J. Y. Mary, J. E. Laberenne, Y. Bouhnik, M. C. Morin, A. Ocmant, C. Velly, J. F. Colombel, and C. Matuchansky. "Reliability of Antitransglutaminase Antibodies as Predictors of Gluten-free Diet Compliance in Adult Celiac Disease." *American Journal of Gastroenterology* 98, no. 5 (2003): 1079–87.

Valentino, R., S. Savastano, A. P. Tommaselli, M. Dorato, M. T. Scarpitta, M. Gigante, G. Lombardi, and R. Troncone. "Unusual Association of Thyroiditis, Addison's Disease, Ovarian Failure and Celiac Disease in a Young Woman." *Journal of Endocrinological Investigation* 22, no. 5 (1999): 390–94.

Vañó-Galván, S., S. Aboín, S. Beà-Ardebol, and J. L. Sánchez-Mateos. "Sudden Hair Loss Associated with Trachyonychia." *Cleveland Clinic Journal of Medicine* 75, no. 8 (2008): 567–68.

Veale, D., G. Kavanagh, J. F. Fielding, and O. Fitzgerald. "Primary Fibromyalgia and the Irritable Bowel Syndrome: Different Expressions of a Common Pathogenetic Process." *British Journal of Rheumatology* 30, no. 3 (1991): 220–22.

Ventura A., G. Magazzù, and L. Greco. "Duration of Exposure to Gluten and Risk for Autoimmune Disorders in Patients with Celiac Disease. SIGEP Study Group for Autoimmune Disorders in Celiac Disease." *Gastroenterology* 117, no. 2 (1999): 297–303.

Ventura, A., E. Neri, C. Ughi, A. Leopaldi, A. Città, and T. Not. "Gluten-dependent Diabetes-related and Thyroid-related Autoantibodies in Patients with Celiac Disease." *Journal of Pediatrics* 137 no. 2 (2000): 263–65.

Venuta, A., P. Bertolani, R. Casarini, F. Ferrari, N. Guaraldi, and E. Garetti. [Coexistence of Cystic Fibrosis and Celiac Disease. Description of a Clinical Case and Review of the Literature.] [In Italian.] *Pediatria Medica e Chirurgica* 21, suppl. no. 5 (1999): 223–26.

Verbeek, W. H., B. M. von Blomberg, V. M. Coupe, S. Daum, C. J. Mulder, and M. W. Schreurs. "Aberrant T-lymphocytes in Refractory Coeliac Disease Are Not Strictly Confined to a Small Intestinal Intraepithelial Localization." *Cytometry Part B: Clinical Cytometry* 76, no. 6 (2009): 367–74.

Verdu, E. F., D. Armstrong, and J. A. Murray. "Between Celiac Disease and Irritable Bowel Syndrome: The 'No Man's Land' of Gluten Sensitivity." *American Journal of Gastroenterology* 104, no. 6 (2009): 1587–94.

Verdu, E. F., M. Mauro, J. Bourgeois, and D. Armstrong. "Clinical Onset of Celiac Disease After an Episode of Campylobacter Jejuni Enteritis." *Canadian Journal of Gastroenterology* 21, no. 7 (2007): 453–55.

Vereckei, E., A. Mester, L. Hodinka, P. Temesvári, E. Kiss, and G. Poór. "Back Pain and Sacroiliitis in Long-standing Adult Celiac Disease: A Cross-sectional and Follow-up Study." *Rheumatology International* 30, no. 4 (2010): 455–60.

Vermes, I., E. N. Steur, G. F. Jirikowski, and C. Haanen. "Elevated Concentration of Cerebrospinal Fluid Tissue Transglutaminase in Parkinson's Disease Indicating Apoptosis." *Movement Disorders* 19, no. 10 (2004): 1252–54.

Vernia, P., M. Di Camillo, and V. Marinaro. "Lactose Malabsorption, Irritable Bowel Syndrome and Self-reported Milk Intolerance." *Digestive and Liver Disease* 33, no. 3 (2001): 234–39.

Villalta, D., M. G. Alessio, M. Tampoia, E. Tonutti, I. Brusca, M. Bagnasco, G. Pesce, and N. Bizzaro. "Diagnostic Accuracy of IgA Anti-tissue Transglutaminase Antibody Assays in Celiac Disease Patients with Selective IgA Deficiency." *Annals of the New York Academy of Sciences* 1109 (2007): 212–20.

Vilppula, A., K. Kaukinen, L. Luostarinen, I. Krekelä, H. Patrikainen, R. Valve, M. Mäki, and P. Collin. "Increasing Prevalence and High Incidence of Celiac Disease in Elderly People: A Population-based Study." *BioMedCentral Gastroenterology* 9 (2009): 49.

Visser, J., J. Rozing, A. Sapone, K. Lammers, and A. Fasano. "Tight Junctions, Intestinal Permeability, and Autoimmunity: Celiac Disease and Type 1 Diabetes Paradigms." *Annals of the New York Academy of Sciences* 1165 (2009): 195–205.

Vogelsang, H., G. Oberhuber, and J. Wyatt. "Lymphocytic Gastritis and Gastric Permeability in Patients with Celiac Disease." *Gastroenterology* 111, no. 1 (1996): 73–77.

Vojdani, Aristo. "The Role of Mucosal Immunity in Complex Diseases: Essential Biomarkers Panel." Slide 66. http://www.glutensensitivity.net/VojdaniDiagrams.htm (accessed November 26, 2010). Click on: Presentation slides for Role of Mucosal Immunity lecture.

Vojdani, A., T. O'Bryan, J. A. Green, J. McCandless, K. N. Woeller, E. Vojdani, A. A. Nourian, and E. L. Cooper. "Immune Response to Dietary Proteins, Gliadin and Cerebellar Peptides in Children with Autism." *Nutritional Neuroscience* 7, no. 3 (2004): 151–61.

Vojdani, A., T. O'Bryan, and G. H. Kellermann. "The Immunology of Gluten Sensitivity Beyond the Intestinal Tract." *European Journal of Inflammation* 6, no. 2 (2008): 1721–27.

Volta, U. "Pathogenesis and Clinical Significance of Liver Injury in Celiac Disease." *Clinical Reviews in Allergy and Immunology* 36, no. 1 (1983): 62–70.

Volta, U., R. De Giorgio, A. Granito, V. Stanghellini, G. Barbara, P. Avoni, R. Liguori et al. "Anti-ganglioside Antibodies in Coeliac Disease with Neurological Disorders." *Digestive and Liver Disease* 38, no. 3 (2006): 183–87.

Volta, U., R. De Giorgio, N. Petrolini, V. Stangbellini, G. Barbara, A. Granito, F. De Ponti, R. Corinaldesi, and F. B. Bianchi. "Clinical Findings and Anti-neuronal Antibodies in Coeliac Disease with Neurological Disorders." *Scandinavian Journal of Gastroenterology* 37, no. 11 (2002): 127.

Volta, U., A. Fabbri, C. Parisi, M. Piscaglia, G. Caio, F. Tovoli, and E. Fiorini. "Old and New Serological Tests for Celiac Disease Screening." *Expert Review of Gastroenterology and Hepatology* 4, no. 1 (2010): 31–35.

Volta, U., A. Granito, C. Parisi, A. Fabbri, E. Fiorini, M. Piscaglia, F. Tovoli et al. "Deamidated Gliadin Peptide Antibodies as a Routine Test for Celiac Disease: A Prospective Analysis." *Journal of Clinical Gastroenterology* 44, no. 3 (2010): 186–90.

Volta, U., R. Lazzari, F. B. Bianchi, M. Lenzi, A. M. Baldoni, F. Cassani, A. Collina, and E. Pisi. "Antibodies to Dietary Antigens in Coeliac Disease." *Scandinavian Journal of Gastroenterology* 21, no. 8 (1986): 935–40.

Wahnschaffe, U., R. Ullrich, E. O. Riecken, and J. D. Schulzke. "Celiac Disease-like Abnormalities in a Subgroup of Patients with Irritable Bowel Syndrome." *Gastroenterology* 121, no. 6 (2001): 1329–38.

Waldo, Rick T. "Iron-deficiency Anemia Due to Silent Celiac Sprue?" *Baylor University Medical Center Proceedings* 15, no. 1 (2002): 16–17.

Walkowiak, J., A. Blask-Osipa, A. Lisowska, B. Oralewska, A. Pogorzelski, W. Cichy, E. Sapiejka, M. Kowalska, M. Korzon, and A. Szaflarska-Popławska. "Cystic Fibrosis Is a Risk Factor for Celiac Disease." *ACTA Biochimica Polonica* 57, no. 1 (2010): 115–18.

Wallace, D. J., and D. S. Hallegua. "Fibromyalgia: The Gastrointestinal Link." *Current Pain and Headache Reports* 8, no. 5 (2004): 364–68.

Wasilewska, J., E. Jarocka-Cyrta, and M. Kaczmarski. [Gastrointestinal Abnormalities in Children with Autism.] [In Polish.] *Polski Merkuriusz Lekarski* 27, no. 157 (2009): 40–43.

Watt, J., J. R. Pincott, and J. T. Harries. "Combined Cow's Milk Protein and Gluten-induced Enteropathy: Common or Rare?" *Gut* 24 (1983): 165–70.

Wauters, E. A., J. Jansen, R. H. Houwen, J. Veenstra, and T. Ockhuizen. "Serum IgG and IgA Anti-gliadin Antibodies as Markers of Mucosal Damage in Children with Suspected Celiac Disease upon Gluten Challenge." *Journal of Pediatric Gastroenterology and Nutrition* 13, no. 2 (1991): 192–96.

Wax, M. B. "The Case for Autoimmunity in Glaucoma." *Experimental Eye Research* 93, no. 2 (2011): 187–90.

Weil, Andrew. "Q and A Library: How to Handle Sticky Blood?" http://www.drweil.com/drw/u/id/QAA326585 (accessed March 12, 2011).

Weinstock, L. B., A. S. Walters, G. E. Mullin, and S. P. Duntley. "Celiac Disease is Associated with Restless Legs Syndrome." *Digestive Diseases and Sciences* 55, no. 6 (2010): 1667–73.

Weisbrot, D. M., A. B. Ettinger, K. D. Gadow, A. L. Belman, W. S. MacAllister, M. Milazzo, M. L. Reed, D. Serrano, and L. B.Krupp. "Psychiatric Comorbidity in Pediatric Patients with Demyelinating Disorders." *Journal of Child Neurology* 25, no. 2 (2010): 192–202.

Weizman, Z., J. R. Hamilton, H. R. Kopelman, G. Cleghorn, and P. R. Durie. "Treatment Failure in Celiac Disease Due to Coexistent Exocrine Pancreatic Insufficiency." *Pediatrics* 80, no. 6 (1987): 924–26.

Welander, A., K. G. Prütz, M. Fored, and J. F. Ludvigsson. "Increased Risk of End-stage Renal Disease in Individuals with Coeliac Disease." *Gut* 61, no. 1 (2012): 64–68.

Werder, S. F., "Cobalamin Deficiency, Hyperhomocysteinemia, and Dementia." *Neuropsychiatric Disease and Treatment* 6 (2010): 159–95.

West, J., R. F. Logan, C. J. Smith, R. B. Hubbard, and T. R. Card. "Malignancy and Mortality in People with Coeliac Disease: Population Based Cohort Study." *British Medical Journal* 329 (2004): 716.

West, J., R. F. Logan, P. G. Hill, and K. T. Khaw. "The Iceberg of Celiac Disease: What is Below the Waterline?" *Clinical Gastroenterology and Hepatology* 5, 1 (2007): 59–62.

Westerberg, D. P., J. M. Gill, B. Dave, M. J. DiPrinzio, A. Quisel, and A. Foy. "New Strategies for Diagnosis and Management of Celiac Disease." *Journal of the American Osteopathic Association* 106, no. 3 (2006): 145–51.

Westerholm-Ormio, M., J. Garioch, I. Ketola, and E. Savilahti. "Inflammatory Cytokines in Small Intestinal Mucosa of Patients with Potential Coeliac Disease." *Clinical and Experimental Immunology* 128, no. 1 (2002): 94–101.

Whitworth, J. A. "2003 World Health Organization (WHO)/International Society of Hypertension (ISH) Statement on Management of Hypertension." Journal of Hypertension 21 (2003): 1983–92.

Wilhelmus, M. M., S. C. Grunberg, J. G. Bol, A. M. van Dam, J. J. Hoozemans, A. J. Rozemuller, and B. Drukarch. "Transglutaminases and Transglutaminase-catalyzed Cross-links Colocalize with the Pathological Lesions in Alzheimer's Disease Brain." *Brain Pathology* 19, no. 4 (2009): 612–22.

Williams, S. F., B. A. Mincey, and K. T. Calamia. "Inclusion Body Myositis Associated with Celiac Sprue and Idiopathic Thrombocytopenic Purpura." *Southern Medical Journal* 96, no. 7 (2003): 721–23.

Winter Del, R. J. L., N. L. Gabrielli, D. Greig, G. Inchauste, F. Quezada, M. J. Torres, and G. P. Castro. [Dilated Cardiomyopathy in Celiac Disease: Report of One Case.] [In Spanish.] *Revista Medica de Chile* 137, no. 11 (2009): 1469–73.

Wolber, R., D. Owen, and H. Freeman. "Colonic Lymphocytosis in Patients with Celiac Sprue." *Human Pathology* 21, no. 11 (1990): 1092–96.

Woollons, A., C. R. Darley, B. S. Bhogal, M. M. Black, and D. J. Atherton. "Childhood Dermatitis Herpetiformis: An Unusual Presentation." *Clinical and Experimental Dermatology* 24, no. 4 (1999): 283–85.

Wright, D. H. "The Major Complications of Coeliac Disease." *Baillieres Clinical Gastroenterology* 9, no. 2 (1995): 351–69.

Yachha, S. K., and U. Poddar. "Celiac Disease in India." *Indian Journal of Gastroenterology* 26, no. 5 (2007): 230–37.

Yeruham, I., Y. Avidar, and S. Perl. "An Apparently Gluten-induced Photosensitivity in Horses." *Veterinary and Human Toxicology* 41, no. 6 (1999): 386–88.

Yoon, S. S., Y. Ostchega, and T. Louis. "Recent Trends in the Prevalence of High Blood Pressure and Its Treatment and Control, 1999–2008." *Centers for Disease Control and Prevention* no. 48 (October 2010).

Yucel, B., N. Ozbey, K. Demir, A. Polat, and J. Yager. "Eating Disorders and Celiac Disease: A Case Report." *International Journal of Eating Disorders* 39, no. 6 (2006): 530–32.

Zamani, F., A. Amiri, R. Shakeri, A. Zare, and M. Mohamadnejad. "Celiac Disease as a Potential Cause of Idiopathic Portal Hypertension: A Case Report." *Journal of Medical Case Reports* 3 (2009): 68.

Zanchi, C., G. Di Leo, L. Ronfani, S. Martelossi, T. Not, and A. Ventura. "Bone Metabolism in Celiac Disease." *Journal of Pediatrics* 153, no. 2 (2008): 262–65.

Zelnik N., A. Pacht, R. Obeid, and A. Lerner. "Range of Neurologic Disorders in Patients with Celiac Disease." *Pediatrics* 13, no. 6 (2001): 1672–76.

Zerem, E., M. Zildzić, D. Sabitozić, J. Nurkić, and A. Susić. [Atypical Manifestations of Celiac Disease in an Adult Woman.] [In Bosnian.] *Medicinski Arhiv* 60, no. 1 (2006): 70–71.

Zhernakova, A., E. A. Stahl, G. Trynka, S. Raychaudhuri, E. A. Festen, L. Franke, H. J. Westra et al. "Meta-analysis of Genome-wide Association Studies in Celiac Disease and Rheumatoid Arthritis Identifies Fourteen non-HLA Shared Loci." *PLOS Genetics* 7, no. 2 (2011): e1002004.

Ziegler, A. G., S. Schmid, D. Huber, M. Hummel, and E. Bonifacio. "Early Infant Feeding and Risk of Developing Type 1 Diabetes-associated Autoantibodies." *Journal of American Medical Association* 290, no. 13 (2003): 1721–28.

Zipser, R. D., S. Patel, K. Z. Yahya, D. W. Baisch, and E. Monarch. "Presentations of Adult Celiac Disease in a Nationwide Patient Support Group." *Digestive Diseases and Sciences* 48, no. 4 (2003): 761–64.

Zofková I. [Celiac Disease and Its Relation to Bone Metabolism.] [In Czech.] *Casopis Lekaru Ceskych* 14, no. 11 (2002): 1271–74.

Zwolińska-Wcisło, M.D., Galicka-Latała, P. Rozpondek, L. Rudnicka-Sosin, and T. Mach. "Frequency of Celiac Disease and Irritable Bowel Syndrome Coexistance and Its Influence on the Disease Course." *Przeglad Lekarski* 66, no. 3 (2009): 126–29.

Dictionaries Consulted

TheFreeDictionary: http://www.thefreedictionary.com

Merriam-Webster: http://www.merriam-webster.com

MedlinePlus: http://www.nlm.nih.gov/medlineplus/

MedicineNet: http://www.medicinenet.com/script/main/hp.asp.

Index

B

C

D

E

F

K

L

M

N

O

P

R

S

T

U

V

W

Z

About the Author

Anne Sarkisian has become an ardent advocate for celiac-disease and gluten-intolerance (CD/GI) awareness since it was diagnosed within her own family. To that end, she has attended numerous conferences as well as read more than 2000 abstracts and research studies, numerous books, and constantly looks for new information on anything related to gluten and its issues.

Disturbed by the slow pace among medical professionals, Sarkisian passionately charts a gluten-free path to greater health, energy, and vitality that could be life changing for you.

Follow her website and blog at www.toxicstaple.com and see the video for more information on *Toxic Staple*, more life-changing testimonials, new research strengthening the link between gluten and a plethora of ill health, a few tasty recipes, and more information on the book and author.

If you have a powerful success story to share please send it in the body of an e-mail to anne@toxicstaple.com. Kindly keep it concise and do not send it in a document.

Website and blog: www.toxicstaple.com

E-mail: anne@toxicstaple.com

CPSIA information can be obtained
at www.ICGtesting.com
Printed in the USA
FFOW03n2119111215
19434FF